BIBLICAL/
MEDICAL
ETHICS

BIBLICAL/ MEDICAL ETHICS

The Christian and the Practice of Medicine

Franklin E. Payne, Jr., M.D.

BIBLICAL/MEDICAL ETHICS

Designed by Leonard George Goss and Joyce Bohn
Copyedited by Leonard George Goss, Michael Pearce Pfeifer and Ruth Schenk
Typeset by Karen White, Suzanne DePodesta and Joyce Bohn

First Edition

Printed in the United States of America
ISBN 0-88062-068-4

To Jeanne
God's helpmeet who makes possible
anything of value that I accomplish

Table of Contents

Foreword

When we first met several years ago, Dr. Ed Payne asked me about the possibility of working together with him on a major treatment of medical ethics from a biblical, Christian perspective. He fet that such a work was badly needed by the evangelical community because he had strong misgivings—which I share—about many ostensibly Christian approaches to medical ethics, including some from respected figures in the religious world. "Medical ethics" as a subject of special interest to the religious community was pioneered by Dr. Joseph Fletcher, at that time a professor at the Episcopal Theological Seminary in Cambridge, Massachusetts, a man who has little in common with evangelical Christianity. A number of other writers with a more recognizably Christian orientation followed Fletcher into the field of medical ethics, but most of them objected only to the nature and extent of his specific proposals rather than to his method—the application of utilitarian considerations instead of the Bible or traditional Christian ethical principles to the solution of contemporary ethical dilemmas. More often than not, the medical ethics that first appeared under such nominally Christian auspices turned out to be a justification of previously abhorred medical practices, including abortion, infanticide, and euthanasia, involuntary as well as voluntary. (Three outstanding exceptions to this trend are the German Helmut Thielicke, an Evangelical Lutheran at the University of Hamburg, and the Americans Paul Ramsay, a United Methodist at Princeton, and George H. Williams, a Congregationalist at Harvard.) Unfortunately, as evangelical Protestants began to take an interest in medical ethics, many of them failed to follow these outstanding exceptions, and instead chose to follow Fletcher and other utilitarians, even if at a distance, often expressing biblical standards as their general principles, but vitiating them in practice with a host of prudential and utilitarian concerns. Even the Christian Medical Society, an association of evangelical Christian physicians and other health professionals, turned out to differ little from secular professional associations in the practical guidance it offered to its members. (This situation and the leading actors in its development are ably discussed by Dr. Payne in the text.)

From within the medical community, Presbyterian layman C. Everett Koop, M.D. (then an eminent pediatric surgeon, now United States Surgeon General) joined forces with the outstanding evangelical thinker, Francis Schaeffer (1912-1984), in a far-reaching effort to recall Christians to fully biblical values concerning the nature and meaning of human life: their film series, *Whatever Happened to the Human Race?*, has stirred millions of previously complacent

American Christians into action. Nevertheless many evangelical leaders seemed more interested in accommodating themselves to the prevailing ethics (or lack of ethics) of secular society and liberal Christianity rather than in applying biblical principles soundly and consistently to newly emerging ethical problems. Evangelical Protestantism began to take an interest in sophisticated ethical issues, but instead of making the distinctive contribution that it ought to have made, on the basis of its distinctive commitment to the Holy Scripture as the authoritative Word of God, the only perfect rule of faith *and* practice, it simply joined the utilitarian trend, making occasional modifications but not trying to challenge basic assumptions.

All this meant that Dr. Payne's initiative was very timely. It might have seemed logical for a medical school professor and medical practitioner to join forces with an evangelical theologian, as Dr. Payne originally proposed. Unfortunately the thousands of miles separating us made it difficult for me to work actively with him; my collaboration finally involved little more than reading much of the manuscript as he wrote it and making suggestions. Now, with the final version before me, I would love to be able to claim co-authorship, as Dr. Payne's final product is a multi-dimensional work which combines scientific detail, medical and psychological sensitivity, and theological and ethical sophistication. It could easily pass for the work of a team of experts, but in fact is almost entirely his own. A work that began as a series of objections and protests against some widespread misconceptions and occasional medical malpractice has developed into a major statement combining medical and theological knowledge with Christian compassion—at least for suffering patients. (The author is less than indulgent towards those supposedly Christian ethicists whose major contribution seems to be finding sophisticated rationalizations for violations of the old Hippocratic Oath.) It will be a valuable handbook for physicians, pastors, counsellors, and indeed for all Christians who want to bring the principles of God's Word to bear in a consistent way on the complex dilemmas of modern medical life.

Harold O. J. Brown
Klosters, Easter, 1985

(Harold O. J. Brown, Th.M., Ph.D., is pastor of the Evangelical Reformed Church of Klosters, in the Canton of the Grisons, Switzerland. Currently on leave from his post as Professor of Biblical and Systematic Theology at Trinity Evangelical Divinity School, he was co-founder with C. Everett Koop, M.D., Sc.D, of the Christian Action Council.)

Acknowledgements

I would be impossible to acknowledge all the people who have contributed to my ideas for this work. Where my memory is clear, I have made appropriate reference. Others, however, have been lost to memory, as our thinking is shaped by all whom we meet and read and hear. This shaping is the work of the Holy Spirit in our individual and corporate consciousness. Ultimately, the glory for all that is right goes to Him, and all the errors to me. Would that we had greater wisdom to discern the difference!

Dr. Hilton Terrell read first, second and sometimes third editions with extensive notes in response (which were not always in agreement!). His serious reflection and balanced wisdom were invaluable and without which I would have made some regrettable blunders. Dr. Jay Adams also reviewed much of the manuscript with some notes in response. But his greatest contribution has been to my personal life in the application of biblical principles, in personal counsel, and in the content of specific parts of this book. Dr. Edward M. ("Ted") Hughes likewise reviewed portions of this project, and offered written comments.

To Dr. Harold O. J. Brown goes particular thanks: for the encouragement to write this book; for writing most of the chapter on Abortion; for his review of much of the material; for his Foreword; and, for introducing me to Mott Media.

My pastor, Rev. John W. P. Oliver, has probably contributed more than both of us realize. His gifted exposition of the Scriptures gave me occasional ideas, but more importantly kept by thoughts balanced and consistent.

Several secretaries did the typing, for subsequent editing by the editors of Mott Media, but the major help came from Karen Widmar whose greater task was to have to work with me!

Introduction

Even though the visible church appears healthy, American Christianity is troubled. Gallup's latest religious survey counted sixty-five million adults who believe that the Bible is inerrant. Thirty-one million claim to be evangelicals (those who believe the inerrancy of the Bible and the basic doctrine concerning Jesus Christ). Evangelism is widespread, missionary endeavors are extensive and monetary giving is on the increase. Yet, the nation has never indulged in such immorality, nor has Christianity ever been the enemy of the state.

Since the gospel of Christ is "the power of God unto salvation" and history has demonstrated that morality and social stability are consequences of a true spiritual reformation within a society, why is America and the church in a spiritual decline? Although there are many causal factors, the major problem among evangelicals is a severence of principle and practice. Biblical teaching is to be consistently and effectively demonstrated here and now. Principles *must* become practice in order to produce fruit.[1]

God has created men and women such that behavior is always based upon some principle. Unfortunately, most practice results from subconscious behavioral attitudes which have been established randomly during one's total life experience. Experiences are garnered from the world; most Christians conform to worldly principles except for a few specifically "Christian" activities. Paul's call for a "renewed mind" (Rom. 12:2) means Christians *must* establish peace and joy within, righteousness without, and reconstruct a moral society. This is achieved by (1) determining *consciously* scriptural principles, (2) adopting a practical plan to apply those principles, and (3) practicing their implementation.

My purpose is to describe the invasion of wordly (even satanic) principles into the practice of medicine, into the believer's life and his church; and to develop values and guidelines for patients and physicians which will enhance patients' health, establish the authority of the family and the church, design a more consistently biblical medical practice, and further God's kingdom on earth.

An attack on medicine is not my primary concern; rather I wish to sponsor reform where biblical direction seems clear. Moral degeneracy in society has affected physicians. Most physicians favor current abortion legislation and practice; infanticide is common; teenagers may be treated without parental knowledge or approval; psychiatry and psychology boast they have the answers to man's problems; and man is regarded as a randomly evolved animal without purpose or destiny. Tragically, many physicians neglect their own families in caring for their patients. Does the Bible address these issues? I intend to demonstrate that it does.

I write with some hesitation. Bringing together the disciplines of theology, ethics, philosophy, psychology, and medicine is a great responsibility, yet someone must step out and begin from an evangelical perspective. Excellent work has been done in the areas of abortion, infanticide and euthanasia. However, a more comprehensive approach is needed. The practice of medicine makes contact with the biblical world view at many points and there is much evidence that optimal health results from a spiritually committed life. Preventive measures such as diet, exercise, and not smoking are secondarily effective and medical measures are third in importance.

Some will regard *Biblical/Medical Ethics* as another irresponsible criticism of medicine. My Christian goal, however, is accuracy, not over evaluation or under evaluation. One does not fear truth because God is truth. Most assertions are fully documented from medical or Christian literature for reader examination. I believe that Christian health professionals have a great opportunity to help, to heal, and to promote health, *if* they believe that biblical authority takes precedence over any other authority, including the science of medicine.

I have covered many areas and several physicians and theologians have reviewed the earlier preparation of my work. Having practiced medicine in a variety of locations and counseled for ten years on a Christian basis, I would hope my critics would involve themselves comparably before they disagree.

Biblical principles necessarily cause departures from traditional medical thinking. At the same time where agreement does occur, overnight implementation of every principle is not expected. God calls us personally and professionally to effect profound changes in our lives. He does not expect immediate accomplishment. Neither do I expect immediate fulfillment of these biblical distinctives in myself or others. Some changes are accomplished easily and quickly; others require long-term efforts and creativity.

The many traits that distinguish each of us as individuals and those opportunities that present themselves to us will result in differing priorities and methods of implementation. (To assist in establishing these principles and priorities early in one's career, it would be well to have training programs for medical students and residents.) Thus, my goal is to determine those biblical principles that apply to medical ethics and practice, not to overwhelm anyone who is convicted by these principles but finds himself far from them. Our primary failure as Christians has been to discern the principles. As I develop my own methodology, the ideal (principle) is influenced by the real (practice). Without clear-cut values, and guiding principles, goals are unclear and virtually any behavior can be labeled "ethical."

Biblical authority provides the skeleton, or foundation, for all issues in life. The sciences and humanities add flesh to the skeleton but in no way do they alter its structure. Where the Bible clearly restricts, rejection, not accommodation, must occur. Where the Bible is silent, freedom exists. To be sure, to discern the Scriptures one must have thorough knowledge of its contents and have understanding for proper interpretation. As with the Trinity, many concepts are not precisely named but are clearly presented in Scripture. The absence of a word in the text does not necessarily mean that the Bible is silent about that word or its denoted concepts.

A specific goal in my writing is the establishment of a comprehensive foundation. Regretably, much information is presented succinctly, even though I tried to cover all crucial points. As one author has written, thoughts should be aired, even if prematurely, in order to present a needed message and allow for the evaluation and contributions of others. Another said:

> When one tries to state his position briefly he seems to come out sounding like Archie Bunker, Spiro Agnew, or the friendly neighborhood storm trooper.

Is it right for an author to ask for deliberate consideration? Perhaps not. I would ask your patient consideration of my writing and encourage others to respond so comprehensive biblical answers are given to modern medical-ethical dilemmas. The Christian community is confused and deceived. Principled direction must be given, and those principles must be practiced to correct our dilemma. As we discuss, study, and practice, a fuller development can occur. Excitedly, I anticipate the contributions that many will make. My prayer is that this work be used by God for His glory.

1 | Current Medical Ethics

Imagine you are the obstetrician for a forty-year-old patient whom you have been treating since the beginning of her pregnancy. Prior testing indicated that she is carrying twins. Routinely, you perform amniocentesis (a procedure in which a six-inch needle in inserted into the sac which surrounds the baby and fluid from within the sac is drawn out) for genetic screening because there is an increasing percentage of genetic abnormalities with the increasing age of the pregnant woman. The procedure is uneventful but the geneticist's report concludes that there is one normal baby and one baby with trisomy 21 (Down's syndrome or mongolism). When the patient is informed, she states that she "desperately" wants the normal child but cannot face the burden of caring for an abnormal child for the rest of her life. She relates a case report in which one twin's life had been "terminated" by the insertion of a needle into its heart while the other twin was delivered successfully after completion of pregnancy. She is determined to abort both fetuses if the same procedure is not made available to her. What are you to do? Kill one to save the other or let both die?

This actual case history represents only one example of the moral dilemmas being faced today by patients and physicians. Does being a Christian make a difference? Is the physician often caught between two apparent "wrongs"? Is the Bible relevant since it rarely speaks explicitly to modern medical procedures (for example, the word abortion does not occur in the Bible as a medical procedure)? Are not moral issues decided among physicians and between themselves and their patients?

These questions are difficult and crucial to our overall understanding, and a biblical/medical ethic *is* possible and necessary for the Christian whether he or she is a medical professional or a patient. However, before a full discussion, a brief review of changes in medical ethics, and what Christians are proposing as answers will better prepare us to evaluate the answers. The issue of abortion will be a common theme in this chapter because:

there is no other issue on the horizon in which the Law of God, as understood from the Bible, and the laws of man in America are so clearly in conflict. . . .if evangelicals do not react in overwhelming number to this challenge, it is difficult to imagine another to which they might rise.[2]

Historical Changes

A major emphasis of the Western *zeitgeist* or spirit of our time, especially in ethics and morals, is the relativity of all things. Nothing is considered so sacred that it should not be questioned, and eventually changed. Any absolute or authority is almost by definition something to be ridiculed and disobeyed. The "unthinkable" behavior of the past has become the norm of the present. Does it seem unreasonable to think that man can so easily cast off the past? Has man's thinking been so errant for hundreds of years that he has only "arrived" today? Serious consideration ought to be given to traditional standards which have prevailed for years, have benefited mankind, and have provided the foundation for modern society.

For two thousands years the Hippocratic Oath has been an ethical standard for physicians and has remained virtually unchanged until the last two decades. Clearly, the changes occurred because of the inclusive statement, "I will not give a woman a pessary to cause abortion." Recently, that statement was omitted from the oath which many medical schools use for their graduation exercises. In some cases the entire oath has been omitted. Reacting to Nazi atrocities, another ethical standard, The Declaration of Geneva, was developed. Concerning prenatal life, it states, "I will maintain the utmost respect for human life, *from the time of conception.*" Thus in Western society, abortion (except where the life of the mother was in danger) has been proscribed specifically in medical oaths.

Further, the American Medical Association (AMA) in its Transactions of 1859 voiced its condemnation of abortion:

> That while physicians have long been united in condemning the act of abortion, *at every period of gestation*, except as necessary for preserving the life of the mother or child, it has become the duty of this association, in view of the prevalence and increasing frequency of the crime, publicly to enter an earnest and solemn protest against such warrantable destruction of human life.[3] (emphasis mine)

Today, the official position of the AMA and other medical organizations has shifted from abortion as a *crime* to an aggressive sanction of the *morality* of abortion as a medically necessary procedure. In late 1982, in response to one of the recurring legal attempts to limit abortion, the AMA, the American College of Obstetricians and Gynecologists (ACOG), the American Academy of Pediatrics (AAP), and the Nurses Association of the American Academy of Obstetricians and Gynecologists (NAAAOG) filed a brief with the Supreme Court against any "obstacles to sound medical practice" (read as obstacles to limit abortion).[4] The ACOG president-elect said that "the medical organizations were not interested in debating the philosophical, religious and ethical issues involved with abortion." Subsequent to these attitudes, abortion has become the most common surgical procedure in the United States.

Abortion was the first major change in medical ethics which led to the inhumanities of Nazi Germany.[5] Later, "agitation for euthanasia began to appear more frequently in the writings of medical doctors."[6] That situation compares to contemporary America.

> What emerges from the (historical) material with striking clarity and persistence are the numerous similarities between killing in Nazi Germany and killing in contemporary society. . . .Among the similarities found, the most pervasive and distressing of all is the extensive role played by physicians in the destructive processes of both countries.[7]

Perhaps, there is some overstatement—certainly a comparison of physicians in the United States today and those of Nazi Germany is preposterous. Or is it? To examine current medical practices, we refer back to the dilemma which opened this chapter. For those involved, the situation did not involve a dilemma.

> The position of the heart of twin B was localized. . . .Under local anesthesia, 40 ml. (1.3 ounces) of amniotic fluid was removed . . . with a No. 18 spinal needle. The needle was then advanced into the fetal chest but missed the heart. A second insertion led to cardiac (heart) puncture and exsanguination (removal) of 25 ml. (slightly less than one ounce) of blood. . . .movements of the affected fetus and (its) cardiac activity ceased.[8]

Following that procedure, the pregnancy continued uneventfully and the normal twin was born healthy. The authors concluded, "It was a very gratifying experience in such an endangered pregnancy to follow the normal fetus to full term and vaginal delivery." Perhaps one could expect some reluctance or remorse by the physicians who were involved, but not a "very gratifying experience!"

"Baby Doe" had Down's syndrome and required simple surgery: the closure of a small opening (3 x 6 millimeters) between the esophagus and the trachea, the opening of the blocked esophagus, and the connection of the two portions of the esophagus which were separated by 5 millimeters.[9] Instead, Baby Doe was allowed to die slowly by dehydration and starvation in spite of the fact that several families offered to adopt him. Phillip Becker is another child with Down's syndrome who at the age of thirteen has been denied life-saving surgery because his life is "inherently not worth living," according to his parents.[10]

It does not require much reflection to identify the parallels between the disregard for human life and the progression of medical atrocities in Nazi Germany and the United States today. On the one hand, principles and practices of physicians simply reflect prevalent attitudes of their society. Families must cooperate and the courts must make such acts legal. On the other hand, physicians are relied upon for their medical expertise and leadership both ethically and legally. Some examples of their aggressive leadership have already been given. Others could be cited but the underlying philosophy must not be overlooked. Occasionally, it is quite clearly stated:

> . . . the new ethic of relative rather than of absolute and equal values will ultimately prevail . . . as (man seeks) to achieve his desired quality of life and living. . . .The part which medicine will play as all this develops is not yet entirely clear. That it will be *deeply involved* is certain. Medicine's role with respect to changing attitudes toward abortion may well be a *prototype* of what is to occur. . . .One may anticipate further development of these roles as the problems of birth control and birth selection are extended inevitably to death selection and *death control* whether by the individual or by society. . . .It is not too early for our profession to examine this new ethic . . . and prepare to apply it in a rational development for the *fulfillment* and *betterment* of mankind in what is almost certain to be a biologically-oriented world society.[11]

Such an attitude is expressed somewhat differently in another recent editorial:

> . . . we will not regard as sacrosanct the life of each and every member of our species . . . If we compare a severely defective human infant with a non-human animal, a dog or a pig, for example, we will often find the non-human to have superior capacities . . . that can be considered morally significant. . . .Species membership alone, however, is not morally relevant. Humans who bestow superior value on the lives of all human beings, solely because they are members of our own species, are judging along lines strikingly similar to those used by white racists.[12]

These conclusions epitomize the ethics which result from evolutionary cosmology and the misdirected focus on the quality of human life.

Relative to Christianity, a historical glance may illumine a possible conflict with such a ''god-like'' attitude.

> . . . as far as Christianity can be compared at all to any of the Greek and Roman cults, the Aesclepius ideal seems nearest to the ideal of Christ. The Greek god of medicine was the most accomplished precursor of the god of a higher Gospel that paganism last brought forth. . . .Of all the Greek gods he persisted longest in exercising his full and undiminished power (against the spread of Christianity in the first few centuries following Christ). . . .For he had been the embodiment of the highest expectations which men cherished, of the highest values which they had known.[13]

One modern book, *Confessions of a Medical Heretic* by Robert S. Mendelsohn, has developed the analogy that medicine is a religion. Indeed, medicine has its rituals and many such ''rituals'' have a tenuous or nonexistent empirical basis. The analogy in the present and the conflict with Aesclepius in the past are appropriate considerations for Christians today.

Only God knows the future, but *Winterflight*, fiction written by Christian author Joseph Bayly, projects a continued deterioration of medical ethics. He portrays mandatory death at seventy-five years of age, bodies kept alive solely to provide organs for transplantation, and imprisonment for those physicians who do not cooperate. The possibilities are frightening. Nazi Germany demonstrated that it can happen to a "civilized" Western nation. We must learn the lessons of the past.

Ethical Positions: Secular and Christian

Both Christian and secular interest has developed in medical ethics. In secularism, scholarly presentations and papers are prevalent. Within the Christian Medical Society, ethical positions are being formally adopted for the first time in its fifty years of existence. But is all this activity worthwhile and productive? To answer this question it is essential to review the situation in medical literature which is primarily secular, and then focus on Christian efforts.

Ethical opinion and emphasis ranges from a call to traditional values to nebulous "new insights and new ways of viewing things." Emphasizing the former, a contemporary Jewish writer perceptively observed:

> It is no accident that the prime examples of humane medicine in the West are to be found in hospitals run by religious groups because the people working these hospitals have been imbued from infancy with a respect for the sanctity of life and for the dignity of human beings. . . .We are too frequently left adrift without an accepted ethical concensus. . . .Our societies must come to grips with this problem, because the problem transcends medicine; it threatens the very fabric of Western societal structure and its future.[14]

Regrettably, a more common emphasis is exemplified by the following:

> I hope and trust we shall go no further with our narcissism and will actively work to find an individual and collective meaning capable of reconnecting our citizenry with each other and with our society. Some of our time honored and traditional values will help, but surely we shall have to develop new insights and new ways of viewing things.[15]

Although world view and philosophy will be discussed in depth later, it should be pointed out here that these examples reflect the frustration of modern man. On the one hand, it is unsettling to see traditional values and standards fall away. On the other hand, it is anticipated that something new can be found to answer all these questions. According to the Bible, man was created with an understanding of absolute truth (Rom. 1:18-20). Contrary to this, evolutionary theory postulates that man is evolving; answers lie in the future and in "freedom" from absolutes. Thus man is frustrated. God created him to have stability based upon certain absolutes, but man sought temporal and relative gratification. Today, he is unsettled by the absence of absolutes, but he cannot find satisfaction in the theories of the moment or the mists of future theory.

Occasionally, a non-Christian understands his dilemma and frustratedly cries out:

> I cannot make peace with the randomness doctrine: I cannot abide the
> notion of purposelessness and blind chance in nature. And yet I do not
> know what to put in its place for the quieting of my mind.[16]

Thus, an emphasis is placed upon the *process* of medical ethical reflection rather than final answers. Ethical decisions should be seriously weighed, but the actual decisions made are of secondary importance. Rarely is an appeal made to traditional values and standards, and doubtfully has any recent appeal been made to absolutes. The thinking Christian should have little difficulty realizing that such emphasis on process rather than the ultimate rightness or wrongness of decisions is the antithesis of God's demand for holiness.

Articles by Christian authors occasionally appear in the medical literature, but their arguments fail to present any distinctive Christian position. Possibly, this failure may result from the unacceptability of such principles to secular editors. It is more likely that such failure results from a lack of understanding of biblical principle and practice, since their work in specifically Christian contexts is little better than the secularists.

Although categories are never precise, it may be helpful to identify groups with general characteristics. Thus, Christian medical ethicists may be divided in these categories: liberal, Catholic, Protestant and evangelical.[17] Liberals are those who consider that the Bible has little or no relevance, even though they profess to be Christians. One example is Joseph Fletcher who is widely known for his situational ethics. Since liberals do not believe that the Bible has special relevance, they are really in the same category as the professed secular relativists.

Catholics have a long history of principles in medical-ethical issues and have developed them extensively. In the battle to restrain abortion, they have been active and vocal. Some Catholic ethicists are respected within the medical profession both by practicing and teaching physicians. There are, however, two profound reasons that prevent their work from being compatible with an evangelical approach. First, their ethical principle is infrequently connected directly to, or derived from, Scripture or scriptural principles, even though it may be consistent with a biblical position. Second, revelational authority is not limited to the Protestant Bible but extends to the Pope (when he speaks *ex cathedra*), to the Roman Catholic magisterium, to its church tradition, and to the Apocrypha of the Catholic Bible. Thus, Catholicism and evangelical Christianity are irreconcilable at the foundation because of their differing conception of revealed truth. Although Catholic ethicists approximate scriptural principle, functionally they do not differ from the secularists and liberals since man remains the final arbiter of that truth from which ethical principle may be derived.

Unfortunately, Protestant ethicists are little different. The most obvious example is Paul Ramsey. His ethics are generally worth studying and are usually consistent with a biblical position; also his insights into medical-ethical situations are incisive. However, similiar to the Catholic ethicists, his arguments are usually not biblically derived or biblically referenced. As such, he can make no authoritative claims for the Christian and his works must be scrutinized for biblical compatibility.

Evangelicals have two inseparable absolutes which epitomized the Protestant Reformation: *sola Scripture* and *sola fide*—the Bible is the only infallible rule of faith and practice. Its understanding and acceptance is limited to those whose faith is a gift of God (Eph. 2:8,9). To the contrary, true faith is incompatible with the nonacceptance of the Bible in this way. Concerning medical ethics, however, two divisions of this category are necessary: evangelicals who function consistently and thoroughly with this biblical position and those who do not. Evangelical ethicists may be judged by the extent to which they give evidence of being under the authority of Scripture.

The Christian Medical Society (CMS) is an organization which falls into the latter division. Their statement of belief includes "the divine inspiration, integrity, and final authority of the Bible as the Word of God" and the remainder of that statement is basically evangelical. Nonetheless, articles in the *CMS Journal* and its ethical positions are inconsistently and incompletely evangelical. Specifically, the CMS Statement on Abortion (Figure 1) is biblically unacceptable in its weak denunciation of abortion and its failure to defend a biblical position. The statement skirts the issue that abortion is immoral and unbiblical. For example, the current legal statutes are not "woefully inadequate" but unethical, unbiblical, and a violation of God's law. Their statement on abortion and the journal articles to be discussed in chapter 9 represent common failures of CMS in its work to be evangelical. Although evangelical by label and its statement of belief, CMS functions on the border of neo-orthodoxy.[18]

To some extent CMS reflects the work of Lewis P. Bird, the Eastern Regional Director of CMS. He was on the commission which drafted the Statement on Abortion and is an editor of the CMS Journal. He is identified as an evangelical, as his articles have appeared in evangelical publications. Such identity, however, is questionable. His method in one article was to identify distinct principles "which have universal appeal" from various codes of medical ethics. Then he states that these "are readily compatible with a thorough-going Christian ethic."[19] The evangelical begins with Scripture, not compatibility from secular sources. His "universal appeal" sounds like utilitarian ethics. In another article his "urgent task" in confronting the abortion issue revolves around the definition of "human personhood." The debate, he says, "may" have to be conducted upon "sociopsychological grounds" or "an exercise in medical metaphysics."[20] What happened to his reference to the values "formulated from a biblical baseline under the continuing guidance of God's Spirit?"[21]

A final category for review concerns the work of evangelicals whose profession and function are biblically consistent. C. Everett Koop (M.D.) and

Francis A. Schaeffer in *Whatever Happened to the Human Race* and their other publications are not only consistent as evangelicals, they develop the philosophical and metaphysical world view that no answers for purpose or ethics can be found apart from the biblical position.[22] Their methodological clarity and means of expression clearly identify them as biblically consistent.

Even so, their work and that of most evangelicals is somewhat limited in scope. A great deal of solid work has been done concerning abortion, and some writing has been done on infanticide and euthanasia, but an approach to medical ethics which seeks biblical answers to every area of medical practice is yet to be written. A collection of articles and presentations by Martyn Lloyd-Jones began a comprehensive approach, but its direct biblical reference and its overall breadth are limited.[23] Nevertheless, to date it is the best evangelical work available.

Biblical/Medical Ethics seeks to develop a biblically consistent and comprehensive approach to medical ethics. Our hope is two-fold: to educate evangelicals in the broad biblical approach that is needed in medical ethics and to stimulate others to expand and deepen what has already been done.

Figure 1

CMS Statement on Abortion

WE LAMENT the casual and often callous attitude society holds toward abortion whereby traditional moral values are deemed irrelevant.

Though by legal statute abortions may be performed for any reason, we feel this minimal criterion is woefully inadequate for responsible clinical practice.

The indiscriminate practice of abortion is contrary to respect for the sanctity of human life; sexual responsibility; traditional codes of medical ethics; and the historic Judaeo-Christian faith.

WE BELIEVE that biblical Christianity affirms certain basic principles which condition any intrusion on human gestation; namely, the ultimate sovereignty of a loving God; the transcendent value of human life; the responsible alleviation of human suffering; and the moral stewardship of human sexuality.

WE RECOGNIZE the right of clinicians and nurses to follow the dictates of individual conscience under the authority of Scripture.

WE ARE FIRMLY OPPOSED to abortion on demand, and urge the active development of alternatives.

WE RECOGNIZE that certain difficult moral choices in medical judgment may need to be made where the values of human life, justice, compassion, and distress appear to collide.

NOTES

1. Evangelical is not the same as evangelistic. Evangelical refers to a Christian who believes the essential truths about Jesus Christ (His Virgin Birth, His sinless life, His being of one essence with the Trinity, His substitutary Atonement, etc.) and the Bible as the only infallible inerrant revelation of God. Evangelistic refers to an enthusiasm to persuade others to one's beliefs. Thus, a mormon could be evangelistic but not evangelical.

Confusion arises because "evangelical" is being increasingly used by those who are clearly not evangelicals. In fact, several authors in one book have argued that the evangelical position is consistent with an erroneous Bible. Their errors are discussed in a brief book by Gordon H. Clark, *The Concept of Biblical Authority* (Presbyterian and Reformed, 1980).

2. Harold O. J. Brown, "Protestants and the Abortion Issue: A Socio-Religious Prognostication," *Human Life Review* 2 (4) 1976:131-139.

3. Transactions of the American Medical Association XII: 75-8, 1859. "Report on Criminal Abortion" In: *Human Life Review* 8 (1) 1982:93-96.

4. *American Medical News* (September 10, 1982) pp. 1-2.

5. William Brennan, "Exterminative Medicine in Nazi Germany and Contemporary America," in *Medical Holocausts* Vol. I, (Boston: Nordland Publishing International, Inc., 1980), p. 79.

6. Ibid., p. 80.

7. Ibid., pp. 5-6.

8. T. D. Kerenyi and U. Chitkara, "Selective Birth in Twin Pregnancy with Discordancy for Down's Syndrome," *New England Journal of Medicine* 304 (June 18, 1981), pp. 1525-1527.

9. J. E. Pless, "The Story of Baby Doe," *New England Journal of Medicine* 309 (Sept. 15, 1983), p. 664.

10. George F. Will, "The Case of Phillip Decker," *Newsweek* (April 14, 1980), p. 112.

11. Editorial. "The Traditional Ethic," *California Medicine* 113 (Sept. 1970), pp. 67-68. [Also in *Human Life Review* 8 (1) 1982:90-2].

12. Peter Singer, "Sanctity of Life or Quality of Life," *Pediatrics* 72 (July, 1983), pp. 128-9.

13. Emma J. Edelstein and Ludwig Edelstein, *Ascelepius: A Collection and Interpretation of the Testimonies* (Baltimore: John Hopkins Press, 1945), p. 138.

14. S. M. Glick, "Humanistic Medicine in a Modern Age," *New England Journal of Medicine* 304 (April 23, 1981), pp. 1036-1038.

15. R. J. Bulger, "Narcissus, Pogo, and Lew Thomas' Wager," *Journal of the American Medical Association* 245 (April 10, 1981), pp. 1450-1454.

16. Ibid.

17. See footnote 1.

18. Carl F. Henry, ed., *Baker's Dictionary of Christian Ethics* (Grand Rapids: Baker Book House, 1973), pp. 452-453.

19. Lewis P. Bird, "Medical Ethics," in *Baker's Dictionary of Christian Ethics*, ed. Carl F. Henry (Grand Rapids: Baker Book House, 1973), pp. 413-416.

20. Lewis P. Bird, "Dilemmas in Biomedical Ethics," in *Horizons of Science*, ed. Carl F. Henry (San Francisco: Harper and Row Pub., 1978), p. 142.

21. Ibid., p. 133.

22. C. Everett Koop and Francis A. Schaeffer, *Whatever Happened to the Human Race* (Westchester, Ill.: Crossway Books, 1983), pp. 125-158.

23. D. Martyn Lloyd-Jones, *The Doctor Himself* and *The Human Condition* (London: Christian Medical Fellowship Publications, 1982).

REFERENCES

Bayly, Joseph. *Winterflight*. Waco: Word Books. 1981.

Brennan, William. *Medical Holocausts*. Vol. I "Exterminative Medicine in Nazi Germany and Contemporary America." Boston: Nordland Publishing International, Inc., 1980.

Brown, Harold O. J. "Protestants and the Abortion Issue: A Socio-Religious Prognostication," *Human Life Review* 2 (4) 1976:131-139.

Bulger, R. J. "Narcissus, Pogo, and Lew Thomas' Wager," *Journal of the American Medical Association* 245 (April 10, 1981):1450-1454.

Edelstein, Emma J. and Edelstein, Ludwig. *Ascelepius: A Collection and Interpretation of the Testimonies*. Baltimore: John Hopkins Press, 1945, p. 138.

Editorial. "The Traditional Ethic," *California Medicine* 113 (Sept. 1970):67-68. [Also, in *Human Life Review* 8 (1) 1982:90-92.]

Glick, S. M. "Humanistic Medicine in a Modern Age," *New England Journal of Medicine* 304 (April 23, 1981):1036-1038.

Kerenyi, T. D. and Chitkara, U. "Selective Birth in Twin Pregnancy with Discordancy for Down's Syndrome," *New England Journal of Medicine* 304 (June 18, 1981):1525-1527.

Mendelsohn, Robert S. *Confessions of a Medical Heretic*. Chicago: Warner Books, Inc., 1980.

Pless, J. E. "The Story of Baby Doe," *New England Journal of Medicine* 309 (September 15, 1983):664.

Singer, Peter. "Sanctity of Life or Quality of Life," *Pediatrics* 72 (July 1983): 128-9.

Transactions of the American Medical Association XII: 75-8, 1859. "Report on Criminal Abortion." In: *Human Life Review* 8(1) 1982:93-96.

Will, George F. "The Case of Phillip Becker," *Newsweek* April 14, 1980, p. 112.

2 | Theism or Naturalism?

Jane had come for counseling because the cost of her medical care became excessive. Over several weeks she had seen a dentist, an otolaryngologist (ear, nose, and throat physician), a neurologist, an internist, a psychiatrist, and a psychologist who specialized in biofeedback for relaxation. Her symptoms included headaches, jaw pain, incapacitating anxiety and sleeplessness. Jane was receiving minimal help, and since she was a Christian, decided to see whether spiritual problems were contributing to her symptoms. An added incentive was that as a ministry of a church, the counseling was free. Sessions with Jane revealed an almost complete absence of spiritual activity, with little church attendance, Christian fellowship, or Bible study. Daily activities in her household were unscheduled, unplanned, and disorderly. In a word her symptoms were due to her disordered life and lack of spiritual activities. Her counselor, through biblical counseling, offered to assist her in strengthening her spiritual life and to order her daily activities. She reacted with incredulity, ''I have seen five physicians and a psychologist at the cost of hundreds of dollars. You are saying that it is probable that I could overcome these symptoms and not need medical and psychological care?'' Indeed, her dilemma was deeper than she had perceived. The physiological symptoms, in reality, involved a question of belief. Medical and psychological science had directed her one way and her counselor advised her another. Which diagnosis was accurate? Who could be trusted?

This anecdote illustrates moral choice in a medical situation. An apparent contradiction existed between the direction and explanation of the counselor and the direction and explanation of medical ''science.'' At the deepest level of contradiction is the issue of truth (world view) from which morality is derived. The deeper issue is our immediate concern; but more comprehensively, the specifics of this case illustrate the general content of biblical/medical ethics: the interdependence of the *psyche* (mind or soul) and *soma* (body), the reliability of modern medicine, the ''science'' of psychotherapy, the ethics of the Christian and the church, and the theology of medical practice.

Truth and World View

"Why Is the Search for the Foundations of Ethics So Frustrating?" asked Alasdair MacIntyre in an article in a Hastings Center Report on medical ethics.[1] Indeed, the situation is frustrating when there *are* so many factions in medical ethics, even within groups which are identified by common interests and beliefs: Christian, non-Christian, pro-life, pro-choice, denominational, medical, and legal. An understandable explanation is that moral issues are not always seen to be secondary to philosophical issues. On the one hand, agreement on a philosophical level enhances the possibility of agreement upon moral issues. On the other hand, agreement on an ethical or moral level without agreement on a philosophical level is not true agreement. Complete agreement requires agreement within a defined, systematic world view.

Truth determines principle (ethic) and principle determines practice (morality). These levels may be linked in a comprehensive definition of the discipline of ethics:

> Ethics deals with the voluntary conduct (practice) of individual men insofar as it is judged to be good or bad in reference to a single, inclusive, and determinative principle of moral value grounded in and validated by ultimate reality.[2]

Ultimate reality, world view, and truth are used as synonyms and defined as "what is." World view is the preferred term because it is more descriptive of the totality of one's orientation. Since ethics and morals can have various interchangeable definitions, they need some clarification to retain consistency.

(1) ethics (ethic, ethical) - (a) the set of principles derived from one's world view
                                    (b) one of those principles
                                      (c) the discipline of ethics (above). The context should denote which is being used.

(2) moral (morality) - the application of ethics (principle) to cognitive or behavioral practice, whether actual or theoretical.

The study of "ultimate reality" in philosophy is called metaphysics and may be further defined as that reality which is beyond physical nature and therefore cannot be perceived by the human senses. One's reasoning begins as he is conscious of his own existence and the existence of those things which are perceived by his senses; touch, taste, vision, hearing, and smell. At this point reality seems quite simple because it is dependent only upon self-attestation. Soon, however, the individual will wonder or someone will ask whether anything metaphysical is real. He has only this choice: a metaphysical reality exists (supernaturalism) or it does not exist (naturalism).[3] The choice is *entirely arbitrary* since *by definition* such reality is imperceptible to the senses; "proof" is irrelevant. "What?" you say, "Evidence can help one decide between the two possiblities." All right, let's consider some evidence.

The Christian, as a supernaturalist, might point to his changed life as evidence of God's supernatural effect in his life. The naturalist's response would be that an emotional, psychological or biochemical change took place. The phenomenon (evidence) is the same but the interpretations of cause are entirely different. At the crossing of the Red Sea the Israelites believed that God had delivered them and established an annual celebration of His deliverance. In modern times, however, higher critics have different interpretations of cause. Theologians use "revelation" to refer to the supernatural (metaphysical) process by which God penetrated man's senses to give him an external, objective world view. The cause of this phenomenon, however, is presupposed.

> All proof must begin with certain assumptions. This is true in science, philosophy, or religion. Some ideas or facts must be accepted as *postulate*— that is, must be taken for granted.[4]

(Synonyms for postulates would include presuppositions, assumptions, *a priori* judgments, first principles, biases, and absolutes.)

Interpreting the Evidence

The interpretation of evidence involves methodology or epistemology, i.e. how one knows what he knows. What may be overlooked, however, is that one's epistemology is dependent upon one's methodology, and methodology is dependent upon one's metaphysical presuppositions.[5] This reasoning is tautological because any individual can only build his world view (system of truth) within and upon his presuppositions. There is an unavoidable interdependency.[6] That everyone bases his reasoning upon presuppositions is crucial to an understanding of the different interpretations of truth and value, from which one's ethics (principles) and morals (practice) are derived. Each part is contained within a whole; each part stands or falls together. Proof is relative to the system. In this sense true statements or value judgments are relative; the relativity, however, is *within* the whole system not *between* systems. Since correspondence and coherence are tests of trust, the more clearly that identity of each part coheres and corresponds (is internally consistent) to the whole, the more assurance one will have that one's ethics and morals are right.[7]

One example may prevent this discussion from being too abstract and unrelated to a natural science which appears to be totally objective. The second law of thermodynamics states that "there is a tendency for any system to become less organized."[8] As energy is used, some is transformed into nonusable heat energy and as such is unavailable for future energy exchanges. There is no other scientific law supported more fully and certainly by more numerous and meaningful lines of evidence. This law is, however, inconsistent with the theory of evolution which states that life systems are becoming *more organized*. Logically, this law and this theory cannot be maintained. They represent antithesis. Christian-theism, with its account of the Fall, however, finds this law consistent with its concept of decreasing order. Thus, the second law of thermodynamics illustrates the relevancy of presuppositional philosophy to objective science. The two are not inseparable and must be tested for their consistency.

Making the Choice—Theism or Naturalism

The importance of this internal identity is enhanced by a further distinction between these two world views: order and disorder (Figure 1). The logic is simply that any order, no matter how limited, must have an Orderer (theism). If there is no order, only disorder is left. The naturalist who holds to disorder cannot be consistent. Communication itself requires complex *order*, that is, letters are symbols which are grouped together to form words, each of which has a limited number of definitions. Consistency within naturalism would require that communication occur with a disorderly arrangement of symbols which, themselves, could have no recurring pattern. *The naturalist must presuppose and use an ordered system just to be able to communicate his view of basic disorder!* Disorder may seem to be a sufficient explanation of the origin of complex design but it is insufficient to accomplish simple communication. To one who thinks presuppositionally, epistemology (methodology) and metaphysics are obviously inconsistent.

This communication by the naturalist is one reason for my philosophical discussion. The naturalist functions and communicates predominately upon a "common ground" with the theist. This commonality is deceptive because their presuppositional foundations are contradictory. Although neither is fully consistent (no one ever is or can be) to theism, the naturalist has never committed himself to attempt consistency, so he may freely choose any rationale for his arguments without hesitancy. In fairness he usually does this unconsciously but the result is the same. Since his function and communication appear rational (orderly) predominantly, his inconsistency is usually unnoticed by himself or the theist. The former considers that he has made a rational judgment; the latter wonders why he has failed to convince. For each, rationality is defined differently: the theist is committed to the rationality of a theistic world view which is an ordered, defined system; the naturalist is committed to the rationality of a world view of disorder which allows him to choose any rationale since a disordered universe does not require ordered (logical) choice. Each will consider the other to be irrational because their bases (presuppositions) are entirely opposite.

> A Christian (theist) and a non-Christian (naturalist) may frequently *do* the same things; they may also frequently *approve* of the same things; but they are not likely to act and judge as they do *for the same reason* with reference to the same ideal, in obedience to a command understood in the same way. Here, in their deep-level orientation to duty, they are set apart from each other. And here where one is close to the center of ethics, the reality of the distinction between a Christian and a non-Christian discloses itself.[9]

On a rare occasion, a naturalist recognizes his position. Sir Julian Huxley acknowledged that somehow or other—against all that one might expect—a person functions better if he acts as though God exists, that is, lives a lie.[10] Albert Camus stated, "There is but one truly serious philosophical problem, and that is suicide."[11]

History of Naturalism

Historically, the "rationality" of the naturalist is apparent. With the Renaissance, secular Western society decided that it did not need God.[12] It had no other explanation, however, for origins. Thus, Deism was conceived. Origins were accounted for, but God's lack of personal involvement with men and with the universe allowed man to do as he pleased morally. When Darwin proposed an explanation which excluded the need for Deism, Western thought was ripe for its acceptance. Science and philosophy were agreed, man was progressing physically and morally. World Wars I and II shattered the reality of moral progress, so man's objective value, the highest form of evolution, was rejected in favor of subjective existentialism which is primarily concerned with the individual self or personal subjective choice. Alasdair MacIntyre is quoted in Paul Brownback's book, "Rational first principles have been replaced by criterionless choices."[13] Existentialism does not work, however, because no one will pay a salary to, or otherwise provide support for, someone who comes and goes as he pleases. ". . . to survive, he must get up in the morning, go to work, and do what the boss tells him [but]. . . .Whenever he can and to whatever extent he can, modern man assumes the existential approach to life."[14] The description clearly represents the naturalist who cannot live consistently with his world view. He picks and chooses between the naturalist and theistic base only in reference to his desires, even though these choices are mostly subconscious.

Knowledge or Belief?

Let us briefly examine how this mixture of world view affects communication and argumentation. The Christian (theist) is often challenged that he *believes* that God exists but the naturalist can *prove* that God doesn't exist. Since Descartes and Kant, this false distinction in Western thinking has occurred between knowledge, fact and belief.[15] The naturalistic scientist considers that he "knows" rather than he "believes." This distinction, however, (as we have shown) is presuppositional; the naturalist has presupposed the possiblity of his empirical investigation: an orderly universe. Further, when he applies empirically-derived concepts to metaphysical reality, *by definition* he has left science (empirical investigation) and entered metaphysics. Therefore, "belief" is the foundational argument for all philosophies *and* empirical sciences. Even, "I don't know" is a belief that the choice of more specific belief is not an imperative. The concept of presuppositional belief is important where evidences for the Christian faith are presented. It is not that the evidences (phenomena) are inconclusive but that the evidence is interpreted (consciously or subconsciously) by another belief system.[16] The presuppositional concept is important, also, when the esteem of modern science is considered. The wonder of scientific technology must not obscure its metaphysical beliefs. Exclusion of any metaphysical or supernatural reality *is* a metaphysical position. (A closer look at the epistemology of science occurs in chapter 3.)

The Search for Objectivity

By now the difficulty which is involved in the discernment of truth should be more apparent since it has been seen to be limited by chosen presuppositions. This limitation is further seen in a discussion of objectivity and subjectivity. Because the naturalist believes in disorder at his deepest philosophical level and evolution tells him that he is the highest intelligence on earth, the discernment of truth becomes dependent upon the individual. Although objection may be offered that truth may be discerned by a group of men, there exists no external objective standard by which the naturalist may decide that his yielding to a group's judgment is any better than one individual's judgment. The decision to do so would be entirely arbitrary. Thus, objectivity and subjectivity merge into indistinction within the individual. Objectivity is dependent upon individual interpretation (subjectivity). The naturalist is ''free'' to choose what truth is from his mixture of world view (order and disorder). From this choice he will derive his principles and practices. Thus, *no naturalist has any compulsion to give credence to any principles and practices that differ from his own.*

It is fascinating that theistic presuppositions lead to a merger of objectivity and subjectivity also. ''What is truth?'' Pilate asked when his answer stood before him. Jesus had previously said, ''I am the way, the *truth*, and the life'' (John 14:6). Thus, theism views truth as a Person, and Jesus Christ as one with the Triune God. *In this sense* truth is ultimately subjective, since subjectivity is the reality which a person perceives or experiences. This Person, however, is unique. He is all-knowing, makes no mistakes, and does not misperceive. Therefore, He is fully objective.[17] Truth, as objectivity and subjectivity, is unified. Any search for truth as totally objective (for example, the search of the naturalistic scientist) will fail. Any search for truth as totally subjective (for example, the existentialist) will fail because the truth is determined by another person. Philosophers and particularly scientists search for total objectivity, but their quest is doomed to failure by this dual nature of truth. This subjectivity in no way limits objectivity; rather, the latter is established. God's characteristics (attributes) become the characteristics of truth: absolute, eternal, ultimate, and complete rather than relative, temporary, derived, or partial.[18] Further, He has promised that (regenerated) man can know the truth (John 8:31-32). On the one hand, He is the guarantee that objective truth exists and that man can know it. On the other hand, the acceptance of such objectivity (which is one operation of the Holy Spirit; John 16:13 and I Cor. 2:9-16) cannot be known apart from the Person (John 14:6).

Thus, it has been shown that reasoning and persuasion, whether within an individual, or between individuals, is inseparable from individual world views.

Presuppositions, epistemology, interpretation of evidence, knowledge—belief, and objective-subjective judgments are limited, even determined, by the whole system. The choice between theism and naturalism is a decisive watershed.

Ethics and morals are dependent upon world view. To proceed to them without a recognition that they cannot be isolated from a whole is to fail entirely because naturalism and theism are contradictory and antithetical to each other. Without agreement at the deepest level of philosophy, ethics and morals disagree, even where agreement may exist on the more superficial level of a particular issue.

Revelational World View

Our attention turns to revelation as *the* ''single, inclusive and determinative principle of moral value'' for Christian theism. Although Christians may agree on theism as a world view, a decision that is crucial to subsequent methodology must be made: it concerns the values given to revelation and to empirical knowledge. One hears, ''All truth is God's truth.'' As we have shown, however, a concept of truth is internally dependent. So the statement itself is simple *and true*, but its usefulness is anything but simple. Some method must be established by which ''all truth'' can be recognized. Without this method, ethics and morals cannot be judged right or wrong where disagreement exists. Where two or more positions exist on a moral issue, only one can be right with all others being wrong. In our day the emphasis is often on the process rather than the final decision, but to fail to distinguish between right and wrong involves something other than ethics. By traditional and current definition, ethics is *the discipline* designed to help us arrive at right and wrong. Process must be careful and thorough, but the final decision is *right* or it is *wrong*; *it cannot be both.* Let us see how Christians may proceed to such conclusions.

How Can Truth Be Determined?

For our purposes, empirical knowledge will be defined as all knowledge which is derived without biblical interpretation. In theological language, such knowledge is ''natural revelation.'' As we have seen, the naturalist must assume some theistic presuppositions before he can think, act, or communicate without his commitment to formulate a consistent theistic world view. Thus, the reliability of any statements, propositions, or research which is proposed as truth by the naturalist, cannot be accepted without thorough inspection by the theist. The necessity of this inspection does not mean that such knowledge is useful; anyone who denies the usefulness of modern technology or the beauty of (some) non-Christian art would be foolish. It must be thoroughly inspected, however, because the world view from which it is derived has no commitment to internal consistency. It cannot be truth from the wholistic concept of truth because it includes a mixture of naturalistic and theistic presuppositions. A beautiful mansion covers over its foundation—which may either be shifting sand or solid rock. The Christian theist knows the foundation of all unbelievers;

for him to buy the house while knowing about its unsound foundation is an extreme error of judgment.

The error is greater when the Christian does not inspect the sources of other Christians who write and speak. Many Christians use a great deal of non-Christian sources. The possibility that they will deceive other Christians is more likely than when a naturalist speaks because many Christians tend to accept without criticism what another Christian presents as truth. Many Christians, even trained theologians, have an amazing naivete in this uncritical acceptance, especially from a Christian who is a professional in one of the natural sciences.

How then do we determine truth? If truth is "what is," how is it recognized? Within the context of this chapter the answer determines the whole thrust of this book, as principles (ethics) result from a study of truth (world view), and practices (morals) are derived from principles. Again, the answer is epistemological or methodological. In the progression from deepest presuppositions to casuistry, the whole system becomes more clearly identifiable and consistent as the parts are related within the whole. Within naturalism the whole can never be identified because each individual is free to choose further means or methods by which he may recognize truth. Thus, naturalism produces as many world views (concepts of truth) as the number of individuals who have ever lived. Within theism God is the final Interpreter of truth, but He must give man an objective standard which is available to the senses of all individual theists or else the theist has no practical (moral) advantage over the naturalist. Both are limited physically to the products of their senses, that is to empirical data. An external objective standard, however, is an immense advantage since contrast and comparison of competing truths to it is possible.

The Importance of Special Revelation

At this point we establish a clear identity with Christian-theism as a world view. The foregoing discussion is, however, particularly relevant because **the Christian without an objective standard is as limited in his determination of principles and practice as the naturalist.** He is left with his individual empirical self as the standard. Precisely at this point the greatest division in Christendom occurs: the Bible as the final source (standard or authority), or the Bible as *a* source (Figure 1).[19] This division is *presuppositional* because "the Bible is eternal, religious truth known only to faith."[20] Of course, coherence and correspondence of evidence will strengthen or weaken one's position with a change of position possibly resulting from the latter. Even so, the initial decision about the Bible is presupposed; it cannot involve evidence because the method by which evidence is interpreted is presupposed also.

For example, a Christian is to "confess with [his] mouth Jesus as Lord, and believe in [his] heart that God raised Him from the dead" (Rom. 10:10). But then, which Christ does the Christian confess: the de-mythologized Christ of higher critics, the nonhistorical (mythological) Christ of modern theology, or the historical Christ of evangelical theology?[21] These Christs *are not the same*;

the differences result from presupposed methodologies. The "higher critics" *assume* that myths about Christ are present in the gospels; modernist theologians *assume* that a reliable history of Christ is unnecessary to faith in Him; and evangelicals *assume* that the gospels without addition or subtraction present the truth about Christ. The first two positions *assume* man's competency to judge what in the Bible is to be included or excluded; the third position *assumes* the whole and interprets, rather than includes or excludes.

The Law of Contradiction

This example is one of many which could illustrate a serious objection from the discipline of logic to any method which allows for different concepts about the same subject: the law of contradiction. If one statement about a subject is true, no statements which contradict that statement can be true. All three Christs may be false *or* one may be true, but all three *cannot* be true. To take the position that all three may be true reduces language to meaninglessness.[22] Then, any statement becomes meaningless; communication or argument becomes meaningless; all becomes meaningless. The seriousness of this particular issue is more apparent when the earthly happiness and eternal destiny of every person is at stake according to the Christ in whom each believes. An error here results in damnation in both spheres of existence!

Biblical World Views

There is another serious objection to any method which does not specifically consider the biblical division of two contrasting world views, identified as light and darkness (John 1:4, 5), foolishness and wisdom (1 Cor. 1:18-25), flesh and spirit (Gal. 5:17), life and death (Rom. 6:23), falsehood and truth (1 John 1:6), and love and hate (1 John 3:11-15). The world view which is contrasted with theism is represented in three ways: personally, as Satan; collectively, as the world; and individually, as unbelievers. Satan is the god of the temporal sphere (2 Cor. 4:4) whose effects closely approximate what God does (2 Cor. 11:13-15). The world's thinking is the enemy of Christian thinking (John 15:18-16:4; Rom. 12:2; John 4:4). The unbeliever is the enemy of God and His people (Rom. 1:30, 3:9-18, 5:10). Thus, the Bible describes "a gigantic battle between good and evil which splits the universe."[23] Coherence and consistency with a Christian-theistic position would seem to require this identifiable contrast wherever Christians are attempting to discern truth since the Bible is very clear on this point, and no one can reasonably deny that the Bible is the major source of truth for all Christians.

The Christian who tries to identify truth but consciously or unconsciously ignores the law of contradiction and the biblical description of opposing world views proceeds against formidable (impossible) limitations. Thus, the simple statement, "All truth is God's truth," is misleading because it says nothing about a methodology which considers these two principles. The issue is *recognition of truth*, not that all truth is derived from God. The same problem exists whenever anyone speaks of the integration of the Bible with other sources of truth. Where contradictions occur, logic demands resolution which further demands that one view be authoritative over the other. The biblical description of opposing world views demands extreme caution because every issue is *for* one world view and *against* the other. Statements and propositions by Christians are no guarantee that they have already exercised these methodological precautions.

Natural Revelation and Tests of Truth

Because final authority must be given to biblical or extrabiblical knowledge, particularly at recognizable points of conflict, let us return for a closer look at extrabiblical (naturalistic) knowledge. What are the results when internal consistency (coherence and correspondence) is applied to naturalism as a system? The naturalist and particularly the naturalistic scientist claims objectivity and avoidance of belief as part of his system. The evidence, however, is not convincing. There is nothing in the empirical world that demonstrates order resulting from disorder. For example, no one is paid a salary for doing whatever he wants, whenever he wants, but schedules are designed to meet objectives; explosions (extreme disorder) destroy life and property whereas precise construction is necessary to build productively; and finally, disorder is not the method of scientific experiments, but rather the opposite as scientists strive for exactness and orderliness in their procedures and records. Now the naturalist believes that order resulted from disorder "in the beginning," but his way of life and experimental design reflect a failure to cohere and correspond to his stated belief. Actually, his life and designs reflect his deepest, subconscious belief of assumed theism.

Even so, doesn't another test of truth, pragmatic value, give credence to naturalism, especially in light of the achievements of modern science?[24] Yes, it does, where experimentation and application are almost totally objective. A positive answer is questionable, however, in areas that involve subjectivity, that is, human experimentation and application. For example, no naturalistic philosophy has shown men how to have a happy life or give them hope. Public education has declined in its effectiveness for the past twenty years as orderliness and discipline have declined in the classroom. Music has become noise. Art has become bizarre. Legal systems are increasingly inconsistent in decisions and liability suits are rampant. Marriages and families are disintegrating. If nontheism works so well scientifically (objectively), where are its accomplishments for man as a person? Nontheistic thought prevails because the lack of an orderly systematic approach (theism) does not immediately impact in nonscientific areas. In the natural sciences, failure would be immediate without assumed theism because it requires detailed precision. In the humanities the result is not immediate because no objectivity exists for comparison and contrast.

Biblical Theism vs. Naturalism

This closer look at naturalism according to the commonly accepted criteria for truth has clarified the second decisive watershed in a presuppositional methodology by which truth can be discerned and from which principle and practice can be derived: biblical theism, that is, the complete Bible, is the final authority for all truth.[25] On the one hand, such a position does not mean that the Bible speaks with equal clarity or equal content to all areas of human endeavor. For example, it was not written to be a detailed science textbook. On the other hand, any subject about which it is concluded that the Bible is limited or is silent must have had the application of sound hermeneutics and a thorough consideration of biblical information. Medicine is one area where Christians have lacked such application and consideration. The entire thrust of this book is to correct that problem.

Serious problems with knowledge which is obtained from naturalists have been shown. Their only real area of competence is in the scientific realm. (Although, beyond the little which has been mentioned here, other methodological problems exist for the natural sciences—chapter 3.) Even here, however, science cannot give ethical principles for moral application.

> . . . Scripture unerringly identifies the good (moral) whereas empirical science cannot do so. And if we do not know the good, the value even of our scientific insights is unsure.[26]

Naturalism is dependent upon the autonomy of the individual man. Biblical theism is dependent upon the autonomy of God who has given special revelation, objectively, and His Spirit, subjectively, in order for His people to know truth. A great distance separates the Christian who gives equal authority to natural revelation and special revelation in his determination of truth and the Christian who accepts the latter as the final authority for truth. Essentially, the former falls into the same world view as the naturalist: the self arbitrates truth. There is no other objective standard which is not itself arbitrary.[27] The biblical theist (Christian-theist) *interprets* truth from the whole which has been posited by God Himself (the Holy Spirit). Arbitrariness and interpretation become opposed methodologies.

This division does not to minimize certain realities. (1) My discussion here has its own presuppositions. Thus, an acceptance of its conclusions will likely occur only in those who hold a similar world view. My hope has been to educate others concerning the limitations of one's presuppositions. The Christian theist must become aware that truth does not exist independent of world view, even though communication and cooperation can occur because of "common ground." The world view of the naturalist or the Christian naturalist and the Christian theist are as antithetical as darkness and light. (2) All Christian theists do not agree on interpretative methods (hermeneutics) or final interpretation (next chapter). We are fallen and finite, even though redeemed. Neither of these realities, however, minimizes the greater gulf between Christian theists and Christian naturalists. These realities may result in denominational and other interpretive differences, but these problems are one step removed from the fundamental metaphysical problem of a system of truth (world view).[28]

In Summary

Ethics or principles from which morality can be derived are dependent upon one's view of ultimate reality (world view), a presuppositional choice or position of faith. Initially, two incompatible options are possible: naturalism (disorder) or theism (Orderer). Communication and cooperation are possible only because those who place their faith in chance are inconsistently theists in their methodology without any commitment to consistency with theism as a world view. Thus, theists must scrutinize "knowledge" derived from naturalists. Theists (Christians) who wrongly use such knowledge are often more dangerous than naturalists because a theistic (Christian) audience almost always assumes that the theist speaks consistently with theism as a world view.

Even a commitment to theism, however, results in a different conception of truth. A standard must be chosen because truth cannot be identified without some objective standard. The only alternative is truth that is individually subjective (existentialism). The choice of the Bible as an objective standard is biblical-theism (Christian-theism). The choice of individual subjectivity is theistic-naturalism (Chrisitan- naturalism). The biblical evidence of antithetical world views and the law of contradiction separates the two options by a great gulf. Indeed, the separation is as complete as that of theism and naturalism, since truth is dependent upon, and decided by, the individual self.

The Christian-theistic position does not prevent disagreements, but these are entirely different from the two presuppositional divisions of naturalism (Christian and non-Christian) and Christian-theism. In Christian-theism the standard for truth is settled; the problem becomes interpretation and application (hermeneutics.)

Some professing Christians may discontinue their reading or automatically discount anything further which is said. Such actions would be consistent with what has been discussed. Without an agreement on a source of truth any individual is free to disagree upon any point, resulting in a stalemate since every individual may choose his own truth. A committment to Christian-theism, however, requires diligence to reconcile our differences because God is unity. Of two or more positions of disagreement, either one must be right, or another not yet considered must be right. God's nature requires that two contradictory positions cannot be right. We must strive toward final agreement in principle and in practice because we have agreed upon the Source of truth *and* His Revelation.

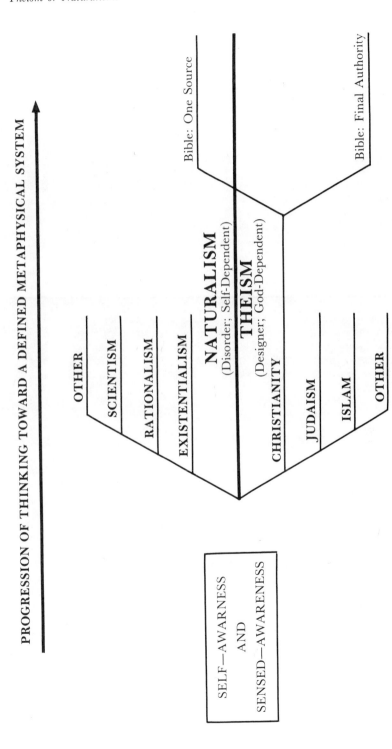

FIGURE 1. Division of World Views
(Christianity further divided according to biblical position)

NOTES

1. Alasdair MacIntyre, "Why Is the Search for the Foundations of Medical Ethics So Frustrating?," *Hastings Center Report* 9(4) (August, 1979), pp. 16-22.

2. Henry Stob, *Ethical Reflections* (Grand Rapids: Eerdmans Pub. Co., 1978), p. 24.

3. An understanding of these terms will become apparent in the following discussion, even though philosophy has many words to describe metaphysical positions: positivism, atheism, dualism, secularism, relativism, etc. Of particular note, however, is a departure from the common philosophical use of "naturalism." In this book it will be expanded from its designation that reality is limited to the empirical world to include the reality of the mind or thought. The latter is usually designated by such terms as rationalism, idealism, or *a priori* reasoning. Since supernatural connotes a metaphysical being, naturalism seems an appropriate choice for all other philosophies.

4. Harold H. Titus, Marilyn S. Smith, and Richard T. Nolan, *Living Issues in Philosophy*, 7th ed. (New York: D. Van Nostrand Company, 1979) p. 200.

5. Gordon H. Clark, *A Christian View of Men and Things: An Introduction to Philosophy* (1952; reprint ed., Grand Rapids: Baker Book House, 1981), p. 26.

6. My critics may accuse that my present methodology is based upon personal presuppositions. In this criticism they would be correct. Neither of us will be convinced of the other's views because our world views are incompatible. My reasoning is directed primarily to two audiences: the Christian who is unaware of the interdependency of truth, and to the person (Christian or non-Christian) who is willing to consider whether Christian-theism fulfills the tests for truth more comprehensively and consistently than naturalism.

7. Titus, Smith and Nolan, *Living Issues in Philosophy*, pp. 202-205.

8. Henry M. Morris, *Studies in the Bible and Science* (Philadelphia: Presbyterian and Reformed Publishing Co., 1966), p. 113.

9. Henry Stob, *Ethical Reflections*, p. 23.

10. C. Everett Koop and Francis A Schaeffer, *Whatever Happened to the Human Race* (Westchester, Ill.: Crossway Books, 1983), p. 140.

11. Ibid., p. 144.

12. Paul Brownback, *The Danger of Self-Love* (Chicago: Moody Press, 1982), p. 27ff.

13. Ibid., p. 31.

14. Ibid., p. 34.

15. David W. Beck, "A Response to Truth: Relationship of Theories to Hermeneutics," Paper written for Summitt II of the International Council on Biblical Inerrancy. (Chicago: November 1982), p. 11.

16. This realization fits with the biblical concept that Christian belief must be preceded by regeneration (rebirth), one result of which is the change of attitude towards the existence of supernatural beings and phenomena.

17. To avoid the criticism of pantheism, let me state that the material world, as God created it, exists entirely separate from Himself.

18. John Murray, *Principles of Conduct* (Grand Rapids: Eerdmans Pub. Co., 1978), p. 123.

19. The evangelical Protestant accepts biblical evidence that the Holy Spirit superintended the selection of the books of the Bible. The church did not decide which ones to include and exclude, but it was unerringly guided to select the books which are contained in the Protestant Bible. This position differs markedly from the Roman Catholic position in which the church had God-given authority to choose which books were included or excluded. The former position is totally dependent upon the Spirit; the latter had delegated responsibility. Thus, orthodox Protestants do not accept the additional books of the Catholic Bible.

20. David W. Beck, "A Response to Truth," p. 10.

21. Harold O. J. Brown, *The Protest of a Troubled Protestant* (1969, reprint ed., Grand Rapids: Zondervan Pub. Co., 1971), pp. 165-187.

22. Gordon H. Clark, *A Christian View of Men and Things*, p. 292 ff.

23. Harry Blamires, *The Christian Mind* (1963; reprint ed., Ann Arbor: Servant Books, 1978), p. 70.

24. Titus, Smith and Nolan. *Living Issues in Philosophy*, p. 206ff.

25. At this point I must be careful. No person can judge whether another person is a true believer; only God is able to discern true faith. The acceptance of the Bible as final source *may* not be necessary to saving faith, but the possibility that it is, deserves to be raised. The Bible is Spirit-expired (2 Tim. 3:16); the Spirit is truth and guides the believer into "all truth" (John 16:13); the Bible is truth and believers are sanctified by the truth (John 17:17); the Spirit inhabits the believer (2 Cor. 1:22; Eph. 1:13). The Bible, the Spirit, and the believer have a necessary intimate relationship. It seems inconceivable that the indwelling Spirit would not confirm to the believer what He had written. This lack of confirmation is understandable in a believer who is immature in knowledge and Christian experience because he is moving from darkness to light, and the darkness from which he comes is powerful and deceptive (2 Cor. 11:13-15). It is less understandable in, and likely incompatible with, an experienced, biblically knowledgeable Christian. It is the nature of Christian growth that the believer increases his identity with Jesus Christ. An absolute essential of that identity is having the mind of Christ (1 Cor. 2:10-18).

26. Carl F. H. Henry, "The Ambiguities of Scientific Breakthrough," in *Horizons of Science*, ed. Carl F. Henry (San Francisco: Harper and Row Pub., 1978), p. 103.

27. Neither the skeptic nor the relativist can escape absolutes. If one says that nothing is true (or variations thereof), there are no absolutes, truth does not exist, all is relative, one cannot know, he has made an absolute statement (upon which he rests his destiny). As a believer, I find this inability to avoid absolutes fascinating: God has so structured logic that at least one absolute cannot be avoided. For a more definitive study of how absolutes cannot be avoided, see *The Necessity of Ethical Absolutes* by Erwin Lutzer.

28. It is amazing, however, how extensive the agreement is among those who are committed to this position and develop it consistently and diligently. Such commitment includes a subjective relationship with Jesus Christ in which an increasing awareness of personal sin and God's attributes grows. It could be stated that there is a commitment to both the science of interpretation—objectivity—and personal Christian growth—subjectivity (Brown, 15-28, 45-55). Historically, cold, sterile Fundamentalism resulted from emphasis upon the former; Pietism (and currently, Pentecostalism) has resulted from excessive emphasis upon the latter. Both should proceed from Christian-theism. As a balanced emphasis is achieved by individuals and groups, many areas of agreement are found. This agreement is convincing and encouraging evidence that such a methodology is correct and that unity does exist, often extensively, among true believers (see note 5). This agreement demonstrates that such committment is presuppositional; that is, truth is known only to Christian faith, personally and propositionally (Harold O. J. Brown, *The Protest of a Troubled Protestant*, pp. 173ff). Many disagreements among professing Christians may arise because this starting point (whether consciously or unconsciously) is not true faith.

REFERENCES

Beck, David W. "A Response to Truth: Relationship of Theories of Truth to Hermeneutics." Paper written for Summitt II of the International Council on Biblical Inerrancy, Chicago, November 1982.

Blamires, Harry. *The Christian Mind*. 1963. Reprint.Ann Arbor: Servant Books, 1978.

Brownback, Paul. *The Danger of Self-Love*. Chicago: Moody Press, 1982.

Clark, Gordon H. *A Christian View of Men and Things: An Introduction to Philosophy*. 1952. Reprint.Grand Rapids: Baker Book House, 1981.

International Council on Biblical Inerrancy. "Hermeneutics: The Chicago Statement: Affirmation and Denials (Articles I-XXV)." International Council on Biblical Inerrancy, P.O. Box 13261, Oakland, CA, 94661.

Koop, Everett C. and Schaeffer, Francis A. *Whatever Happened to the Human Race*. Westchester, Ill.: Crossway Books, 1983.

Lutzer, Erwin. *The Necessity of Ethical Absolutes*. Grand Rapids: Zondervan Publishing House, 1981.

MacIntyre, Alasdair. "Why Is the Search for the Foundations of Medical Ethics So Frustrating?" *Hastings Center Report* 9(4) Aug. 1979: 16-22.

Morris, Henry M. *Studies in the Bible and Science*. 1966. Reprint. Philadelphia: Presbyterian and Reformed Publishing Co., 1966.

Titus, Harold H., Marilyn S. Smith and Richard T. Nolan. *Living Issues in Philosophy* (7th ed). New York: D. Van Nostrand Company, 1979.

3 | The Credibility of Science

A counselee came to my office because of continual depression over the previous eighteen months. Originally, she had seen another physician and related her symptoms of fatigue coupled with an inability to manage housework and other daily responsibilities. Her doctor's medical workup failed to reveal any physiological basis for her symptoms. He diagnosed depression, prescribed an anti-depressant drug, and told her the depression would continue throughout her life. She and her husband would have to adjust their lives accordingly. She sought other counseling because such a dismal and ineffective life was not what she believed the Christian life should be. Prior to our first visit she had discontinued the drug because there were no noticeable benefits.

At our first session, it was clear she had a substantive and knowledgeable Christian faith. I agreed that her current experience was abnormal for a Christian and discussed the biblical alternative of hope (1 Cor. 10:13; James 1:2-4). A revised plan included a schedule and a list of prioritized responsibilities. After following our plan, her first visit showed a smiling and joyous Christian. This simple plan for organization, based upon her commitment to her faith, was effective. Only one additional session was necessary and over my forty-two months of follow-up, her disposition showed steady improvement.

This case simply illustrates that traditional medical practice may fail in its assessment of patient problems. Of course, the failure may be due to the art and/or the science of medicine. Most would acknowledge occasional or even frequent error because medicine is partly an art practiced by imperfect human beings. Few would admit that a frequent cause of error is the "science of medicine;" primarily because accounts of medical triumphs appear in the news media daily. Since scientific methods are the objective foundation of medicine, one must analyze science generally to determine the degree of its limitations. If the "objective" sciences have limitations, medical science which is much less objective, can be seen as more subject to limitations.

The idea that science is the major source of fact and truth is perhaps *the* greatest obstacle to a biblical/medical ethic. "Centuries ago it may have been possible to ignore science . . . but today its successes are so phenomenal that it is usually accorded the last word in all disputes"[1]

This "last word" is valued by both Christians and non-Christians because:

> The scientist tries to rid himself of all faiths and beliefs. He either knows or he does not know. If he knows, there is no room for faith or belief. If he does not know, he has no right to faith or belief.[2]

With this attitude the scientist easily assumes himself to be an authority on ethics and morals.

> . . . even philosophers are coming to see that, in a metaphysical study of reality, the methods and results of science are the **best** available evidence, and that new realism, if possible at all, must be built up by **their** means.[3]

Within the medical profession this authoritative posture is seen in the activities of medical organizations that remove abortion from the list of moral problems and relate it to "medical" considerations.

Science cannot be divorced from faith. Indeed, the natural sciences have distinct limitations that ultimately rest upon one's world view and position of faith. Ask yourself—"What immediately comes to mind when I think about the word "science?" Most likely, your images are related to the natural sciences, e.g. biology, chemistry, physics, or medicine. Etymologically, the word "science" meant the systematic knowlege and understanding of *any area* acquired through study or empiricism.[4] For example, "Theology is called the science of the knowledge of God."[5] This meaning has changed, so today science generally refers to a natural science and connotes precision, sophistication, and accuracy. If something is "science" or "scientific," its factuality or truthfulness is considered above question. However "there is no universal agreement, even among scientists, as to what is meant by the words "scientific method.""[6] It is more accurate to speak of "scientific *methods*" as the numerous processes and steps by which the various sciences are built up. These methods include theory development, experimental design, and collection of relevant and available data. Thus, a unique "scientific method," which is *the* standard for empirical investigation, does not exist.

Faith and Science

The contemporary mindset incorrectly divorces knowledge from belief; they are intimately related yet distinct. Belief determines the specific content of knowledge which is valued to the extent that one is willing to conform his behavior to that particular knowledge. Although scientists prefer to avoid faith, the naturalistic scientist's starting point and foundation involves a faith commitment no less than any other discipline (including religions).

Faith and belief are synonyms; they are used interchangeably; they are used generically to apply to content which is not religious. This broader use, however, does not alter the observation that the described characteristics of faith are applicable to religious contexts. It extends to concepts such as presuppositions, assumptions, axioms, *a priori* judgments, biases and first principles.

A starting point of the reasoning process can be individual self-consciousness; from this self-consciousness, most people are certain that they exist and an external world exists.[7] This certainty is grounded in personal faith. Thus, *any* and all verification involves the senses. Entirely objective (external) proof does not exist and our most (subjectively) valued beliefs are infallibly revealed by what we say and do (objectively)! Since entirely external proof does not exist, certainty of personal existence and action is grounded in presuppositions (faith). The mind is isolated from everything external to itself; its final verification is self; it is self-dependent for knowledge of its own existence.

All empirical observations and demonstrations of objective (external) reality are dependent upon the assumption of existence of the individual mind or self-consciousness. Such empiricism is science. Therefore, all science is ultimately dependent upon the belief in one's own existence and in the reliability of one's senses. It is a fatal mistake to think or argue that science and supernatural religions proceed from different starting points. Does this realization clearly place science and faith upon equal ground? The supernaturalist should not give any more credibility to the scientist than he does to himself. Either may have more fully and consistently developed his "faith" (world view), but their foundations are similiar.

Where does this foundation leave faith relative to knowledge? Knowledge is distinguished from faith at the point of action. The Christian may extensively *study* the Koran but he will not *act* upon its knowledge. On the one hand knowledge does not always result in commitment. On the other hand, faith is never blind; that is, it is never divorced from some degree of knowledge, consciously or unconsciously. In summary, faith is subjective, determining the objective knowledge upon which concrete speech or behavior will be based; but it lacks direct correlation to the quantity or quality of the knowledge. There is an organic relationship, but one controlled by the subjective element.[8] An increase of knowledge may result in a change of commitment, but faith not the knowledge, allows or directs change. Further, the most significant personal acts may be based upon little knowledge.

Disconcertingly, knowledge and belief are commonly interchanged as synonyms. A person may say, "I know," when he means, "I believe." This use is common even in the scientific literature. To the credit of scientists in general, it should be stated that their published research is usually quite clear about their acknowledgement of incomplete information and assumptions. To their discredit, however, this acknowledgement does not usually extend to their willingness to allow supernatural foundations for ethical principles or moral practices. Thus, the uncertainty and incomplete explanations which are present in the scientific literature are absent in the ethics of scientists. To illustrate our point Norman MacBeth shows that, privately, evolutionists lack confidence in their "theory" but will not admit their doubt to the public.[9]

Faith is central to, and facilitates, every area of human life. Most decisions are made with little or no empirical investigations; indeed we cannot empirically investigate all the decisions necessary to daily existence. In short, faith is fundamental and necessary to every human endeavor. Modern society has been brainwashed to think that science is fundamental and ultimate when it is actually secondary to and predetermined by faith.

It is this universal belief in self-existence that allows science! If individuals did not believe their senses, observation, experiment, and communication of the results would not be possible. Further, science has faith in its ability to determine what research will be done and how it will be applied. Its results cannot be guaranteed in advance and its "progress" is often ambiguous and costly. Science is thoroughly enmeshed in faith. Science has not earned the right to issue any challenge to the supernatural. Scientists, as well as others, demonstrate that science is no deterrent to belief in the supernatural.[10]

Faith establishes the priority and authority of revelation (the Scriptures) over scientific investigation through a simple *acceptance*. Naturalistic scientists and Christians begin at the same starting point—self-consciousness; however, Christians realize the priority and authority of revelation because of the Revealer's presence within the believer to understand that revelation (1 Cor. 2:10-16). This scriptural position is the major tenet of a biblical approach to medical ethics and a Christian's goal is to ascribe value according to Scripture and not mundane concepts. Many judgments concerning science today improperly value empiricism; and Christians have often accepted this improper evaluation. Science is limited in the answers it can provide because of its own characteristics: its assumed premises, its mutability, its subjective choices, its lack of universality, its exclusion of metaphysics, its inability to establish value, and its examination of parts rather than wholes.

The Limitations of Science

These limitations of science concern its ability to determine truth (ultimate reality or world view), and therefore ethical principles and moral practice. It should be remembered that presuppositions proscribe what one accepts as truth. In science, presuppositions are called axioms, premises, postulates, fact, hard data, proofs, law or other similar names. The one presupposition upon which they all rest, however, is rarely named: a predictable or orderly universe. This one presupposition, as well as all others, involves assumption or belief. Thus, science is subordinate to faith and cannot be an arbiter of truth because it must presuppose principles upon which it experiments. It has no special claim on truth and should not be perceived to do so.

Faith is (foundationally) prior to science or any other knowledge. The reliability of scientific methods is not necessarily greater than knowledge which is derived by other means, and the nature of science is such that it cannot make moral judgments, so the priority of faith further underscores any effort by science to make such judgments. This priority covers medicine, as well.

Physicians who conclude that a certain treatment, such as abortion, is a valid medical procedure are stating a medical possibility *not* its morality. Many Christian physicians recognize this fact concerning abortion, euthanasia, and other ethical issues, but they must *extend* this fact to all medical practices. *No hope of a thoroughly biblical ethic is possible until the principle that no medical practice is inherently moral is used as a starting point by Christian physicians.*

No ultimate conflict of truth exists within a Christian world view. All knowledge has one Source. A problem of terminology and interpretation may exist between science and the Bible but the only difficulty is man's inability to resolve the problem, *not* any conflict of truth. Science cannot derive truth, but Scripture claims truth. The superior credence for Scripture over science is clear. In the creation debate Francis Schaffer has spoken to this necessary authority for Scripture and is "convinced that the outcome of the discussion will determine the value of the heritage we leave to our children and grandchildren."[11]

> . . . it may not always be possible to correlate the two studies (science and the Bible) . . . yet if both studies can be adequately pursued, there will be no final conflict. . . . Science by its natural limitations cannot know all we know from God in the Bible, but in those cases where science can know, both sources of knowledge arrive at the same point, even if the knowledge is expressed in different terms. . . . there is no automatic need to accommodate the Bible to the statements of science. . . . there is the danger of evangelicalism becoming less than evangelical, of its not holding to the Bible as being without error in all that it affirms.[12]

Medical "science" excludes the biblical world view, bases its interpretation of man and medical science upon a naturalistic philosophy and evolutionary process. The practice of medicine is saturated with, and founded upon, principles that are *antithetical* to the Christian world view. Christians *must* understand this situation. This antithesis explains in part why the "spotlighted" ethical issues have occurred. The Christian physician is *not* in friendly territory within his profession. It would seem obvious that upon this basis alone, the Christian would not readily accept *any* medical practice without an attempt to discern its scientific validity, and more importantly, its moral (biblical) implications. Realistically, well-studied and discerning Christians are needed in *every medical specialty* to discern those practices that are soundly scientific and clearly biblical. The task is enormous but the exciting possibility of a truly Christian practice of medicine awaits such endeavor.

NOTES

1.Gordon H. Clark, *A Christian View of men and Things: An Introduction to Philosophy* (Grand Rapids: Baker Book House, 1981), p. 198.

2. Ibid., p. 200.

3. Harold H. Titus, Marilyn S. Smith, and Richard T. Nolan, *Living Issues in Philosophy*, 7th edition (New York: D. Van Nostrand Company), p. 239.

4. Abraham Kuyper, *Principles of Sacred Theology* (1898; reprint ed., Grand Rapids: Baker Book House, 1980), pp. 59-68.

5. Harold O. J. Brown, *The Protest of a Troubled Protestant* (1969; reprint ed., Grand Rapids: Zondervan Pub. Co., 1971), p. 15.

6. Titus, Smith, and Nolan, *Living Issues in Philosophy*, p. 223.

7. Certainty, here, extends to the degree that a person speaks or acts (puts into practice), regardless of any remaining ambiguity in his mind. Greater certainty is really not needed. The absence of ambiguity would bring internal peace, but peace itself would not change the speech or behavior that is put into practice. Further, these actions reflect one's certainty about the existence or non-existence of supernatural reality, even if that reflection is subconscious because such reflection includes metaphysically-derived purpose and motive; that is, the person's own *raison d'etre*.

8. One would expect evolutionists (naturalists) to deny clearly that science can derive truth. Evolution involves continual change. Such change prevents any absolute or true statement. Nothing can be known for sure because it may change tomorrow. Theists, however, should expect to find constancy since God created all things and continues to sustain them (Heb. 1:3). Thus, the theist should more easily discern that changing concepts result from such limitations of science as are being presented here. Indeed, the case has been developed that it was the rise of a clearer and more complete Christian theism that allowed the development of modern science (R. Hooykaas, *Religion and the Rise of Modern Science*. Grand Rapids: Eerdmans, 1972).

9. Norman MacBeth, *Darwin Retried: An Appeal to Reason* (Ipswich, Mass.: Gambit, 1971), p. iii-iv.

10. Harold O. J. Brown, *The Protest of a Troubled Protestant*, p. 207.

11. Francis A. Schaeffer, *No Final Conflict* (Downers Grove, Il: InterVarsity Press, 1980), p. 9.

12. Ibid., p. 44-48.

REFERENCES

Clark, Gordon H. *A Christian View of Men and Things: An Introduction to Philosophy*. 1952. Reprint. Grand Rapids: Baker Book House, 1981.

Custance, Arthur C. *Science and Faith*. Doorway Papers, vol. 8. Grand Rapids: Zondervan Publishing House, 1978.

Macbeth, Norman. *Darwin Retried: An Appeal to Reason*. Ipswich, Mass.: Gambit, 1971.

Schaeffer, Francis A. *No Final Conflict*. Downers Grove, IL.: InterVarsity Press, 1980.

Titus, Harold H., Marilyn S. Smith, and Richard T. Nolan. *Living Issues in Philosophy*. 7th ed. New York: D. Van Nostrand Company, 1979.

4 | Empirical Uncertainties of Modern Medicine

That which has been is that which will be, and that which has been done is that which will be done. So, there is nothing new under the sun.

Ecclesiastes 1:9

And a woman who had had a hemorrhage for twelve years, and had endured much at the hands of many physicians, and had spent all that she had and was not helped at all, but rather had grown worse . . .

Mark 5:25-26

* * * * * *

. . . the care of a poor woman who had continued pain in her stomach . . . they (physicians) prescribe drug upon drug without knowing a jot of the matter concerning the root of the disorders . . . they cannot cure. . . .Whence came this woman's pain? . . . from fretting for the death of her son.

John Wesley, 1759

This chapter must be read with a conscious awareness of its intended goal: a systematic analysis of the empirical foundations of modern medical science. My focus may appear to be negative because the real and impressive achievements of science in general, and medicine in particular, have resulted in common practices which are in many cases empirically uncertain. To present a consistently biblical approach to the practice of medicine, these scientific weaknesses must be evaluated critically. The effectiveness of medicine is not assumed here.

It is not my purpose to do away with medicine but to maximize its effectiveness, minimize its harm, make its hopes realistic and more consistently biblical. Since Christian physicians have an understanding of reality unavailable to secular doctors, they have the opportunity to enhance their patient care and affect medicine generally. Further, they have the opportunity to be used of

God and to effect a spiritual "cure". Even though their care of the physical body can be a true Christian ministry, the best medical care will only delay the inevitable: disease and/or death of the body. The application of biblical ethics within the practice of medicine which results in saving faith or spiritual growth in a patient is a permanent "cure," since it holds promise for the present life and also for the life to come (1 Tim. 4:8).

It is to be hoped that an increasing number of Christian physicians will become able to individualize medical care with a more complete application of the spiritual and physical dimensions of health. Christian laymen and pastors may be part of that hope by discipling Christian physicians to analyze medical science and to apply biblical principles in medical practice.

One precaution should be observed by nonphysicians. Specific disease and treatments will be discussed largely from research data. No effort will be made to present these comprehensively, since the primary intent is to establish general concepts and not to arrive at conclusions about specifics of diagnosis and treatment. These concepts should not be applied to personal problems without medical advice.

How Effective is Medical Care?
Highly-Rated? or Overrated?

> More of your patients are alive and well than might have been in 1970 or 1980. Your increasing knowledge made it possible. A lot of things have been going wrong lately but American health care is not one of them. . . . This is simply amazing, a record of success unmatched by any other segment of society or the economy. Indeed, without such success in health care, our country might be in more dire straits than it is. . . . To your health, doctor—and everybody's.[2]

This recent editorial in the *American Medical News* represents the professional and lay perception of the efficacy of modern medicine.

The news media is constantly announcing the latest scientific discoveries, each of which is heralded to be the great breakthrough that is needed with a particular disease. In this atmosphere a gigantic growth in expenditures has occurred. In 1970 sixty-nine billion dollars were spent for health care. This figure grew to 287 billion dollars in 1981. In relationship to the Federal Budget, in 1970 the Health and Human Services Department comprised 24.8 percent of the total budget. For 1983 this figure has risen to 36.2 percent. These total expenditures do not include those funds which were spent for research, health promotion, and administration of governmental agencies which do not provide direct health care (Centers for Disease Control, Food and Drug Administration, etc.). Neither does the total include the nonmedical products, or cost and services of medical fringe benefits which are provided to employees and their families. These huge expenditures clearly reflect a strong belief in the effectiveness of medical care.

Such effectiveness, however, is not so apparent.

> A dangerous misconception . . . is that the influence of its personal physi-
> cians on a society's health can be measured by the mortality statistics of
> that society. In reality, such statistics are almost wholly unrevealing as to
> what it is the physician does or does not do . . . incredible as it may seem,
> there is no certain way to measure the health benefits of most of our society's
> multi-billion dollar expenditure for health.[3]

The author explains his conclusion on the basis of the inseparable and complete interactions of one's genetic characteristics, the public health system (im-
munizations, sanitation, etc.), personal care by physicians, and personal health
practices. The editorial from the *American Medical News* contrasts sharply with
this analysis. The gigantic growth of medical care by physicians has been *assumed*
to be the cause of our increasing longevity, even though no method exists by
which the office and hospital care of patients by physicians can be isolated in
order to demonstrate its contribution to the health of the American people.
Another dimension is provided by the following estimates:

> That health statistics do not particularly reflect what doctors do in the
> hospital or office should not cause much consternation or even surprise.
> . . . Let us assume that 80 percent of patients have either self-limited
> disorders or conditions not improvable, even by modern medicine. . . .
> In slightly over 10 percent of cases, however, medical intervention is
> dramatically successful . . . in the final 9 percent, give or take a point or
> two . . . the patient ends up with iatrogenic (physician-caused) problems.
> So the balance of account ends up marginally on the positive side of zero.
> . . . Perhaps the role of the doctor as reliever rather than healer should
> be accentuated . . . health statistics appear somewhat irrelevant to the or-
> dinary purposes of patient care, which deal with the hope of an individual
> human being that his trouble will be ameliorated.[4]

Two points should be noted: the small net effect of medical care and the author's
emphasis upon the nonphysician (spiritual) dimension, "hope."

Another dimension is provided by an analysis of what may be the most sought
after cure in medicine.

> What would happen if cancer were to be wiped out overnight? Much of
> our fear, pain, and suffering might be eliminated . . . but the surprising
> answer, at least statistically, is "probably not much." Dr. Conrad Tauber,
> Associate Director of the Center for Population Research at Georgetown
> University's Kennedy Institute of Ethics, analyzed the questions and found
> the medical costs would increase slightly (from treating other conditions),
> and life expectancy might rise by a year and a half for the typical 65-year-
> old. Lifespan would not be stretched dramatically; he says we'd simply
> die of other diseases.[5]

Dr. Tauber's conclusions contrast with the usual intensive promotion of cancer
research as though a cure would dramatically improve man's health. The

biblical truth is that man suffers from a spiritual disease which has physical manifestation. Many diseases cause just as much suffering and disability even though cancer is more dreaded. If cancer were eliminated, other diseases would continue to wreak havoc in similar ways that cancer does now.

Medicine may create and perpetuate the very problems which it seeks to cure.

> Medicine, for example, with its tremendously enlarged capabilities, really moves in a vicious circle. Whatever it does to preserve diseased life threatens at the same time to deteriorate the hereditary mass. . . . That which he has created actually turns on him.[6]

A demonstration of this effect appeared recently:

> An international hunt is on for thousands of young women treated in childhood for phenyl-ketonuris (PKU) and others with mild cases who were not treated. . . . Phenylketonuria in pregnant women who no longer stick to diets free of phenylalanine may be a far more serious cause of retardation than rubella.[7]

Dr. Thielicke is saying that the increasing effectiveness of medical care and other measures will result in an increasing number of genetically-defective children because they will become mothers and in turn bear children who would not otherwise have been born. Again, the inevitability of physical disease and death is clearly evident in spite of effective medical treatment. It seems that medicine simply rearranges diseases but it is limited ultimately in its overall effectiveness upon diseases and death.

> If we are not struck down prematurely by one or another of today's diseases, we live a certain length of time and then we die, and I doubt that medicine will ever gain a capacity to do anything much to modify this. . . . At a certain age, it is our nature to wear out, to come unhinged, and to die, and that is that.[8]

Health is relative to a definition which is based upon one's anthropological understanding. For example, mortality statistics do not include prenatal life. The Bible and scientific evidence defines life to begin at conception. If abortions are added into mortality statistics, longevity would be severely reduced, the age factor for unborn babies being zero. With two million deaths each year, 1.5 million abortions would increase the mortality rate by almost 50 percent! This simple adjustment dramatically demonstrates how much statistics are *relative* according to definitions.

Still another dimension is the personal morality of the physician. It used to be taken for granted that doctors were primarily concerned with patients' welfare. Now there is suspicion that their own self-interest has become dominant. Some illustrations of this suspicion follow:

> Physicians' slowness to respond to consumer needs has resulted in increasing governmental involvement.

One of the most immoral trends in medicine in recent decades has been the steady immigration of physicians from "have not" to "have" countries. What does it say of the physician's professional motivation when it is said that medical care would deteriorate if the method of payment were changed?[9]

Examples of physicians' primary self-interest is apparent from even a superficial review of common medical publications. To be fair, this decline in physicians' attitudes only reflects proportionally an increase in self-interest among people in our society.

In conclusion, the overall effectiveness of medical care cannot be assumed. Most problems which present to the physician are self-limited but even a suddenly available cure for all cancers would not greatly extend longevity or alleviate morbidity. Effective treatment of hereditary disorders may even contribute to a general deterioration of the health of mankind. The application of different definitions of life and of health would markedly alter health statistics. Finally, physicians are less patient-oriented and more self-oriented than in the past.

Medical Research: Less Than a Firm Foundation

"The first significant advance in the diuretic field in more than a decade" read a pharmaceutical manufacturer's advertisement. "It may prove to be the preferred diuretic and first step antihypertensive drug for patients. . . ."[10] "It" was marketed in May 1979 and was recalled in Janurary 1980. In consultations between the FDA and the manufacturer, there was strong evidence that deaths resulted from severe hepatic injury as a secondary effect of the drug. The severity of this effect went unrecognized prior to its release, even after extensive experimentation, a necessity for a new drug to be released by the FDA. In spite of recall, "officials are not sure (that) deaths are drug-caused."[11] What went wrong with initial expectations? Why did uncertainty continue? Why is the drug still marketed in Europe? Answers to these questions will become more evident as we proceed.

Medicine, as a science of "living things" is highly subjective, not objective. Consequently, degrees of confidence are arbitrarily selected. Subjective variables are based solely on the judgment of the researchers who, by human nature, cannot eliminate personal biases. The use of numbers is necessary for experimental design but the subjective correlations upon which those numbers are based, is obscured by the objectivity of mathematical computations. Many empirical conclusions ignore that original subjectivity. Studies of studies reveal the effects of this objective-subjective imprecision.[12] In a six-month period in one of the more reputable heart journals, 44 percent of 142 scientific articles were found to contain errors in their *statistical* techniques.[13] Thirty-nine percent contained *no* statistical analysis, and 27 percent used one type of analysis *incorrectly*. A similar review of other reputable medical journals showed two-thirds to contain faults in research design and interpretation that were serious enough to *invalidate* their conclusions![14] One author commented:

This (his personal) study emphasized our need to avoid passive acceptance of statistically significant results and to maintain a healthy skepticism regarding their clinical applicability until they have been replicated by other studies. There are so many studies published in an increasing array of journals that we tend to depend on a small number of journals whose quality is maintained by editorial selectivity and completion. *The above study questions the validity of these as well.*[15]

Medical research has problems with its frequently used methodologies of design, as well.

Randomized Controlled Trials

The randomized controlled trial (RCT) enjoys a reputation as the most reliable experimental technique for evaluating therapies . . . when Dr. Chalmers and his associates examined the quality of 159 randomized trials published from 1975 through 1976 in *Lancet* and the *New England Journal of Medicine* (two of the leading medical journals), they couldn't find a single one that could be rated "excellent." Only a third of the studies qualified as "well done" by their scoring system.[16]

Death Certificates

Data from death certificates frequently is used for epidemiologic study of disease . . . it is reasonable to conclude that for us in statistical study, any statistical data referable to disease as obtained from death certificates must be carefully evaluated. In their particular study, they concluded (that) . . . these registered death certificates . . . indicate that the data would contribute no scientific information.[17]

Matched Controls

In reading the medical research literature, one often sees reference to or use of matched controls . . . it is important to remember that one should try to avoid matching on a basis that is directly related to the factor being investigated. . . . What is not so obvious and is not uncommon is the selection of matched controls in such a way that there is indirect, partial matching of the putative (supposed) factor.[18]

We must emphasize the seriousness and prevalence of these problems, since these methodologies are the means of validation in medical research. Such problems prevent the isolation of single causes and effects (see previous section) without which uncertainty cannot be overcome.

A specific research study illustrates this difficulty. Table I is a simplified chart from a study of patients in whom drug "X" was evaluated concerning its effect on mortality.[19] The methodology is that in which mortality is compared in adherers to the treatment regimen with nonadherers. Thus, the mortality of adherers to drug X is 15.0 percent compared to 24.6 percent of the nonadherers to drug X, a clearly significant difference. This comparison excludes all the patients who took placebos, but such exclusion seems to be entirely reasonable since a placebo is an inert substance. Further analysis reveals the serious error of such logic. Placebo-adherers and drug-adherers have *identical* mortality rates but in addition, both groups of adherers show a marked difference in mortality rate when compared to both groups of nonadherers: 24.6 to 15.0 and 28.2 to 15.1. Obviously, a drug can only be evaluated if patients adhere to its prescribed schedule. This study, however, indicates that adherers, that is, people who followed their prescribed therapy as a group, have an increased likelihood of survival over nonadherers regardless of the potency or impotency of the drug! Patients who follow prescribed regimens seem to be inherently different from those who don't adhere *or* efficacy exists in the adherence itself. Thus, all studies which compare the mortality of a drug group with a placebo group, *must* have the two groups divided further into adherers and nonadherers, a total of four groups. A review of the medical literature will reveal the paucity of drug-placebo comparisons which divide patients into these four areas. Even further, those studies which limit their evaluations to morbidity might be erroneous without these divisions.

TABLE I
FIVE-YEAR MORTALITY—DRUG X VS. PLACEBO[20]

Adherence	DRUG X Number	% Mortality	PLACEBO Number	% Mortality
80%	357	24.6	882	28.2
80%	708	15.0	1813	15.1
Total	1065	18.2	2695	19.4

"Adherence" refers to the patient who did or did not adhere his taking pills at least four out of five times (80 percent). "Percent mortality" refers to the percentage of people who die over the five year period of study. "Numbers" refers to the actual number of patients in each of the four categories: adherence with drug X, nonadherence with drug X, adherence with placebo, and nonadherence with placebo.

An increasing volume of research invalidates previous research both in its design and in its results. This invalidation extends to *most* previous studies by one means or another, yet those studies of medicine are largely delusional, and in our opinion most physicians are not consciously aware of this weak basis for what they do.

Hypotheses, Changes, and Physician Compliance

Recently, a friend sought an impromptu consultation as we were headed to the golf course. He inquired about a diet for his wife who had colitis. He was confused. She had had this problem for several years and her physician had initially instructed her to eat low-fiber foods. Now, they were being told to change to the exact opposite, a high-fiber diet. No wonder he was confused. I had to confess that medical opinion had changed over the past decade from the time when she started treatment. Further, I had to confess that I began to wonder about its validity when "scientific" medical practice was changed, often dramatically. Some of the difficulties were addressed at the 1978 meeting of the Massachusetts Medical Society and were later published. It was entitled, "Annual Discourse-Unproved Hypothesis." In his presentation Thomas R. Dawber, M.D., M.P.H. (Master Public Health) analyzed the research base for four commonly accepted medical hypotheses: (1) the causal relationship of the dietary intake of salt to high blood pressure, (2) the need for tonsillectomy in children, (3) that alcoholism is a disease, and (4) the causal relationship of dietary fats and cholesterol to atherosclerosis (fatty deposits in the arteries which eventually become occluded, block blood supply, and cause heart attacks or death).[21] His extensive arguments devastate these hypotheses:

> The above examples are only a few of the thousands of hypotheses that govern our approach to the prevention and cure of the many diseases that afflict mankind. *Very few* of the hypotheses involving the management of the *bulk* of disorders now affecting the adult population—hypertension, atherosclerotic diseases, cancer, arthritis, degenerative joint disease, and senility—have been adequately tested, or, if so tested supported by unequivocal evidence. Almost *every* therapeutic measure that we take can be challenged. Cast adrift in this Sargasso Sea with no medical compass, the physician can easily convince himself that *whatever* course he advocates can be justified and ask, "Who has anything better to offer?" He should not forget that the proponents of Laetrile may well ask the same question as they look over the results of medically accepted cancer therapy. . . . When various combinations of therapy are considered, whose end component may contribute only a small increment of benefit, the number of study subjects necessary becomes astronomical to the point that any definitive test appears *totally impracticable*. Faced with such a situation we may well ask how scientific medicine may be practiced. . . . No one is unaware that research is the backbone of modern medicine. Less clear is what research is necessary or desirable, what the priorities should be if there are limited funds and manpower (and there are), and who should determine those priorities.[22]

The reader is encouraged to read further into his presentation. It is an accurate, full discussion of these issues.

Another problem with medical science is its changing nature. Medical students are commonly taught that 50 percent of what they learn will be obsolete within five years. Since their training to achieve that knowledge requires five to ten years beyond college, it is apparent that a full-time practice after graduation will not allow the time necessary to stay current.

Examples of changes are prevalent. (1) The change from a low-fiber to a high-fiber diet has been given. (2) The annual physical exam, especially for cancer screening, recently was changed markedly by the American Cancer Society. (3) In the mid-1950s, ligation of the internal mammary artery in the chest was used to alleviate angina pectoria (pain in the chest due to a lack of blood supply to the heart muscle.[23] In one study 38 percent of 213 patients who underwent operations had complete relief, and 65 to 75 percent showed considerable improvement. Another study found 91 percent had symptomatic relief and 64 percent had "objective" improvement on electrocardiography (an electrical graph of the heart). "Despite these enthusiastic reports, many doubted the physiologic basis for ligation of the internal mammary artery," so two studies, which "are among the *few* (emphasis ours) double-blind trials which involved a surgical procedure," were carried out. One set of patients had only the skin incised; the other set had the same incision but the artery was ligated (tied off), as usual. The results showed the ligation of the artery was not better than the skin incision alone. The original evidence was scientific, even objective, but the subsequent evidence proved the original evidence to be unreliable.

New practices are the result of research, yet no one is able to identify those procedures today which will be proven ineffective, or worse, proven to be harmful in the future. In addition surgery and drugs are becoming more potent in their side effects (infra). A science which changes so rapidly should be appropriately tentative in its conclusions, yet the popular and professional literature is usually anything but tentative in its portrayal of the "latest" findings.

Studies also demonstrate that physicians' knowledge and skills are often less than optimal. At one medical school more than one-third of all patients who were admitted to the hospital were placed on antibiotics, but for sixty-four percent of those on antibiotic therapy, the medication was "not indicated or inappropriately administered in terms of drugs or dosage."[24] The article cited other studies with similar results.

Even though we have given evidence that medical studies are not fully reliable, they remain the most objective source of information to the physician. One would hope that physicians would base their prescribing practices upon those studies, but such practice is based more upon ads in medical journals and presentations of detail people.[25] With cerebral vasodilators (drugs which are supposed to increase blood flow to compromised brains) the clinical literature "overwhelmingly" shows that they are not useful. Yet, seventy-one percent of the doctors surveyed believed that such drugs are effective. Of the physicians themselves, sixty-eight percent and fifty-four percent think that drug ads and detail people respectively have little influence on their prescribing habits! Eighty-four percent prescribe an analgesic, propoxyphene, which has been repeatedly shown to be less effective than aspirin. One drug company reports that in excess of fifty million dollars was spent on advertising *one* drug (valium) *only* to physicians. The great extent to which this drug is prescribed is probably proportional to its promotional costs, as reflected in the influence of drug advertisements and detail men upon physicians.

Physicians' performance in ambulatory care was the focus of an university-affiliated public general hospital. "The frequency that abnormal test results were unknown to (i .e., went undetected by) physicians in our study ranged from a low of twenty-eight percent for chest roentgenograms (x-rays) to a high of ninety-three percent for urine colony counts.''[26] Thus, the diagnosis or treatment prescribed did not even take these abnormal test results in consideration..

At a northeastern hospital, peer review was instituted because of a sharp increase in heart pacemaker implantation.[27] After the peer review began, the total number of implantations decreased from 130 to 54. Unexpectedly, patient survival increased 85 percent to 57 percent and symptoms decreased 19 percent to 9 percent! The study demonstrates that physicians without peer review (which is the predominant situation) will not treat patients identically and that a common medical practice may not be the best one, and may even be detrimental to patients' health.

We have reviewed three areas: (1) the vast majority of hypothesis, and thus, therapeutic measures are inadequately supported by research; (2) medical care changes rapidly and radically; and (3) physicians, when their performance is studied, frequently do not comply with their own scientific standards. A fourth area, patient compliance, shows that patients fail to comply with doctors' prescriptions between twenty and eighty-two percent of the time; so both patients and physicians fail to implement prescribed regimens. Uncertainties and gaps do exist in the practice of medicine!

Iatrogenic Disease

"First of all, do no harm" (*primum non nocere*) is taught to all physicians at some point in their training, and even subsequently. The slogan is an appropriate reminder when iatrogenic (physician-induced) disease seems to be increasing.

Mortality rates. For example, the results of a doctor slowdown in Los Angeles County in 1976 were not the catastrophe that might be expected.[28] In an attempt to apply political pressure during the first five weeks of 1976, approximately seventy-five percent of the county's physicians withheld their services, principally in the area of nonemergency surgery. Mortality rates *declined* steadily during those five weeks! Then, they rose abruptly to peak the first week that elective surgery was resumed, then leveled off to predicted rates. Death rates (after the first two weeks) ranged from six percent to twenty-nine percent *less* than those expected from data over the previous five years (see Figure 1). Some conclusions of a study of phenomenon were:

> The data cannot support a conclusion that the strike significantly impacted on the health status . . . of the country population . . . on balance. The Los Angeles County Physicians' strike of January, 1976. was responsible for *more deaths prevented* than lives lost (emphasis added).[29]

Admittedly, all causes and effects are impossible to isolate. The consistency and coincidental timing of the decreases in mortality, however, when the opposite would be expected, are striking in comparison to previous years. The data does demonstrate that in general physician reduction of mortality rates should not be assumed, and in this instance may have resulted in more harm than good. There are other studies to support the conclusion that no remarkable deterioration in health occurs when the available medical care is decreased.[29]

TABLE I

Actual vs. Expected* Deaths in Los Angeles County for the First Seven Weeks of 1976.

Week No. as of 1/1/76	Actual	Expected*	Difference	Standard Error
1	1472	1140	+ 332	157
2	1470	1331	+ 139	154
3	1382	1469	-89	78
4	1208	1432	-224	99
5	1193	1358	-166	115
6	916	1293	-377	124
7	957	1254	-297	104

* The expected number of deaths was determined through use of a moving average method applied to actual deaths for the same weeks over the preceding five years.

Side Effects

In the 1960s, a southern medical school recorded adverse episodes, as "any response to medical care that is unintended, undesirable, and harmful to the patient . . . (which) resulted from, and occurred during, the present hospitalization."[30] Twenty percent of patients had these adverse episodes and almost half were of moderate or major severity. The adversely affected group of patients averaged over seven days longer in the hospital than the unaffected group. A similar study, (although admittedly not identical in design or criteria), was conducted in a northeastern hospital in 1979, fourteen years later.[31] Thirty-six percent of these patients (who were consecutively admitted to a general medical service) had an iatrogenic illness which resulted from a diagnostic procedure or a form of therapy. One-fourth of these events were "considered major in that they threatened life or produced considerable disability." In two percent the iatrogenic illness was believed to be involved in the patient's death. From twenty percent (1965) to thirty-six percent (1979) is almost double over the fourteen years. The latter study concluded that "the current risk is probably greater than ever."

Unnecessary Surgery

In one "Annual Discourse," the author cited 800,000 tonsillectomies in children each year with 300 lives lost to this procedure. These results occurred even though for the ten years previously, it had been documented and widely taught that few indications existed for tonsillectomy.

> It is impossible to be statistically accurate in evaluating the results of an elective procedure such as T and A (tonsillectomy and adenoidectomy) which has no accurately measurable parameter of success or failure . . . we must conclude that no answer to the usefulness of tonsillectomy can be obtained and that it is useless to try to find one. If such a conclusion is justified, the logical answer should be "cease and desist."[32]

Coronary artery bypass graft surgery (CABG) is another example. It was used as an analogy in an editorial in which the authors pleaded for the construction of careful pilot studies with other new techniques. They stated that the premature application of CABG led to a major controversy which confused patients and physicians alike.

> Indeed, although almost a million such operations have now been carried out in the United States alone, there is still considerable debate about the indications for CABG and its value.[33]

Scientific objectivity is lacking when one million operations, at a cost of $15,000 to $20,000 each, are not clearly effective! It took ten to twenty years for tonsillectomy to undergo a significant decline after it had been demonstrated to be needless in most children! CABG and tonsillectomy give evidence that the indications and efficacy of many common surgical procedures remains unanswered, and because of the difficulty to validate efficacy, will continue to be unanswered.[34]

Long-Term Effect of Medications and Procedures

Radiation, when it was first introduced, was used commonly on the skin, tonsils, and other parts of the body until it was recognized that cancer could result from its indiscriminate use. Today, some thyroid cancers are being discovered thirty years later that are due to earlier radiation treatment. A drug, diethylstilbestrol (DES), was once used in pregnant women to prevent miscarriage and no ill effects were noted at that time. Many daughters of these women, however, were found to have an increase in a precancerous disease of the skin and required surgery. Complete effects will not be known until most of them have lived their entire lives. Further, there is a third generation of daughters to consider. What will the effects of DES be in them?

Most medications currently in use are studied for several months, sometimes for a few years, but rarely beyond five years. Some drugs are taken continuously over a long period of time. These include antihypertensives, birth control pills, antidepressants, other mood altering drugs, and heart medications. What will their effect on patients be over several decades *or* in their children? No one knows, but DES has shown the potential for serious problems.

Our concern extends beyond these direct long-term effects for two reasons. (1) In 1953 it was proved DES was ineffective for preventing miscarriage and in 1971 the first report of its effect on the daughters was made. In 1974, however, a survey by the Food and Drug Administration revealed 11,000 prescriptions for DES written specifically for threatened miscarriage or prenatal care![35]

(2) Another estrogen, ethinyl estradiol, is currently undergoing experimentation as a "morning after" contraceptive at one hundred times the dose of the same hormone in birth control pills.[36] Thus, both practicing physicians and medical researchers seem to ignore the long-term complications of high-dose estrogen therapy which was manifested by the effects of DES. Such continued practice and research in the face of substantial evidence for potential harm, is irrational, unscientific, and immoral.

In Summary

> Physicians now began to be in admiration, as persons who were something more than human. And profit attended employ as well as honor; so that they had now two weighty reasons for their keeping the bulk of mankind at a distance, so that they might not pry into the mysteries of the profession. . . .They filled their writings with abundance of technical terms, utterly unintelligible to plain men. . . . How often by this compounding medicines of opposite qualities, is the virtue of both utterly destroyed? Nay, how often do these joined together destroy life, which singly, might have preserved it?
>
> John Wesley[37]

Diatribes against physicians and the formal practice of medicine are nothing new, as can be seen from this quote of John Wesley. Even Hippocrates engaged in sharp criticism of some of his colleagues. Recent books of an antimedical nature usually recommend strategies to avoid the deleterious effects of medical care. Christians, however, should remember that these analyses do not necessarily recognize the spiritual dimension, any more than the orthodox medical profession does. The healthy lifestyle which is advocated is usually unachievable without the change of heart and motivation. For Christians, the Holy Spirit gives motivation, direction, and ability to change in conjunction with biblical principles.

In summary, our purpose is not to place medicine in complete disrepute. I am not advocating a complete rejection of medicine. I am advocating a realistic understanding of its limitations, as well as its potential. Medicine does not deserve the great expectations for health which many of its leaders, physicians, public press, and lay advocates claim. Most importantly, we are advocating a more biblical approach to the practice of medicine that includes God's glory in its ethics and in its real effect upon the physical health of patients. The details of this approach are the directions given throughout this book. Medical literature reflects many physicians and researchers who seek a realistic appraisal of medicine but the lack of any practical implementation is understandable when physicians have invested their lives in the research and practice of orthodox medicine. Many controversial areas could have been included along with appropriate references: the lack of definition of normal and abnormal, the placebo effect, the imprecision of laboratory studies, the restrictions of fiscal resources, the political power of physicians, the personal ethics of physicians, ineffective but commonly used drugs, the application of animal studies to humans, and the transfer of evidence between ethnic groups.

Nonphysician believers who read these evaluations will face a dilemma. If the "science" of medicine is unsure, and so few Christian physicians seem able to discuss the spiritual priorities and empirical weaknesses in medical care, what should be done when medical care is needed? The unbeliever is left with the hope that modern medicine can keep him healthy or restore him to health if necessary. Such hope decreases the likelihood that he will realistically face the inevitability of his own eternal destiny. Medical care and the hospital become the objects in which to place his trust since he believes that both his body and his mind can be effectively treated by those who are there. He will not spare personal or public resources to enhance such care. Interestingly, such hope further removes any personal responsibility which can be effective in the prevention, delay, or reduction of morbidity and mortality. Some unbelievers, however, become aware of the uncertainties of medicine and begin a serious health program in which some succeed and others fail. Those who are successful will have their health enhanced, but the stark reality of death remains. Unbelievers cannot cope with that dilemma which is infinitely greater than any believer's dilemma concerning health or medical care.

NOTES

1. R. L. Parker, ed., *The Journal of John Wesley* (Chicago: Moody, 1974), pp. 230-231.

2. "Highly-Rated or Overrated?" *American Medical News* (December 26, 1980/January 2, 1981), p. 4.

3. Walsh McDermott, "Absence of Indicators of the Influence of Its Physicians on a Society's Health," *American Journal of Medicine* 70 (1981):833-843.

4. E. J. Ingelfinger, "Health: A Matter of Statistics or Feeling?", *New England Journal of Medicine* 296 (1977):448-449.

5. Conrad Tauber, "Cancer: $23 Billion Drain," *Perspective* (Summer, 1981) p. 36.

6. Helmut Thielicke, "Ethics in Modern Medicine" in *Who Shall Live*, ed. Kenneth Vaux (New York: Harper and Row, 1964), p. 148.

7. Helmut Thielicke, *Medical World News* (November 23, 1981), p. 48.

8. David E. Allen, Lewis P. Bird and Robert Herrmann, eds., *Whole-Person Medicine: An International Symposium* (Downers Grove: InterVarsity Press, 1980), p. 26.

9. Merville O. Vincent, "Professional Ethics," in *Baker's Dictionary of Christian Ethics*, ed. Carl F. Henry (Grand Rapids: Baker Book House, 1973), pp. 536-537.

10. *Medical Letter*, (July 27, 1979), pp. 61-62.

11. "Ticrynafen Recall in U.S. Not Being Followed in Europe," *Medical World News*, (Feb. 4, 1980), p.18.

12. Unfortunately, space cannot be taken here to discuss those qualitites which distinguish between reliable and unreliable studies. Examples of such criteria include journal selection, study design, and use of statistical tests. The astute reader will note that we have used studies to refute other studies. Obviously, our bias has entered in. The main purpose of this chapter on the science of medicine, however, is to destroy any myth that medicine is infallible. Until that destruction occurs, medicine will continue to generate its own morality. If its scientific foundations can be

shown to be shaky, necessary moral changes will not come so reluctantly (as though great benefits were being withheld only for moral reasons).

13. S. A. Glantz, "Biostatistics: How to Detect, Correct and Prevent Errors in the Medical Literature." *Circulation* 61 (January, 1980), pp. 1-7. Although this report is dated, there is no reason to doubt the situation has changed recently.

14. S. Schor and M. A. Karten, "Statistical Evaluation of Medical Journal Manuscripts," *Journal of the American Medical Association* 195 (March 28, 1966), pp. 145-150.

15. R. E. Rakel, *YearBook of Family Medicine* (Chicago: Year Book Medical Publishers, 1981), p. 13.

16. "Randomized Trials: Are they Really all that Random?" *Medical World News* (July 10, 1978), p. 12.

17. R. H. Rigdon, "Problems in a Statistical Study of Disease Based on Death Certificates," *Southern Medical Journal* 74 (September, 1981), pp. 1104-1106.

18. W. H. Gullen, "A Danger in Matched-Control Studies," *Journal of the American Medical Association* 244 (November 21, 1980):2279-2280.

19. The actual drug is named in the cited study. Its name is omitted here to prevent confusion by those who may be using it presently.

20. H. Benson and D. P. McCallie, "Angina and the Placebo Effect," *New England Journal of Medicine* 300 (June 21, 1979), pp. 1424-1429.

21. The reader may note a conflict with the position taken in the second chapter, that diet is related to atherosclerotic events (heart attacks, strokes, etc.). This refutation itself identifies the selectivity with which the medical literature can be used to "prove" hypothesis.

22. T. R. Dawber, "Annual Discourse-Unproved Hypotheses," *New England Journal of Medicine* 299 (August 31, 1978):452-458.

23. Benson and McCallie, pp. 1424-1429.

24. M. Castle and C. M. Wilfert. "Antibiotic Use at Duke University Medical Center," *Journal of the American Medical Association* 237 (June 27, 1977):2819-2822.

25. "Doctors Don't See Power of Drug Ads," *Medical World News* (September 13, 1982), pp. 19-20.

26. C. R. Kelly and J. J. Mamlin, "Ambulatory Medical Care Quality: Determination of Diagnostic Outcome," *Journal of the American Medical Association* 227 (March 11, 1974):1155-1157.

27. Atul B. Chokshi and Howard S. Friedman, "Impact of Peer Review in Reduction of Permanent Pacemaker Implantations," *Journal of the American Medical Association* 246 (August 14, 1981):754-757.

28. J. J. James, "Impact of the Medical Malpractice Slowdown in Los Angelos County: January 1976," *American Journal of Public Health* 69 (May, 1979):437-443.

29. R. H. Pantell and C. E. Irwin, "Appendectomies During Physicians Boycott," *Journal of the American Medical Association* 242 (October 12, 1979):1627-1630.

30. J. T. McLamb and R. R. Huntley, "The Hazards of Hospitalization," *Southern Medical Journal* 60 (1967):489-492.

31. K. Steel and P. M. Gertman, "Iatrogenic Illness on a General Medical Service at a University Hospital," *New England Journal of Medicine* 304 (March 12, 1981):638-642.

32. T. R. Dawber, "Annual Discourse-Unproved Hypotheses," *New England Journal of Medicine* 299 (August 31, 1978):1336-1340.

33. Ibid.

34. A dubious distinction in the area of controversial surgery is the fact that abortion (the destruction of life) is now the *most common surgical procedure* in the United States, and probably in the world. One would think that surgery was to extend life, not to end it!

35. *Medical World News* (August 23, 1976) pp. 44-56.

36. Garret W. Dixon and James J. Schlesselman et al. "Ethinyl Estradiol and Conjugated Estrogens as Postcoital Contraceptives," *Journal of the American Medical Association* 244 (Sept. 19, 1980):1336-1340.

37. John Wesley, *Primitive Remedies* (Santa Barbara: Woodbridge Press Publishing Company, 1975), pp. 13, 16.

REFERENCES

Benson, H. and D. P. McCallie. "Angina and the Placebo Effect." *New England Journal of Medicine* 300 (June 21, 1979):1424-1429.

"Cancer: $23 Billion Drain." *Perspective*, Summer 1981, p. 36.

Castle, M., C. M. Wilfert, et al. "Antibiotic Use at Duke University Medical Center." *Journal of the American Medical Association* 237 (June 27, 1977): 2819-2822.

Chokshi, Atul B., Friedman, Howard S., et al. "Impact of Peer Review in Reduction of Permanent Pacemaker Implantations." *Journal of the American Medical Association* 246 (Aug. 14, 1981):754-757.

Coronary Drug Project Research Group. "Influence of Adherence to Treatment and Response of Cholesterol on Mortality in the Coronary Drug Project." *New England Journal of Medicine* 303 (Oct. 30, 1980):1038-1041.

Dawber, T. R. "Annual Discourse—Unproved Hypotheses." *New England Journal of Medicine* 299 (Aug. 31, 1978):452-458.

Dixon, Garret W., Schlesselman, James J., et al. "Ethinyl Estradiol and Conjugated Estrogens as Postcoital Contraceptives." *Journal of the American Medical Association* 244 (Sept. 19, 1980):1336-1340.

Glantz, S. A. "Biostatistics: How to Detect, Correct and Prevent Errors in the Medical Literature." *Circulation* 61 (Jan. 1980):1-7.

Gullen, W. H. "A Danger in Matched-Control Studies." *Journal of the American Medical Association* 244 (Nov. 21, 1980):2279-2280.

Ingelfinger, E. J. "Health: A Matter of Statistics or Feeling?." *New England Journal of Medicine* 296 (1977):448-449.

James, J. J. Impact of the Medical Malpractice Slowdown in Los Angelos County: January 1976." *American Journal of Public Health* 69 (May 1979):437-443.

Kelly, C. R., J. J. Mamlin. "Ambulatory Medical Care Quality: Determination of Diagnostic Outcome." *Journal of the American Medical Association* 227 (March 11, 1974):1155-1157.

McDermott, Walsh. "Absence of Indicators of the Influence of Its Physicians on a Society's Health." *American Journal of Medicine* 70 (1981):833-843.

McLamb, J. T., R. R. Huntley. "The Hazards of Hospitalization." *Southern Medical Journal* 60 (1967):489-492.

Muller, J. E., P. H. Stone, et al. "Let's Not Let the Genie Escape from the Bottle Again." *New England Journal of Medicine* 304 (May 21, 1981):1294-1296.

Pantell, R. H., C. E. Irwin. "Appendectomies During Physicians Boycott." *Journal of the American Medical Association* 242 (Oct. 12 1979):1627-1630.

Parker, R. L. (ed.). *The Journal of John Wesley.* Chicago: Moody, 1974, pp. 230-231.

Rakel, R. E. In the Introduction to: *Year Book of Family Medicine.* Chicago: Year Book Medical Publishers, 1981, p. 13.

Rigdon, R. H. "Problems in a Statistical Study of Disease Based on Death Certificates." *Southern Medical Journal* 74 (Sept. 1981):1104-1106.

Schor, S. and M. A. Karten. "Statistical Evaluation of Medical Journal Manuscripts." *Journal of the American Medical Association* 195 (March 28, 1966): 145-150.

Slee, U. N. "Appendectomies during Physicians Boycott (Letter)." *Journal of the American Medical Association* 243 (June 27, 1980):2483.

Steel, K., P. M. Gertman, et al. "Iatrogenic Illness on a General Medical Service at a University Hospital." *New England Journal of Medicine* 304 (March 12, 1981):638-642.

Wesley, John. *Primitive Remedies.* Santa Barbara: Woodbridge Press Publishing Company, 1975.

5 | Biblical/Medical Ethics

Bobbie had lived a stressful life for all of her thirty-three years. Her first husband had a chronic disability caused by a brain tumor. He suffered with this for two years before his death and left her with five young children to raise. Her meager income from his insurance and a job as a department store salesperson barely provided essentials. Confused and troubled, she married a man who was only occasionally employed and absent from the home for weeks at a time. Bobbie was well-known by physicians in the area because her numerous visits and weekly phone calls presented problems which rarely had a discernible physical basis.

One of these physicians began to counsel her. Further information revealed she was not fully caring for household responsibilities and was leaving the children to care for themselves. She professed to be a Christian but did not practice her faith in any regular way. Bobbie was admonished to become responsible at home, begin daily devotions, attend church regularly and study biblical solutions to her problems. Through much direction she was able to change her thinking and behavior, even though financial problems continued and other situational problems occurred within her family which were beyond her personal responsibility.

In the beginning, since she had physical symptoms, she assumed her problems were physical. During doctor visits she received medication with little clinical explanation. Through counseling she realized the connection between her irresponsibility and her symptoms. Progress was made only after an approach which integrated counsel for the biblical *psyche* and medical care for the *soma*. Bobbie's reduced number of phone calls and fewer visits indicated real progress which has continued for eight years. The majority of her medical visits are now related to real physical problems.

Integrating Faith and Medicine

Many Christians are rightly interested in the integration of their profession with their Christian faith. It is a worthwhile and vital goal if Jesus Christ is to be "Lord of all" and if one wants to avoid an artificial separation of the sacred and secular. A right intention must be accompanied by a proper methodology. Even with the best of intentions, a wrong result is wrong and misleading.

Concerning behavioral scientists, Robertson McQuilkin has said:

> . . . that in the next two decades the greatest threat to biblical authority is the behavioral scientist who would in all conscience man the barricade against any theologian who would attack the inspiration and authority of Scripture while all the while himself smuggling the context of Scripture out the back door through cultural or psychological interpretations![1]

His statement involves two principles consistent with our concern for medical ethics. First, right belief can be undermined by wrong methodology. Second, behavioral science *is* having a profound effect upon medical care. From these two principles and the preceding chapers, we can briefly review a proper methodology which should integrate medical practice with the biblical faith.

Integration implies the synthesis of equals. Regardless of the reason, Christian scientists are often more influenced by science than by biblical principles or concern for biblical practice. God's revelation in the Scripture must control any attempt at integration. All truth is God's truth but an arrival at that truth may be variable and subjective. Scripture is objective truth. All other truth must be subject to it. Empirical science has demonstrated the effectiveness of biblical principles and attitudes as the most likely means by which optimal physical health can be achieved and maintained. Spiritual problems cannot be separated from physical problems. Most people think that spiritual problems, more frequently called psychological or psychiatric problems, are primarily managed by psychologists or psychiatrists, but every physician is significantly involved with problems that are primarily spiritual. "More than seventy percent of psychotropic drugs are written by nonpsychiatrists, and there is concern that far too many prescriptions are being written for such conditions as insomnia, anxiety, and depression."[2] It is estimated that up to fifty percent of patients' visits to primary care physicians, those physicians whom patients see initially, are due to psychosocial rather than biomedical causes.[3]

Physicians' training now gives more attention to the connection of the mind as understood by secularists, and the body, ". . . psychiatrists, along with other behavioral scientists, continue to be in the best position to familiarize students and young physicians with the psychosocial knowledge basis for all of medicine."[4] Observance of practicing physicians has shown that they invariably refer nonmedical problems to psychiatrists. Thus within the medical profession, the psychotherapist has become the normative standard for value judgments concerning patients. Within the Christian world view this situation is antithetical to true integration—it ignores God, His revelation, and all the principles of a biblical ethic. Christians in these professions have generally not helped to clarify or correct the situation.

Thus, the importance of a biblically-based medical ethic is underscored. The treatment of the *soma* cannot be treated without consideration of the *psyche*, and the current general direction of Christian professionals is not from the position that biblical principles are practical and foundational to a healthy body. This understanding is not dependent upon modern empiricism since John Wesley was able to recognize it two hundred years ago.

> Why then do not all physicians consider how far bodily disorders are caused or influenced by the mind, and in those cases, which are utterly out of their sphere, call in the assistance of a minister; as ministers, when they find the mind disordered by the body, call in the assistance of a physician? But why are these cases out of their sphere? Because they know not God. It follows, no man can be a thorough physician without being an experienced Christian.[5]

A modern Christian ethicist has made this recognition as well, "To treat man only as a body is to treat him abstractly."[6]

Dr. McQuilkin has stated "that the functional control of Scripture over any discipline will vary in direct proportion to the overlap of that discipline with the substance of biblical revelation."[7] From this thesis he develops five levels into which the various disciplines may be placed. These range from the level with the greatest overlap, containing theology and Christian philosophy, to the level with the least overlap, including manual skills. He places the behavioral sciences—psychology, sociology, and anthropology—into the second level where extensive overlap of the basic substance of biblical revelation, the nature of man and his relationship occurs; although subject matter may be "extended by empirical research and experimentation." Medical practice is placed in the second level because it is a highly subjective science, extensively influenced by naturalistic psychotherapy, at least as much an art as a science, and its most effective means to health must involve biblical principles and practice. The ineffectiveness of medical care, its harm, its ethical misdirection and its failure even to determine a standard by which it may be measured reflect the omission of biblical principles from the development of medical theory and practice. If Christians are to integrate their faith with medical practice, "functional control" of their methodology must be evident and extensive.

McQuilkin's second thesis concerns evidence that evangelicals are under the authority of Scripture. From my observations and reading, evangelicals have differed little in their principles and practice from the naturalists.

McQuilkin's third thesis is that the functional authority of Scripture "must be achieved through the integration of biblical and extrabiblical ideas in one person's mind" through his "dual competence" in the two areas that are being integrated. He continues that "it will not do" for this integrationist "to be a giant in his empirical research and theorization and a pigmy in the knowledge of Scripture." To demonstrate dual competence, he required that such a person "teach at least one Bible study or course in Christian doctrine each year" at the college or seminary level.

If he does not have the knowledge and credentials to do so, (not that he
does necessaily) I am calling into question his credentials to make the
integration of scriptural truth and empirically derived truth with the Bible
in functional control.[8]

This criterion alone would not automatically prevent the loss of functional control by the Scripture, but it would challenge those who currently attempt integration and call for their withdrawal if professional competence is not matched
by biblical competence. Integration involves a thorough knowledge of the difficulties inherent in the determination of truth. Medical care is extensively
overlapped by Scripture and thus functional control by Scripture is absolutely
essential.

Establishing a Biblical/Medical Ethic

Some issues and principles must be introduced to demonstrate this integrative
process. If theologians who are committed to the same basic values and
hermeneutics cannot agree, then a process that is at least one further step
removed has more chance for divergence. The key concept is distinctiveness.
Christian ethics must be *clearly* distinctive from secular ethics. Particular distinctives among evangelicals may vary, but a lack of distinctiveness reflects non-
Christian ethics, or intemperate compromise.

The first principle of a biblical/medical ethic concerns the preoccupation of
Western culture with the physical body.

One of the most culturally powerful forms of idolatry in contemporary
America is that of the body and, more particularly, of the youthful body.
The cult of the body has not a priest but *magus*, the physician-envisaged-
by-the-patient-as magician. This cult inspires the extraordinary financial
and moral investment of our culture in attempts to defeat aging and death,
attempts which express a resentment at the condition of finitude generally,
as well as at mortality, in particular.[9]

Americans' senses are bombarded with advertisements of over-the-counter
medications and prescription drugs. These ads promise health and happiness
and when they fail, the patient is told to consult a doctor. The strong implication
is that the physician is able to eliminate any problem not overcome by drugs.
This conclusion is logical in a naturalistic, materialistic society where only the
physical is real; the body is the most valuable entity with the physician responsible for its care. In 1982 Americans spent 322 billion dollars supporting that
myth.

In contrast, the Bible views man as a whole, who consists of body *and* spirit.
For this reason bodily health is not the sole consideration.

It (healthfulness) quite evidently lacks all absoluteness and universality,
for whether a given mode of conduct is healthful or not, depends upon

a host of variable factors. . . . For it is clear that I am not always required to do the biologically healthful thing. The path of moral duty may lead to the gibbet or to the pyre (e.g., martyrdom). Not health, not even life is an ultimate value. . . . This does not mean, of course, that the virtuous man may ignore his health. . . . It simply means that doing one's duty and keeping one's health are not to be identified; to be good and to be healthy are not the same.[10]

Another example where biblical principle has priority over ''medical'' practice concerns abortion and mental health.[14] One Christian has said:

. . . there are undoubtedly family situations where inadequacy, marital breakdown, financial stringency, unemployment and a host of other adverse social conditions lead to the conclusion that abortion of the unwanted pregnancy is the least tragic of a number of options.[15]

This philosophy compromises the biblical principle of the sanctity of life primarily stated by the Sixth Commandment for ''medical'' reasons.[16] The destructiveness of this compromise is illustrated by the fact that in 1969 seventy-two percent of psychiatrists surveyed ''approved of abortion on request.''[17] Clearly, this necessitates that biblical principle have priority over medical practice.

A third principle concerns the reality of supernatural evil. In many places the spiritual aspects of medicine are beginning to receive more attention as the medical world boasts of its open-mindedness. Such an attitude is quite

A second principle is the priority of the biblical principles for bodily health. Certainly, we are emphasizing the morality of care for the physical body; but even so, biblical principle must take priority. The experiences of two missionary physicians illustrate this point.[11]

With all of these blessings (resources to meet medical needs), I just have to pray constantly that we will not set our hearts and ambitions on the physical and material side of the work. If we can only use all of these added opportunities to win more souls to Him.[12]

I did not at first intend to give up all attention to medicine and the treatment of disease, but now I feel it my duty to have as little to do with it as possible. I shall attend to none but severe cases in future, and my reason for this determination are I think good. The spiritual amelioration of the people is the object for which I came, but I cannot expect God to advance this by my instrumentality if much of my time is spent in mere temporal amelioration.[13]

Thus, evangelism is ultimately more important than medical care. The latter *always* fails at some point; that is, the patient dies. We are not minimizing medical care as a ministry, but even the best medical care, when it is viewed from an eternal perspective, is quite limited in its effectiveness.

deceptive. This "openness" usually disappears when Christ or the Bible are mentioned. But more deceptive to Christian principles is that this welcomes any approach that calls itself spiritual. In April, 1982 over 1000 people in medicine, psychology, education and related areas met in San Francisco under the sponsorship of a medical university for a four-day conference on imagination and the healing arts.[18] The topics seemed appropriate for a medical conference, except for the presence of priests, holy men, and "inner advisers." In one presentation a Christian hymn was used as background music simultaneously with the picture of a priest, but in the absence of any other Christian identity. Such an admixture falsifies the Christian message. Thus, a paradoxical situation exists: the pluralistic mentality of the Western World condones the value system of any religion, including much pseudoreligion and occultism. A Christian world view understands that supernatural evil is introduced into the practice of medicine through such pluralism.

A fourth principle is the destructiveness of evolutionary theory. The Bible states that man is created in the image of God. Evolutionary theory asserts that man is an animal. Further, the Bible states that man has lost his "normality" and has de-volved. Evolution says that man is evolving by chance mechanisms. Since medicine is infiltrated by evolutionary thinking, there is no logical reason to think man should be treated any differently than the other animals. Fortunately, by the grace of God, biblical revelation gives man identity with the living God through a creation which places him a little lower than the angels (Ps. 8:5) and redemption places man above the angels (1 Cor. 6:3; Heb. 2:5-13). Evolution and the Bible conflict. If man is an animal, then he cannot be a child of God! What man is considered to be will determine the manner in which he is treated.

A fifth principle is that Christian physicians are "first and foremost Christians and only secondarily medical men."[19] Physicians, at least as they are represented by their organizations, are opposed to governmental regulation whether it is by the Food and Drug Administration or the "Baby Doe" rules by HEW designed to protect babies with birth defects. The Christian recognizes that God has ordained the state to restrain evil and preserve order.[20]

Common misconceptions in an approach to medical ethics, which relate to the practice of medicine, to biblical principles, or both, are enumerated below:

(1) *Medical ethics is only concerned with certain practices such as abortion and euthanasia.* Certainly, it is not! The argument is both medical and biblical. Well-known medical ethicists clarify this point:

> . . . an ethical or moral reason for refusal (to do an abortion) cannot be separated from the professional judgments of medical personnel, any more than ethical objection can be separated from religious objection. Physicians and nurses make medical moral judgments that are independent of one another.[21]

The act specific to medicine, that which makes it medicine and thereby distinguishes it from both a science and an art, is a decision about what is right and good for a particular patient . . . Once we speak of a *right* and *good* action we are squarely in the realm of morals, the realm of what *ought* to be done. Medicine, therefore, is at its center a moral enterprise.[22]

Most attention is focused upon the more apparent medical dilemmas, but every practice of the physician is moral or immoral. Thus, it is not sufficient to limit concern and discussion.

Theologically, the term "adiaphora" is used of matters which are indifferent. Indifference, however, refers to the external act only.

It does not mean that there are some things we do which in the doing have an amoral quality. There is no conscious voluntary human behavior that does not possess a moral quality, and everything that we do we do in dedication to God, in the way of his service, to his praise and glory, or not.[23]

Certainly, this position is biblical (Ecclesiastes 12:13-14; 1 Cor. 10:31; 2 Cor. 5:10). Thus, both medically and biblically this book has a broad approach because no medical practice be considered *a priori* above such evaluation.

(2) *The patient comes first.* One's first response is to commend this position since a patient by definition is distressed or diseased and needs help. However, there are many fallacies here. The doctor cannot neglect his family, his church, or biblical responsibilities in order to care for his patients. Nowhere does the Bible allow that. Neither are all requests by patients moral: the patient who requests medication which he clearly does not need; the patient who wants to die because he is no longer willing to struggle with his problems; or the patient who wants medical disability even though his physical evaluation is quite normal. Christian allegiance is to God first and secondly to neighbors. Certainly, the physician should have deep concern for his patients because that is his responsibility. This concern must fit into the "whole" life as defined by biblical principles.

(3) *If it is legal, it is moral.* Abortion is legal, but it is not moral. Legality can be subtly erroneous.

If an act is once established as legal, even though not everyone will necessarily proceed to perform it, the natural tendency is for people to grow accustomed to it and eventually to accept it.[24]

Paul Ramsey calls this result, "legal positivism."

From no legal "is" can a moral "ought" be drawn—either in medical or in general ethics . . . It is only to say that from the fact of it—or even from the legal rightness of it—no conclusion follows for morality or for the ethical practice of medicine.[25]

Two historical examples will suffice. In the United States, slavery was legally permissable and popularly condoned, however, few Americans would espouse slavery. More recently in Germany, Hitler "legalized" millions of inhumane atrocities. Clearly, by biblical standards societal law is not the standard for morality.

(4) *Technical ability or competence is moral license.* Few who advocated this principle would state it in this way, but its wording does not change its meaning.

> He (the physician) is a scientist, and as a scientist he is by training and practice tempted more than most individuals to equate know-how with knowledge and technical mastery with wisdom.[26]

A blatant example of such practice was the killing of a Down's fetus.[27]

(5) *Decisions about medical ethics is the province of the medical community alone.* Again, this erroneous principle may not be recognized when stated this way, but nevertheless the meaning is the same. The World Health Organization has said that:

> Health is a state of complete physical, mental and social well-being and not merely the absence of disease.

On the one hand, such a definition for health is needed because health is not merely a physical consideration. On the other hand, this definition opens the door for medical professionals to determine what factors enhance or inhibit health. Since these factors are inclusive of all areas of life, medical professionals assume "responsibility for the full range of human moral considerations."[28]

Evidence for this practice is prevalent. Abortion decisions are almost exclusively left to the patient and her physician with the result that over ninety-five percent of abortions are performed for nonphysical reasons. Are these decisions "medical judgments?" Several medical organizations recently protested legal restrictions on decisions not to care for handicapped newborns on the same grounds that these were medical judgments.[29] It is obvious that in a majority of cases medical professionals determine what is and is not moral, but those decisions are disguised under "medical judgments." Medical ethics cannot be isolated from other societal ethics; because whether naturalistic or biblical, medical care is only part of the whole. Further, whether naturalistic or "Christian", a medical ethic which neglects the role of the church neglects God's primary instrument for the care of His people.

(6) *The value of a person is determined by what he "does" rather than what he "is."* Although it may not be known, physicians for some time have had to "ration" medical procedures. How has such rationing been determined? Usually, it is the functional ability of the patient: his value to his profession or to the community, his total physical ability, and his mental stability. Decisions based upon this functional ability, often called "personhood" by both Christians and non-Christians, are most prevalent and blatant with aborted babies and handicapped infants. The Bible states clearly that the individual does not have to meet any arbitrary requirements of personhood, because he is *imago Dei.* He is neither at his own disposal nor at the disposal of a physician or surgeon.[30] Failure to uphold this ethic "leaves the weak and powerless to die."[31]

(7) *The greatest good is that which is good for the greatest number.* This principle has not only been misapplied to ethical issues but it is the major factor upon which medical research and practice is based. Side effects and other untoward

results occur with any medical treatment and sometimes these will be worse than the original problem. In other words the method of medical practice is that some harm is allowable so the majority will be helped. The method *per se*, not its morality, is our concern here because it is identical to the utilitarian ethic which dominates medical ethic discussions. Since the method of medical practice and the current medical ethic are identical, the promotion of individual moral considerations becomes extremely difficult. The "flow" is toward the greatest good for the greatest number. Since pleasure is the goal of utility, medicine is inclined to be another servant of a hedonistic society.[32]

(8) *The exceptional case determines ethical princple.* Ethicists and others, both Christian and non-Christian seem compelled to remove guilt from all moral dilemmas. In this process they allow the unusual, rare, or difficult case to establish ethical principle. For example, arguments about abortion frequently focus on the "defective" fetus, the threat of death to the mother, rape, incest and the horrors of the "black-alley" abortionist. Yet, if *all* these were added together the result would be less than ten percent of all pregnancies. Thus, the argument is distorted by the failure to reveal the infrequent incidence of these cases and this lack of relevance to the great majority of abortions. No one wants to be known as a cruel, unfeeling person who fails to appreciate the emotional difficulty of such cases. The Christian, however, should realize that we live in a world distorted by sin and as a result, these dilemmas occur. Kindness, love, and mercy are necessary in hard cases, but not to the compromise of principle. In spite of dilemmas where one must choose between evils, "we shall insist that evil remains evil."[33] Such guilt, as any other, may be removed through the forgiveness available through Jesus Christ. A principle is not changed because dilemmas exist in a fallen world. If it is, sinful practices have become the standard by which ethical principle is measured. This position is obviously untenable for the Christian who accepts the absolute standards of God's revelation.

(9) *Physicians are moral people.* Surveys continue to show that people's trust in physicians remains high, and sometimes it even tops the list. Within the profession itself an AMA committee concluded that "physicians as a group are inherently decent, honest and trustworthy."[34] Such respect, however, is not necessarily warranted. To begin with, physicians generally are neither better nor worse than the rest of society. In our decadent society, however, that statement calls for caution. The evidence bears this out; most physicians favor liberal abortion practices and most pediatricians "would acquiesce in parents' decision to refuse consent for surgery in an infant with intestinal atresia and Down's syndrome."[35]

For Christians who are against abortion and euthanasia, it is apparent that physicians cannot be relied upon to set the standards for these practices, making them suspect for medical ethics in general. In fact, physicians are more concerned with "etiquette parading as ethics" rather than ethics itself.[36] This situation is easily demonstrated by a review of the ethical concerns in medical publications. Practically, the Christian patient does not have to be suspicious of everything that his physician does, but he must realize that he cannot rely upon his physician alone to determine what is and is not moral. The patient himself will thus have to increase his sensitivity to and seek other resources for the possible morality or immorality of medical choices and treatments.

(10) *The efficacy of modern medicine should not seriously be questioned.* One might wonder what the efficacy of medicine has to do with ethics with a whole chapter devoted to its uncertainties later. Categorically, such efficacy does not belong to medical ethics but to medical science. The question of efficacy, however, may be the largest stumbling block to a clear biblical/medical ethic. If the efficacy of most medical practices is assumed *or* is true, every effort should be made to make them widely available. What mother would want to be considered neglectful by missing a "well-baby" check-up for her child or what adult wants to feel guilty about missing an annual physical exam? The efficacy exerts a tremendous pressure which tends to overpower moral considerations. Properly understood, such efficacy cannot be authoritative over Scripture or even societal obligations. Nevertheless, the existence of such pressure is apparent as medical expenditures are being reduced and no one wants to be left out!

If, however, such efficacy is more apparent than real, two immediate results occur. First, the pressure to provide complete medical care for everyone is markedly reduced and its provision can be more objectively considered along with other societal obligations. Second, each medical treatment would undergo scrutiny. Resources for that which is less effective can be given to that which is clearly effective. It is time for Christians to realize that efficacy *is* more apparent than real and to act upon these two results with the Scripture giving authoritative direction for balanced priorities.

(11) *Discussion alone is sufficient for the process of medical ethics.* In other words the applicability of a principle does not have to be considered. Complete casuistry is impossible. Nevertheless, an ethic that cannot be concretely applied is useless. For example, the position that abortion is moral following rape and incest or when the mother's life is in danger, can be applied practically. It is quite specific. When one moves to the position that the mental illness of a pregnant woman may warrant abortion, practicality is lost because mental illness is a broad, general concept that is interpreted differently by professionals and nonprofessionals. Worse, it opens the door for a wider practice than was originally intended. Many Christian ethicists err on this point as they allow this compassion for difficult cases to determine a principle which lacks definable limits and fails to account for the extent to which human nature will stretch a vague principle for personal ends.[37] If biblical principle is retained, its practical value will become apparent.

(12) *If I don't do what the patient asks, someone else will.* Patients can almost always find a physician who will do what they desire. For example, tonsillectomies are rarely indicated today. Yet a patient who is convinced that his child needs this procedure, can find a physician who will do it for more liberal indications.

Two more examples would be the provision of a means of birth control without parental consent and major surgery for which there is not a clear indication. Often, the physician's intention is moral. He may desire to develop rapport with the patient, hoping to eventually win him to the physician's moral position or witness to him. The Christian, however, must be moral in *both* his means and his ends. Specifically, he is acting immorally in the *real* situation if he only has the *possibility* of his attaining his desired end. In those instances where a choice of more than one equally acceptable treatment is possible, the physician may acquiesce to the patient. There is no biblical warrant, however, where biblical principle is clear, to compromise means in order to achieve ends.[38]

A Methodology for Biblical Ethics

A methodology for biblical ethics must be wholistic. Helmut Thielicke wrote, "A succession of isolated tactical actions will not suffice; an overall (wholistic) strategy will have to be developed."[39] The analytical method of a scientific world view fragments wholes into parts. Then, the derived answers for particular questions are applied to the whole, frequently neglecting other parts which were excluded by such analysis. Medical ethics is a part of the whole of society. Contrariwise, the biblical world view is clear that two groups, the saved and the unsaved, exist and interact simultaneously. Ethics and in particular medical ethics, must be seen within these cultural wholes.

The term "biblical ethics" is preferable because "Christian ethics" is not sufficiently explicit. Many professing Christians are more dependent, consciously or functionally, upon naturalism for ethical direction than on God's revelation. Thus, a consensus of Christians is not an appropriate methodology.

> The study of biblical ethics. . . . is not that of surveying empirically the sum-total of the behavior of those who are . . . believers. What such a study would furnish is simply a description of the behavior of believers. . . . there is . . . much sin and inconsistency in the behavior of believers at their best. . . . The biblical ethic is that manner of life which is consonant with, and demanded by, the biblical revelation. Our attention must be focused upon divine demand, not upon human achievement, upon the revelation of God's will for man, not upon human behaviors.[40]

A methodological starting point has to be necessarily evangelical and inseparably two-fold: regeneration (*palingenesis*, Titus 3:5) and inerrant, infallible Scripture.[41] It is dual because regeneration without Scripture is not enlightening and without regeneration Scriptures cannot be understood or obeyed. It is not legitimate to separate the authority of Christ from the authority of Scripture; and one cannot stand in opposition to the other. The point is raised that a person who claims regeneration and does not adopt this scriptural position is likely deceiving himself.

Appallingly evangelicals lack, in their medical ethics, a consistent methodology based upon this two-fold starting point. An intermingling of principles taken both from naturalism and Christian theism, coupled with the failure to distinguish between believers and unbelievers among those who profess to be Christians, confuses the issues and obscures a clear Christian world and life view. One example in medicine is a symposium report in which the majority of the speakers fail to give importance to regeneration as fundamental to health and the Bible as a means to a medical ethic, as well as a healthy lifestyle.

Part of this problem concerns those Christians whose motives are proper but whose methodology, ability, or self-deception disasterously affects their results. In other words their principles are inconsistent with their profession. An ethicist whose worship of and service unto God and whose thorough reliance upon the Scripture is obvious, is more worthy of serious consideration than the ethicist whose spiritual commitment is not readily apparent. It would be naive to consider that final agreement in all areas is possible but we would be amazed at the degree of agreement which could result from a methodology that is identifiably biblical through a clear profession and a consistent process.

Another part of this whole is the knowledge of the universe as God's creation and its relationship to knowledge from His special revelation. The biblical description of the universe includes the material universe that is identifiable by our senses, empirical methods and the immaterial universe which is not sensed but nevertheless has both substance and being. As a part of this dual universe man is a whole, consisting of both a material body and immaterial spirit. A biblical/medical ethic must give consideration to both material *and* immaterial dimensions of the universe and of man.

Consideration must also be given to the division of society into two wholes, Christian and non-Christian. That is not to say that these two societies are clearly identifiable. The true church will always exist on earth and to some extent inseparable from *the remainder of society* (Matt. 13:24-30, 36-43). Though God is the only Person who can finally discern those who are wheat and tares, functional judgments can be made.[42] If both profession and lifestyle are examined, functional judgments can be made relative to palingenesis and such judgments need to be made where possible because the unbeliever does not have the same understanding or ability to act that the believer does. How can the unbeliever respond to this command: "Husbands, love your wives, just as Christ also loved the church" (Eph. 5:25).

Still another component of the wholistic approach is the relationship of the Scriptures of the church and to the believer. From *an ethic* (world view), *ethics* (principles) are derived to direct morality (practice). God in His great wisdom gave us His revelation which consists of history, symbolism, analogy and propositional statements. A critical task of the church throughout history has been the development of its dogma into a systematic form from which its ethics and morals are derived.

Developmental priority must be Scripture, then the church, then systematics, then ethics and morality.[43]

... the Christian ethicist bends every effort to appropriate the theological truth stored up in the Church. Illumined, purified, and enriched through even new addresses to the Word of God by the active theological community, the funded knowledge is the very stuff of ethical reflection and the designated tool for the moralist's reforming work. The truth grasped in the creeds, in the classical treatises on dogmatics, and in the responsible conclusions of contemporary theologians, is all that the ethicist has with which to transform personal and social life. In the last analysis, the good life is the life patterned after God in Christ, the Truth; or alternately, it is the life patterned after what God has done, the fact. And since God and Christ, and what they have done for men, are systematically portrayed in dogmatics, the latter is indispensable to ethics.[44]

On the one hand, the church cannot absolutely be trusted in its formulation of doctrine, or else the Reformation would not have been necessary. On the other hand, within certain traditions a wealth of soundly and thoroughly developed doctrines do exist. For example, *The Westminister Confession of Faith* and *Calvin's Institutes of Christian Religion* exist within the Presbyterian and Reformed traditions. Thus, the Christian has much upon which to build and sound theology[45] does not have to be "performed by every believer personally."[46] Within evangelicalism a great error occurs when moderns arrogantly consider anything not developed within their lifetime as unworthy of consideration. This attitude ignores the historical transmission of God's authority through His church which contains men whom He has gifted (Matt. 28:18-20). "For the church carries the institutional authority of a Body established by God and guaranteed by our Lord as His own Body, the vehicle of his continuing life in time."[47]

Theology should come to the believer primarily through the preaching and teaching of his local church. As we shall see, moral practice is the external essence of the Christian faith, but it is organically part of a whole lifestyle. Thus, it is ". . . objectionable that the isolated local church, out of effective contact with the larger Christian fellowship (including the historical dimension), or that the isolated believer, maintaining personal devotions in independence of a local church, is ethically self-sufficient."[48] The local church, and much less the individual believer, does not have the spiritual and physical resources to become theologically or ethically proficient without building upon the prior and concurrent work of the universal church. Thus, the local church has a crucial role in the ethical process, as it makes more immediate application for the believer through all its functions: the preaching and teaching of the Scripture, the administration of the sacraments of baptism and communion, and the practice of church discipline. A subtle but powerful moral effect occurs in the context of a local, Spirit-directed church.

One form of church teaching, individual counsel, deserves special emphasis.[49] The pastor should be closely aware of, and provide theological underpinning of such counsel, but today's complexity of moral problems is likely to demand more time than he is able to devote because of his other pastoral responsibilites. For medical ethics, a particular passage, James 5:13-18, seems directly applicable. Here, personal counsel in the form of confession is noted (v.16). The elders' responsibility for sound doctrine would include counsel in medical matters. The counselor would not necessarily have to be a physician but a physician would have the advantage of professional expertise. This expertise alone, however, is not sufficient for such a role. The counselor should be an elder (or his equivalent by another denominational title) because *counsel is teaching* one-on-one. He must know the Scriptures well enough that the church recognizes his ability to teach (one criterion of the office of elder: 1 Tim. 3:2; Titus 1:9). This availability of knowledgeable and experienced counsel is a direct means by which the local church can immediately apply the great theology of the historical and modern church to ethical problems.

The final part of biblical ethics is the conscience of the individual believer. Ultimately, God judges whether his thoughts and actions are moral or immoral (2 Cor. 5:10). The finality of the believer's choice and freedom of the believer's conscience were key principles of the Reformation: "unless this be understood there can be no right knowledge of Christ, or of evangelical truth, or of internal peace of mind."[50] Three elements of conscience need definition: liberty, responsibility, and the Holy Spirit. The first two emphasize "an ethic of responsible freedom."[51] At no point in his spiritual life is a believer without the wisdom necessary to make a moral decision (James 1:5-8). At the same time he is responsible to know the judgment of the Scripture (Heb. 4:12-13), which includes the theology of the church. To oversimplify, at one extreme are the pietists whose practice is almost, if not entirely, and individually subjective. At the other extreme are the legalists (Pharisees of Jesus' day) who attempt total casuistry. The concept of counsel is one means by which the extremes may be avoided. It provides the situation where individual considerations are integrated with appropriate biblical principles. The third element is the Holy Spirit who indwells the believer. He works through the studied efforts of the believer to enable him to understand and apply the Scripture, but He does not work apart from biblical knowledge in any of its forms. This balanced emphasis is seen in the Chicago Statement on Hermeneutics:[52]

> We deny that the Holy Spirit ever teaches to anyone anything which is contrary to the teaching of Scripture (IV.b).

> We affirm that the Holy Spirit enables believers to appropriate and apply Scripture to their lives (V.a).

The wholistic characteristic of this methodology from the Scriptures through the church to the believer is God's design to prevent conflict in believers' lives. Since all activities of life are to be performed as a "service of worship" (Rom. 12:1), the sacred and the secular are parts of a whole. The mystical experience of prayer (Phil. 4:6-7) is combined with planning and principle (Phil. 4:8) which culminates in practice (Phil. 4:9). Personal ethics do not conflict with societal ethics. Both obligations are blended into the whole. "None of these matters can be separated. . . . He that seeks righteousness seeks to realize himself, seeks the good will, seeks happiness, seeks usefulness, seeks rewards, seeks the kingdom of God and seeks God Himself."[53] In a fallen world apparent conflicts will arise, but the concept of a whole that is designed to integrate all endeavors makes the moral life realistically practical.

In this process from the universal, historical church through the local church to the conscience of the individual, direct correlation with Scripture must not be neglected. Theology assists believers to understand Scripture and God Himself. Consistent with our emphasis here, it is essential. Although the distance varies, ethics is one step further removed from Scripture. For example, ". . . do not let the sun go down upon your anger" (Eph. 4:26) is quite direct; whereas not playing golf on Sunday is further removed as a viable application of the Fourth Commandment. Thus, the continual linking of the church's theology and ethics to scriptural texts is crucial. The Scriptures are God's complete revelation, not merely theology or ethics: ". . . the points of support may never be looked for in the church."[54]

As the Scriptures are neglected by Christians who develop ethics, God is also neglected. Our two-fold starting point has demonstrated that *the neglect of one is the neglect of the other*: ". . . the question about God is the central question in ethics, and the apprehension of him is or should be the ethicist's chief concern." A Christian says "It is not I who apprehended him; he apprehended me"[55] This position expresses "an entire epistemology." Too often, Christians are caught up with "godly" activities to the neglect of God Himself. God is the ultimate principle of an ethic. The import of this truth is seen by the contrasting force of "the Bible says" versus "God says." Of course for a consideration of ethics they are one and the same.

> It is impossible to segregate the biblical ethic from the teaching of Scripture on other subjects. The ethic of the Bible reflects the character of the God of the Bible. Remove from Scripture the transcendent holiness, righteousness and truth of God and its ethic disintegrates.[56]

Christ gave a worshiping heart as a priority in a right relationship to God over ethics or the right relationships with others (Matt. 22:37-39). The biblical ethicist must be so devoted to knowing God and His attributes that he spontaneously breaks forth into a doxology in a manner similar to Paul (Rom. 11:33-36; 1 Tim. 1:17). His highest ethical goal is the fulfillment of God's will (Rom. 12:2) and the promotion of God's glory (1 Cor. 10:31) which are in their essence the same.

> . . . a holy affinity and a spiritual sympathy with the life of God must be manifest in our spirit, if the revelations of the Holy Scripture are to be real to us and to refer to an object grasped by us as a real object. Both together are the constituent parts of our knowledge of God."[57]

Unique to all other ethics, the Bible states that man is sinful and immoral in his very nature (Roman 5:12-19), and not just in his behavior (Rom. 3:10-18).[58] One's personal acceptance of the sacrificial death of Jesus Christ makes his nature moral (Rom. 3:24) and enables him to live morally (Rom. 8:1-14). "To lead man before the judgment seat of sin, and in so doing to the grace of God in Christ, is the supreme task of the ethical quest."[59] Two principles arise from this gospel message. First, the immoral nature of man's nature demonstrates one of our two-fold starting points, the necessity of regeneration for the Christian ethicist. Second, evangelism is central to all ethical discussion. The unbeliever can do *nothing* pleasing to God because his nature is sinful, and as a result his motives and goals violate the first of Christ's great commandments. Because disease is directly and indirectly related to sin, a Christian physician cannot develop an approach to health without a concern for the conversion of his patients and a desire that they grow in a biblical direction.

Other ethical principles flow from the character of God. (a) He establishes the moral necessity of prayer—one means by which we are dependent upon Him (John. 15:56). (b) He gives unity to the Christian life so that ideally no conflict exists among one's moral responsibilities to God, neighbor and self. (c) He determines what is right and wrong. Without Him no inherent morality exists in the universe; to suppose that it does is a common error of both Christians and non-Christians.[60]

Although Scripture and regeneration are tangible origins for truly Christian ethics, God is *the* starting point, as well as *the* dynamic that actively and immanently directs all things to moral ends.[61] The centrality of God in ethics provides criteria that delineates a true Christian ethicist. Does he clearly manifest a deep concern to obey God rather than please men? Is Christ in the foreground? Does his epistemology give more credence to a naturalistic philosophy than a Christian theistic world view? Are his references and supporting statements more from Christian literature than secular literature? Is evangelism central to all his ethical directions? Does prayer have a defined place?

> A particularly vicious way in which the principle of redemptive mediacy
> is denied appears when men avowedly write works on Christian ethics . . .
> and still do not really bring Christianity (centered in God and the Atone-
> ment) into the picture.[62]

As the individual believer stands objectively in the mainstream of historic Christianity with its biblical doctrines and subjectively in relationship to his God, he faces practical decisions daily. The Bible says little about medical practice *per se*. This omission, however, it is only apparent, not real.

Application of biblical admonitions into real life situations is the most crucial practice which the evangelical Christian must learn and follow during his lifetime. On the one hand, the delineation of the process is quite simple: biblical principle directs biblical practice. On the other hand the process is quite arduous because derivation of biblical principle requires an extensive study of Scripture. Once principles are derived, further application to daily problems must occur.

All activities of Christians should be performed with a conscious awareness of those biblical texts that direct those activities. That involves more than the simplistic quoting of book, chapter, and verse. Biblical principle must stand *within the whole* methodology of biblical ethic. The Chicago Statement on Hermeneutics[63] balances individual and scholarly interpretation: ". . . a person is not dependent for understanding of Scripture on the expertise of biblical scholars," but neither should ". . . a person . . . ignore the fruits of the technical study of Scripture by biblical scholars."[64]

Concerning the Scripture in this process, two characteristics balance each other. First, "minutely detailed obligations" are seldom found in the Bible.[65] Second, Scripture is sufficient to answer all questions of ethical principle and moral practice, if only we learn the act of fitting to our situation that which Scripture offers either in principle or example.[66] The former emphasizes that principles must fit into the whole and the latter emphasizes that God's revelation to us is indeed "whole." Both underscore the conscious connection which needs to exist between biblical texts and Christian practice. One rule, however, is appropriate for our consideration and relates to the sufficiency of Scripture. This rule concerns the spirit of the law and the letter of the law.[67] Jesus illustrated the letter of the law and the spirit of the law in His Sermon on the Mount. "Thou shalt not kill" was extended to cover anger toward one's brother and its result of inappropriate name calling (Matt. 5:21-22). Also, "Thou shalt not commit adultery" was extended to cover the lustful look (Matt. 5:27-28).

Within the theology of the church, another example appears in *The Westminster Confession of Faith*. Question 139 of *The Larger Catechism* asks, "What are the sins forbidden by the seventh commandment?" The answer (in part) is:

> The sins forbidden in the seventh commandment, besides the neglect of the duties required, are adultery, fornication, rape, incest, sodomy, and all unnatural lusts; all unclean imaginations, thought, purposes, and affections; all corrupt or filthy communications or listening thereunto, wanton books, impudent or light behavior, immodest apparel . . . lascivious songs, books, pictures, drawings, stage plays, and all other provocations to, or acts of, uncleanness either in ourselves or in others.

These biblical and doctrinal examples illustrate the extension of the letter of the law to cover the spirit of the law in its many applications. The neglect or extreme emphasis of either letter or spirit results in biblical imbalance. Since we have noted that the New Testament says little that is explicit about the practice of medicine, this principle is crucial to a biblical/medical ethic.

Within the spirit of the law is the unique emphasis in Christian ethics upon motive, "the dispositional character or complex which is the psychological determinant of action."[68] Motives are between the individual and God. Only He can judge the heart, also, it behooves a Christian to judge his own motives.[69] Jesus' interaction with the Pharisees provides a clear illustration of the depth of this issue. He was extremely critical of those who were meticulously concerned to keep the law externally. He never criticized, however, their attention to the law. In fact, He demanded greater perfection of it (Matt.5:20). He criticized *their heart* (Matt. 15:7-9). Thus the biblical ethic must be concerned with motive even more than external action.

A close interdependency exists between principle and practice and from this mutual dependency two principles emerge for our purposes. First, principle directs practice.

> . . . Christian ethics is not left to chart its course of divinely approved con-
> duct by self-reflection alone, or by an immediate spiritual impression traced
> to 'encounter'. . . . The biblically revealed ethic or principle, command-
> ments, examples and application provides such a content.[70]

Even so, the influence of practice upon principle does give a situational aspect to biblical ethics.[71] For example, sexual intercourse with someone who is not a spouse is sin; with a spouse it is not. The external act is similar, but the morality of the situation is different.

Certain foundations remove Christian morality from situationalism: a Christian-theistic world view, palingenesis, the inerrancy and infallibility of the Scripture, the theology of the church, availability of counsel and the conscience of the believer. Situational ethics refuses to accept such conditioning factors.[72]

Although Christian priorities are concrete principles that govern choices within a situation, there is allowance for obvious conflicts. For example, the pregnant mother whose life is threatened by the continuing presence of her baby in her womb may choose to have an abortion, ". . . we shall insist that evil remains evil, even when, being the lesser evil, it appears the right thing to do; we shall do it with a heavy heart, and seek God's cleansing of our conscience for having done it."[73] Practice in an imperfect world will occasionally modify the usual practice which follows from principle. "Life and theory, existence and conviction, love and understanding here stand and fall together . . . such principles as we have we should be constantly enriching with the accumulating wisdom of practical experience."[74] Principle must be practical; the practical exception does not warrant principle. These two are frequent errors within medical ethics.

Even though total casuistry is impossible, Christians must develop principles *which focus the Scripture upon the concrete situation.* Believer's thoughts and actions must continually link biblical principles with daily practice.

Biblical ethics must be founded on the concept of love. Christ summed up the central commandments as the love of God and the love of neighbor. Paul emphasized the essential role of love in all activities (1 Cor. 13:1-3) and described its characteristics extensively (1 Cor. 13:4-13). Biblical love and synonymously Christian love is "the fulfilling of the law."[75] "It is through an objective divine outline alone that he (the Christian) can discriminate between right and wrong (moral) direction of life in action."[76] The practice of biblical morality *is* love. It begins with God who motivates man (John 3:16;

1 John 4:19) to love his neighbor (Matt. 22:39) and his enemy (Matt. 5:43-48). To divorce Christian love from the biblical ethic surrenders Christian truth to the antithetical, subjective relativity of the naturalistic world view.

Harry Blamires speaks of Christian answers resulting from that Christian dialogue which is grounded upon Christian presuppositions.[77] Abraham Kuyper speaks of "the consciousness of our regenerated race. . . . a task which is in process century upon century."[78] From these it may be said that *biblical ethics is developmental*. Through individual study, dialogue, and reflection our experience in the concrete application of biblical principles to the practice of medicine should develop in its breadth and depth. Some individual and collective inconsistency will always be present but increasing development should be evident in both ways. Consistency and development within this world view should result in an increasing *distinctiveness* from the naturalistic world view. If it does not, our salt and light are diminished.

Given our established methodology for a biblical ethic and some diversity, there is extensive agreement among those who are committed to this methodology and develop it consistently and diligently. There does exist commitment to both the science of interpretation objectively and personal Christian growth subjectively.[79] As a balanced emphasis is achieved by individuals and groups, many areas of agreement are found. This agreement is convincing and encouraging evidence that such a methodology can result in unity among true believers.

NOTES

1. J. Robertson McQuilkin, "The Behavioral Sciences Under the Authority of Scripture," *Journal of the Theological Society* (March, 1977), p. 12.

2. For further discussion of the physician as priest, see Rousas Rushdoony, "Healing Priests or Pagan Gods," *Christian Medical Society Journal* 8 (1) 1977:9-16.

3. B. H. Roberts and W. M. Norton. "Prevalence of Psychiatric Illness in a Medical Outpatient Clinic," *New England Journal of Medicine* 245 (1952) p. 82. J. D. Stoeckle, I. K. Zola and G. E. Davidson, "The Quanity and Significance of Psychological Distress in Medical Patients," *Journal of Chronic Disease* 17 (1964):959.

4. George Engel, "The Biopsychosocial Method and Medical Education," *New England Journal of Medicine* 306 (April 1, 1982):802-805.

5. R. L. Parker, ed., *The Journal of John Wesley* (Chicago: Moody, 1974), p. 231.

6. Henry Stob, *Ethical Reflections*, (Grand Rapids: Eerdmans Pub. Co., 1978) p. 227.

7. J. Robertson McQuilkin, "The Behavioral Sciences Under the Authority of Scripture," *Journal of the Theological Society* (March, 1977), p. 3.

8. Ibid.

9. Alasdair MacIntyre, "Theology, Ethics, and the Ethics of Medicine and Health Care: Comments on Papers by Novak, Mouw, Roach, Cahill, and Hartt," *Journal of Medicine and Philosophy* 4 (4) 1979:435-443.

10. Henry Stob, *Ethical Reflections*, pp. 17-18.

11. The complexity of these priorities cannot be detailed here. More will be said in the appendix, but it will not be entirely sufficient either. Certainly, all Christians are not called to abandon necessary functions, such as milking cows, typing letters, diapering children, and building bridges. They are necessary and righteous endeavors. Serious consideration must be given to spiritual gifts, life situations, opportunities and available time. Particulars will vary widely among Christians with similar understanding and commitment. The emphasis here, however, is the neglect by many Christian health professionals to bring biblical principle into their practices.

12. John Pollock, *A Foreign Devil in China* (Grand Rapids: Zondervan Publishing Co., 1971), p.117.

13. Bernard Glensen, *Mr. Burkitt in Africa* (New York: World Publishing Co., 1970), pp. 12-13..

14. Medical is italicized because the conditions specified here are certainly not medical, even though most medical people place them there.

15. D. Gareth Jones, "Abortion: Thoughts on a Perplexing Issue," *Christian Medical Society Journal* 14 (1) 1983:4-8.

16. John Murray, *Principles of Conduct*, (1957; reprint ed., Grand Rapids: Eerdmans Pub. Co., 1978), pp. 107-122.

17. Jonas Robitscher, *The Powers of Psychiatry* (Boston: Houghton Mifflin Co., 1980) p. 307.

18. Stanley Dokupil, "Seizing Power: The Use of the Imagination for Healing," *Spiritual Counterfeits Project Newsletter* 8 (6) 1982, pp. 1-4.

19. D. Martyn Lloyd-Jones, *The Doctor Himself and the Human Condition* (London: Christian Medical Fellowship Publications, 1982) p. 51.

20. Ibid., pp. 56-57.

21. Paul Ramsey, "Medical Ethics Skewed by the Abortion Issue," *Human Life Review*. 2 (1) 1976:74-85.

22. E. P. Pellegrino, "Educating the Christian Physician," in *Whole-Person Medicine*, eds. David E. Allen, Lewis P. Bird, and Robert Herrmann (Downers Grove: InterVarsity Press, 1980), pp. 103-104.

23. Henry Stob, *Ethical Reflections*, p. 160.

24. Harold O. J. Brown "Legal Aspect of the Right to Life," in *Thou Shalt Not Kill*, ed. Richard L. Ganz. (New Rochelle: Arlington House Pub., 1978). p. 114 .

25. Paul Ramsey, "Medical Ethics Skewed by the Abortion Issue," *Human Life Review* 2 (1) 1976:74-85.

26. Henry Stob, *Ethical Reflections*, p. 224.

27. A blatant example of such practice was killing of a Down's fetus. See chapter 1.

28. Paul Ramsey, *The Patient as Person* (1970; reprint ed., New Haven: Yale University Press, 1979), p. 123.

29. Several medical organizations recently protested any legal restrictions on decisions not to care for handicapped newborns on the same ground that these were medical judgments. "Medical Groups Divided on 'Baby Doe' Alternative." *Medical World News* (Sept. 16, 1983), pp. 1-20.

30. Henry Stob, *Ethical Reflections*, p. 225.

31. Carl F. Henry, "The Ambiguities of Scientific Breakthrough," in *Horizons of Science*, ed. Carl F. Henry (San Francisco: Harper and Row Pub., 1978), p. 105.

32. James Hitchcock, "Guilt and the Moral Revolution," *Human Life Review* 7 (4) 1981:79-94.

33. Bruce Kaye and Gordon Wenham, *Law, Morality and the Bible* (Downers Grove: InterVarsity Press, 1978), p. 164.

34. "Impact." *American Medical News* (November 28, 1980), p. 2.

35. "New 'Baby Doe' Rule Similar to Original," *American Medical News* (July 15, 1983), pp. 3, 7.

36. Haddon W. Robinson, "Morality in Malpractice," *Christian Medical Society Journal* 8 (1) 1977: pp. 2-5.

37. D. Gareth Jones, "Abortion: Thoughts on a Perplexing Issue," *Christian Medical Society Journal* 14 (1) 1983: pp. 4-8.

38. J. Robertson McQuilkin, "The Behavioral Sciences Under the Authority of Scripture," *Journal of the Theological Society* (March, 1977), pp. 31-43.

39. Helmut Thielicke, "Ethics in Modern Medicine," in *Who Shall Live?*, ed. Kenneth Vaux (New York: Harper and Row, 1964), p. 178.

40. John Murray, *Principles of Conduct*, (Grand Rapids: Eerdmans Pub. Co., 1978), pp. 13-14.

41. Simply, inerrancy refers to the original writings (autographs) which exist today. Infallibility sometimes refers to the practical application of the Bible, but it is essentially a synonym of inerrancy. For further reading, see Norman Geisler, *Inerrancy*, (Grand Rapids, Zondervan, 1980).

42. Jay E. Adams, *More Than Redemption* (Phillipsburg, N. J.: Presbyterian and Reformed Pub. Co., 1979), pp. 292-293.

43. Relative to whether the church selected the Scriptures, it must suffice here to convey the position of the Reformers: the church was the *agent by which* the Scriptures were selected but it was restricted to those texts that God had predetermined. Thus, the Scripture governs the church because God wrote it and directed the process. This position is an irreconcilable difference between Roman Catholics and orthodox Protestants.

44. Henry Stob, *Ethical Reflections*, p. 40.

45. Theology is used here in its true definition that assumes our two-fold starting point. It is the systematic study of the knowledge of God as He reveals Himself in the Scripture to His regenerated subjects. Thus, theology combines the objectivity of the Scripture with subjective regeneration. Sinful, finite man may err in his scriptural interpretation but such error does not eliminate the fact of God's continuing revelation of truth through the study of the Scripture. See Abraham Kuyper, *Principles of Sacred Theology* (1898; reprint ed. Grand Rapids: Baker Book House, 1980). p. 567.

46. Ibid., p. 567.

47. Harry Blamires, *The Christian Mind* (1963; reprint ed., Ann Arbor: Servant Books, 1978), p. 143.

48. Carl F. H. Henry, *Christian Personal Ethics* (1957; reprint edition, Grand Rapids: Baker Book House, 1977), p. 205.

49. Arbitrarily, I am distinguishing between counsel and counseling. Counsel involves a few sessions whereby a person is assisted in his review of principles and alternatives which are appropriate to a particular decision that he faces. Counseling (see chapter on Psychotherapy) involves repeated sessions whereby a person who is failing in his daily life because of ongoing problems, is helped. Of course, counsel and counseling overlap but this distinction applies in most cases.

50. Henry Stob, *Ethical Reflections*, p. 151.

51. J. I. Packer, *Knowing God* (Douner's Grove: InterVarsity Press, 1973) p. 191.

52. Chicago Statement on Hermeneutics: International Council on Biblical Inerrancy, P.O. Box 13261, Oakland CA 94661.

53. Cornelius VanTil, *"Christian Theistic Ethics,"* in Defense of the Faith. vol. 3 (Philadelphia: Presbyterian and Reformed Publishing Co., 1980), p. 58.

54. Abraham Kuyper, *Principles of Sacred Theology*, p. 577.

55. Henry Stob, *Ethical Reflections*, pp. 38-39.

56. John Murray, *Principles of Conduct*, p. 202.

57. Abraham Kuyper, *Principles of Sacred Theology*, p. 579.

58. Today, many professing Christians prefer some word other than "sin." Certainly there are words in the Scripture that are synonymns for sin. Further, it is sometimes useful to use other words to denote sin for variety in writing and speaking. To depart, however, from a clear relationship between such substituted words and the biblical concept of sin *is to depart from the Christian faith.* Since "The person and work of Jesus Christ are the central focus of the entire Bible" (Intl. Council on Biblical Inerrancy iv.a) His redemptive work is significant only to the extent that the seriousness and depth of human sinfulness, both in man's being and in his behavior, is appreciated. Remove sin and Christ is removed. Thus, knowledgeable believers are not hesitant to use the word, "sin"; neither are they reluctant to call thoughts, words, and deeds, "sin." Such designation brings these things under the forgiving and restoring mercy of God. Morbid preoccupation with sin can and does occur but that results from a failure to grasp the fullness and completeness of Christ's justifying work.

59. Carl Henry, *Christian Personal Ethics*, p. 392.
60. Cornelius VanTil, *Christian Theistic Ethics*, pp. 22, 29-32.
61. Henry Stob, *Ethical Reflections*, p. 101.
62. Cornelius VanTil, *Christian Theistic Ethics*, p. 141.
63. The word, "hermuneutics," may frighten the nontheologically trained Christian but it is necessary to be familiar with the basic principles of interpretation. Recommended sources are:
a. Sproul, R. C. *Knowing Scripture* (Downers Grove: InterVarsity Press, 1977).
b. McQuilkin, J. Robertson. *Understanding and Applying the Bible* (Chicago: Moody Press, 1983).
c. "The Chicago Statement: Articles of Affirmation and Denial." P. O. Box 13261, Oakland, CA, 94661.
64. Article XXIV International. Council or Biblical Inerrancy.
65. Henry Stob, *Ethical Reflections*, p. 156.
66. Cornelius VanTil, *Christian Theistic Ethics*, p. 26.
67. R. C. Sproul, *Knowing Scripture* (Downers Grove: InterVarsity Press, 1977), p. 90.
68. John Murray, *Principles of Conduct*, p. 13.
69. It is here that Christians err in their concept of judging. We *are to judge* the external actions and words of others. For example, we make judgments about the disharmony between us and other believers and take action to remedy the situation based upon that judgment (Matt. 5:23-24; Matt. 18:15-17). Indeed, Christians need to make critical judgments about all things *except* another's motives.
70. Carl Henry, *Christian Personal Ethics*, p. 301.
71. Henry Stob, *Ethical Reflections*, pp. 156-157. John Murray, *Principles of Conduct*, pp. 21-22.
72. Bruce Kaye and Gordon Wenham, *Law, Morality and the Bible* (Downers Grove: InterVarsity Press, 1978), pp. 152-153.
73. Ibid., p. 164.
74. Henry Stob, *Ethical Reflections*, pp. 44, 48.
75. John Murray, *Principles of Conduct*, p. 22.
76. Carl Henry, *Christian Personal Ethics*, p. 301.
77. Harry Blamires, *The Christian Mind* (1963. reprint ed., Ann Arbor: Servant Books, 1978), pp. 42-43.
78. Abraham Kuyper, *Principles of Sacred Theology*, p. 567.
79. Harold O. J. Brown, *The Protest of a Troubled Protestant*, pp. 15-28, 45-55.

REFERENCES

Blaimires, Harry. *The Christian Mind.* 1963. Reprint Ann Arbor: Servant Books, 1978.

Brown, Harold O. J. "Legal Aspects of the Right to Life." In *Thou Shalt Not Kill.* ed. Richard L. Ganz. New Rochelle, N.Y.: Arlington House Publishers, 1978, p. 111.

Brownback, Paul. *The Danger of Self-Love.* Chicago: Moody Press, 1982.

Dokupil, Stanley. "Seizing the Power: The Use of the Imagination for Healing." Spiritual Counterfeits Project Newsletter 8 (6) 1982:1-4.

Engel, George. "The Biopsychosocial Method and Medical Education." *New England Journal of Medicine* 306 (April 1, 1982):802-805.

Glensen, Bernard. *Mr. Burkitt in Africa.* New York: World Publishing Co., 1970.

Hitchcock, James. "Guilt and the Moral Revolution." *Human Life Review* 7 (4) 1981:79-94.

Impact. *American Medical News,* November 28, 1980.

Jones, D. Gareth. "Abortion: Thoughts on a Perplexing Issue." *Christian Medical Society Journal* 14 (1) 1983:4-8.

Kaye, Bruce and Wenham, Gordon. *Law, Morality and the Bible.* Downers Grove: InterVarsity Press, 1978.

MacIntyre, Alasdair. "Theology, Ethics, and the Ethics of Medicine and Health Care: Comments on Papers by Novak, Mouw, Roach, Cahill, and Hartt." *Journal of Medicine and Philosophy* 4 (4) 1979:435-443.

McQuilkin, J. Robertson. "The Behavioral Sciences Under the Authority of Scripture." *Journal of the Theological Society,* March, 1977.

"New 'Baby Doe' Rule Similar to Original" *American Medical News,* July 15, 1983.

Parker, R. L., ed. *The Journal of John Wesley.* Chicago: Moody, 1974.

Pollock, John. *A Foreign Devil in China.* Grand Rapids: Zondervan Publishing Co., 1971.

Ramsey, Paul. "Medical Ethics Skewed by the Abortion Issue." *Human Life Review* 2 (1) 1976:74-85.

Roberts, B. H. and Norton, N. M. "Prevalence of Psychiatric Illness in a Medical Outpatient Clinic." *New England Journal of Medicine* 245 (1952):82.

Robinson, Haddon W. "Morality in Malpractice." *Christian Medical Society Journal* 8 (1) 1977:2-5..

Robitscher, Jonas. *The Powers of Psychiatry.* Boston: Houghton Mifflin Company, 1980.

Sproul, R. C. *Knowing Scripture.* Downers Grove: InterVarsity Press, 1977.

Stoeckle, J. D., Zola, I. K. and Davidson G. E., "The Quanity and Significance of Psychological Distress in Medical Patients." *Journal of Chronic Disease* 17 (1964):959.

VanTil, Cornelius. *Christian Theistic Ethics.* In Defense of the Faith, vol. 3. Philadelphia: Presbyterian and Reformed Publishing Co., 1980.

6 | Pneumosomatic Health and Medicine: Principles and Practice

Ron, age 37, had a seven year history of recurrent spastic colitis whose symptoms included abdominal cramps and vomiting. At times he was incapacitated and spent some nights in the bathroom. His gastroenterologist related that his emotions were likely the most significant cause of his disease and recommended treatment consisted of a bulk-forming agent and dietary changes.

As a Christian, Ron had been active for eleven years in an evangelical church and was serving on its governing board. He realized joy, peace and contentment were absent from his life; he wanted these fruits of the spirit but did not know how to get them. Counseling with his pastor did not help. He was frustrated both physically and spiritually.

Then, significant events occurred. Through close fellowship with other believers it became apparent he harbored a chronic state of anger which was hidden but occasionally manifest by explosive outbursts. Along with this recognition he learned to apply biblical teaching to his daily life, including practical ways to control his anger. These applications included reconciliation (Matt. 5:23-24), confession of sin which resulted from his anger (Matt. 5:22), and immediate handling of problems (Eph. 4:26-27). As inconsistency and reluctance were overcome, joy, peace and contentment resulted.

To Ron's surprise, a marked reduction in the symptoms from colitis occurred. Now, even though six years have passed and he has faced other crises, his colitis is an almost insignificant problem. Until these physical changes had occurred, no connection had been made between his colitis, his psychological state, and his Christian life. Ron's story aptly illustrates the effective resolution of a severe medical problem indirectly through the application of biblical

direction to life situations—problems with the body were resolved *only* following changes in his spirit.

Wholistic medicine and health have become popular among many health
professionals, both Christian and non-Christian. "In the majority of instances,
however, one fears that it is just one more expression of that loose and sen-
timental thinking which has become so characteristic of our time." Further,
". . . Christianity, and Christianity alone can deal with the 'whole man.'"[1] Thus,
D. Martyn Lloyd-Jones has summarized the wholistic popularity. For non-
Christians, the neglect of the spiritual dimension of man is to be expected.
Spiritual (biblical) considerations rank first in importance in health and
medicine; preventive measures are second; and medical care is third. Wholistic
medicine and health must be concerned with man's spirit primarily, not secondarily. "We are first and foremost Christians and only secondarily medical
men."[2] Within a Christian world view, such priority should be expected for
health and medicine, as in any other discipline.

Medical schools place the basic biological related sciences in the early years
because an understanding of the body is necessary to the diagnosis and treatment of disease. Other preparatory study includes psychology and sociology.
The presence of these courses reflects the awareness that disease is often an
environmental influence upon the mind. This perception rarely acknowledges
the anthropological assumptions upon which these studies are based; consequently, health and medicine are based on a naturalistic world view. A Christian approach to wholistic health must be distinct from the predominant theory
and practice in medicine and health today.

> . . . one cannot undertake to make even biological or medical judgments
> unless one is also willing to face up to certain fundamental decisions and
> bring within the focus of his scholarly concern the very nature of human
> existence.[3]

Christian anthropology teaches the origin, nature, and destiny of man,
especially from the perspective of his relationship to God. However, biblically, wholeness existed in man's prefall state and will exist as a future state, but
does not exist in this earthly life. Man's origin occurred in Genesis when "God
created man in His own image, in the image of God He created him; male
and female He created them" (Genesis 1:27). Man was created to be disease
free but disobedience (Genesis 3) resulted in physical disease and death. Thus,
the Bible presents disease and death as consequences of sin and severely abnormal from God's plan for mankind. Spiritual restoration *is* established in
this earthly life (2 Cor. 5:17); physical restoration is primarily future (1 Cor.
15:42-44), but may be experienced on earth. Thus, the effects of salvation are
different *in timing* relative to the body and the spirit.

In unbelievers no correction of the fallen state has occurred, in either body
or soul, so they remain in an abnormal (nonwholistic) condition. In believers
partial restoration of normality (wholeness) has occurred but remains incomplete. Thus biblical wholism is quite distinct from nonbiblical wholism

which states that wholistic health *is* possible—the Bible is clear that limitations remain.

Historically, Christians have debated whether man is dichotomous or trichotomous. The latter, however:

> originated in Greek philosophy, which conceived of the relation of the body
> and the spirit of man to each other after the analogy of the mutual relation
> between the material universe and God.[4]

A third substance, the soul, was considered necessary for the body and the spirit to enter into a mutually vital relationship. Beginning with Augustine the dichotomous view gained prominence, became common during the Middle Ages, and was sustained during the Reformation. Traditionally, the trichotomous view has not met with great favor in the theological world despite its nineteenth century revival.

> The prevailing representation of the nature of man in Scripture is clearly
> dichotomic. . . . The Bible teaches us to view the nature of man as a unity,
> and not as a duality consisting of two different elements, each of which
> move along parallel lines but do not really unite to form a single organism.
> The idea of mere parallelism between the two elements of human nature
> . . . is entirely foreign to Scripture. While recognizing the complex nature
> of man, it never represents this as resulting in a two-fold subject in man.
> Every act of man is seen as an act of the whole man. It is not the soul
> but the man that sins; it is not the body but the man that dies; and it is
> not merely the soul, but man, body and soul, that is redeemed in Christ.[5]

Further, orthodox Christians have believed that between our death and the end times, the soul or spirit will continue to exist entirely separate from the body (2 Cor. 5:8; James 2:26; 2 Peter 1:14).

Too easily, the crucial points concerning man's composition are missed in the dichotomous-trichotomous debate since biblical evidence and reputable theologians can be found to support both viewpoints. Regardless of one's position in this debate, some things are clear. First, man functions as a unit or a whole in his earthly existence. Thus, he must be treated, medically or otherwise as a whole—he must not be parceled out: his body to the physician, his spirit to the pastor, and his mind to the psychotherapist. Secondly, man is composed of immaterial and material substances. If man is only material, he is not responsible for his actions or his attitudes. Neither can he change. Christian advocacy of behaviorism is one example of such an error.[6] Thirdly, biblical directives are applicable to the whole man, not to the spirit only. Thus, the body must not be isolated to the realm of medicine without consideration of relevant biblical principles. Although these three points are interrelated, serious errors commonly occur among Christians because of their failure to emphasize all three. Dichotomy or trichotomy *per se* is less important than an approach which carefully develops and emphasizes these points.

Further clarity is gained by looking at related biblical words. *Pneuma* is translated spirit and may be used in reference to the Holy Spirit (John 3:8). "Soul" (*psyche*) is almost synonymous with spirit, because of "the extreme difficulty of distinguishing between the soul and the spirit, alike in their nature and in their activities."[7] "Heart (*kardia*) . . . is the inner life that one lives before God and himself, a life that is unknown by others because it is hidden from them."[8] These three words may be distinguished:

> the word soul (in one way or another) always depicts the non-material aspect of human nature in relationship to (or in unity with) the material, so the word spirit always refers to the same non-material aspect out of relationship to (or disunited from) the material. Heart, on the other hand, refers to the non-material side of man in contrast to his material side—usually with an emphasis upon the visibility of the latter and the invisibility of the former.[9]

Flesh (*sarx*) is:

> mere human nature, the earthly nature of man apart from divine influence, and therefore prone to sin and opposed to God . . . the entire nature of man, sense and reason, without the Holy Spirit."[10]

"Mind (*phren, nous*) is probably not to be thought of as an entity in itself (like the brain) but as the thought life of the nonmaterial side (or inner life) of man."[11]

Soma, primarily translated "body" in English versions of the New Testament needs to be treated more fully because of a viewpoint that has been prominently represented by Rudolf Bultmann and J. A. T. Robinson who consider that soma is "the most comprehensive term which Paul uses to characterize man's existence . . . Man, his person as a whole, can be denoted by soma."[12] Thus they incorporate man's immaterial component into *soma*.

> This holistic definition has become so widely accepted that virtually all recent handbooks, dictionaries, and studies of Pauline theology take it for granted with little or no felt need for argumentative justification.[13]

The correct biblical description can be summarized as follows:

> The *soma* denotes the physical body. . . . It forms the part of man in and through which he lives and acts in the world. It becomes the base of operations for sin in the unbeliever, for the Holy Spirit in the believer.[14]

> The biblical touchstone for truly human life is not consciousness of the spirit, let alone the material being of a physical object such as the body. Rather, man is fully himself in the unity of his body and his spirit in order that the body may be animated and the spirit may express itself in obedience to God. Both parts of the human constitution share in the dignity of the divine image. The dignity lies in man's service to God as a representative caretaker over the material creation. For such a task, man needs a physical medium of action as much as an incorporeal source for the conscious willing of action. Neither spirit nor body gains precedence over the other. Each gains in unity with the other.[15]

> We conclude then that Paul along with most Jews and other early Christians habitually thought of man as a duality of two parts, corporeal and incorporeal, meant to function in unity but distinguishable and capable of separation.[16]

In summary, man consists of two distinct components; a physical body (material or corporeal) and spiritual (immaterial or incorporeal). These two components are a unity that is the individual person. Each component interacts with the other, yet remains distinct (Hebrews 11:3). So, a biblical physician must realize that health and the medical treatment of the patient entails both components.

> Few medical textbooks set out an understanding of what medicine is. . . .
> This failure to define medicine as a discipline leads to some rather loose construals of medicine.[17]

As with any concept, health, disease, and medicine must be defined so that the limits and scope of the subject are clearly understood. It seems logical to assume that medicine is the treatment of disease and that disease is an absence of health. Thus, to define medicine, a concept of health must be formulated.

Current Concepts of Health and Medicine

The World Health Organization has defined health as "a state of complete physical, mental, and social well-being, not merely the absence of disease or infirmity." Definitions are not that simple. If medicine could be limited to physical diagnosis and treatment, its practice would be clear. But health and therefore medicine, *is not* and *cannot* be limited to the body. Many mental and social factors are involved both directly and indirectly. Some of these derive from a concept of health; others derive from the practice of medicine itself.

If disease is the absence of health, a standard is necessary by which this absence may be recognized. Quite surprisingly, such a standard is quite variable in modern medicine. "There are many views as to what constitutes 'health'. . . . no single concept is fully acceptable."[18] Normality is perhaps the most frequent attempt at a standard but normal and abnormal also have several meanings: conventional, clinical, statistical, optimal or typical. The problem of normality results from individual variation. Further, what is normal for an infant, a young adult or an elderly person is obviously quite variable. Normality primarily concerns individuals and their characteristics: age, sex, race, genetic endowment, and their environment.

Another problem is the absence of complete health in anyone. From the moment of conception disease is present. Gerontologists who study the aging process have clearly demonstrated this phenomenon. One specific example is atherosclerosis. Newborn babies have fatty deposits in the walls of their arteries which will increase in size throughout life, eventually causing a stroke, heart attack, or other damage due to a blocked blood supply to some organ. Autopsies on young soldiers have confirmed the continuing progression of these fatty deposits. Every person has some degree of involvement, yet many will never have any problems from this process; others will die from it. Other processes of deterioration continue throughout life with the same high degree of individual variation. No one is free of disease and no one is entirely healthy.[19]

Mental factors affect health in a variety of ways. For example, psychological states can cause physical disease or aggravate disease that is already present. Lifestyle choices, a function of the mind (will), may result in many severely disabling, chronic, and eventually fatal diseases. Finally, there is the vague concept of "mental health" as defined and described by a wide variety of psychological and psychiatric theories and practices.

The social factor involves the various relationships which promote health, such as marriage and family, churches, and other social groups. Since the mental factor coupled with social circumstance determines these relationships, mental and social cannot be separated. Occupations may promote or detract from health, due to poor lighting, exposure to toxic products, and safety measures. Society, as a whole, is affected by a polluted or nonpolluted environment.

Medicine, as both a science and an art, raises other complexities. Comment has already been made of the relative nature of science in general and the greater relativity of the biological science. The entirely subjective nature of "art" should be apparent. Therefore, the "art" of medicine will vary as widely as the individuality of physicians. Since medical judgments are moral judgments and personal values determine morals, art quite extensively and intensively impacts upon medical practices. Thus, both areas are influenced by subjectivity, the art of medicine much more than the science of medicine. For example, ". . . clinical judgment, which some would delineate almost entirely as an art (is) *insusceptible to explicit analysis.*"[20]

The factor of "mental health" places *all* human thought and behavior under the practice of medicine. Many examples will be given in another chapter to illustrate the extensive degree to which medicine, primarily represented by psychiatrists affects individuals and society. A mental factor which originates with patients themselves is their perception that they have a physical problem because of pain or dysfunction due to what is primarily or entirely mental or social. Once in the physician's office, the patient is susceptible to whatever "treatment" the physician decides is appropriate. The problem may be nonphysical but it becomes "medical" when taken to the physician. Of course, physicians can do little to control patients who come for these reasons, but the medical community has not been reluctant to assume medical management of these problems.

Socially, activities of medicine include laws to govern the spread of infectious agents, screening for the early treatment of disease, safety in industry, and the disposal of toxic wastes. The economic impact is great. Ten percent of the gross national product goes to what has been labeled "medical and health care." This figure does not include "hidden" costs such as employee health and workmen's compensation.

This brief analysis points to the breadth that health concepts and medical practice are present in the lives of individuals, groups, and society. An understanding of this involvement is necessary to an understanding of health, medical practice, and medical ethics. Medicine is not a precisely defined discipline. Indeed, physical, mental, and social well-being encompasses the totality of life. And health and medicine is not a science in the strictest sense. Thus, many concepts of health and the practices of medicine are entirely determined by some world view. Christians have been, and will continue to be led astray if they do not realize this connection. We began this section with a comment by Dr. Pellegrino that medicine was rather "loosely" construed. This brief analysis has demonstrated the variables which have caused this vagueness. A concrete definition of health, medicine and disease is not possible in the modern milieu where worldwide the scope of medicine encompasses the entirety of life.

A Biblical Concept of Health

Thus, "because of variations in the concepts of health and normality, it is essential to clarify the reference sense in which each term is used."[21] This "reference sense" distinguishes a biblical concept of medicine from the current secular concept. The reference sense for modern medicine is evolution which arises from naturalistic world view. Whatever is found empirically is "normal" because nothing else exists outside of natural processes (a closed system, philosophically and scientifically). Biblical anthropology totally opposes such materialism. Although believers will receive a new body, the clear biblical emphasis is on man's spirit. Most importantly, God is spirit but as such He is irrelevant to naturalistic concepts of health and medicine. Abraham Kuyper recognized such ignorance almost 100 years ago. ". . . as long as the medical science confines itself to these independent studies, it still lacks its *higher unity*, and cannot be credited with having come to a clear self-consciousness."[22] The Bible may not say much about medical practices but its main concerns are "mental (the soul or spirit) and social well-being" (man's relationship to God, and self). Optimal physical health flows from these concerns.

"Had there been no sin, there would have been no sickness."[23] The absence of sickness is "normality" or perfect "health." The Bible names three healthy (normal) people and two healthy (normal) situations for man. Adam and Eve were healthy prior to their sin and Jesus Christ lived a sinless life. The healthy situations are the Garden of Eden prior to the entrance of sin and the future state of believers:

> . . . perfect physical health is promised, not for this age, but for heaven,
> are part of the resurrection glory that awaits us . . ."[24]

Thus, the biblical standards of health (true wholism) are unattainable in this earthly life. The believer, however, does have a great advantage for potential health over the unbeliever. Neither should it be overlooked that the health of the unbeliever is greater in his temporal existence than after physical death where God's punishment will be unrestrained (Luke 16:19-31; Matt. 22:1-4).

Biblically, the most fundamental problem in health and medicine is spiritual, not physical. *Since what is spiritual is moral, it could be said that the underlying fundamental problem is moral.* A contrast with the naturalistic approach should be noted. First, science can say nothing about morality—what it is or how to deal with it since morality lies outside the definition and scope of scientific endeavor. In modern medicine, however, scientific means are being used to solve a spiritual/moral problem. Critical to biblical solutions to problems is the recognition of sin for what it is: offense and rebellion against a perfect, sinless Creator.

Dr. Karl Menninger provides an explicit example of this spiritual failure when he defines sin in every way but an offense against God.[25] Sin has "abounding" provision for forgiveness and restoration through God's grace in the substitutionary, sacrificial death of Jesus Christ (Rom. 5:20). If a sin is diagnosed as merely physical, or behavioral, or social, the remedy will always fail. Two examples illustrate this truth. Alcoholism is considered to be a disease by many physicians. The Bible calls it sin. Until it is recognized as disobedience against God's will, its most important dimension has been ignored; even though some physical, psychological and social change may occur. Another example is venereal disease.

> Modern biomedicine might say that the man was cured if the venereal disease organisms were no longer found in his body or that further healing was somebody else's responsibility. A modern advocate of wholistic medicine from agnostic assumptions might say that he was not healed until his marriage was restored to happiness. But to the Christian true healing would also mean that the couple be reconciled to their Creator.[26]

Biblical emphasis always places personal responsibility to God before all other considerations. In reality, medicine and health are secondary considerations.

Another aspect of such priority is discussed in James Parker's article entitled, "Poor Health May Be the Best Remedy:"

> (In His) sanctifying providence God uses chronic pain and weakness as His chisel for sculpting our souls. . . . we certainly should go to the doctor, and use medication, and thank God for both. But equally certainly we should go to the Lord . . . and ask what message of challenge, rebuke, or encouragement he might have for us regarding our sickness.[27]

Thus, a naturalistic anthropology and the inclusion of mental and social well-being has resulted in an increasing departure from biblical anthropology, wholism, and priority. If health, medicine and disease were limited to physical factors, a practical problem would not (and does not, in some areas) exist between secular and biblical analysis. Medical outrages, such as abortion and euthanasia, are symptoms that the root of our modern medical and health dilemmas are philosophical and metaphysical.

Patients sometimes perceive spiritual or moral problems to be physical and will go to a medical doctor. Until a patient has been saved in Jesus Christ, he is not entirely healthy (whole). Such situations and others prevent the limitation of medical practice to the body alone and contrary to modern medicine, spiritual needs do not have to be *provided* by the Christian physician, but they should be made *available* to patients. A doctor can give his primary attention to the treatment of physical problems but he must utilize other resources in providing wholistic care: biblical counseling, preventive health practices, evangelism to all patients, instruction in the "balanced Christian life," and the continuing study of the interface between sin and disease.

Health and its medical management is definable only within a particular world view, so a biblical definition of "pneumosomatic" or wholistic health might be: the physical state which results from the comprehensive and diligent application of biblical, i.e. spiritual, preventive, and medical wisdom to an individual person. "Medical" here refers to empirical knowledge that is less affected by a naturalistic world view, a conclusion that recognizes the cogent place of biblical analysis.

Health and the Balanced Christian Life

For several days Mrs. Jones had severe and incapacitating headaches. She had visited her physician who had prescribed a strong non-narcotic analgesic for pain, and two types of tranquilizers. These gave her no relief. She doubted there was a physical cause for the headaches since she was in the stressful situation of being involved in legal action against her brothers and sisters. She asked for my help as a medical doctor and a counselor. Her Christian lifestyle revealed she had a sound Christian knowledge in general but did not have a consistent devotional life. My directions were simple: structure a thirty minute devotional time in the morning prior to any daily activity and pray weekly for her relatives. Prior to this she could not pray for them without the accompanying stressful thoughts and emotions. I also encouraged her to practice the substitution of constructive thoughts for those which were stimulated by the intense emotion from her situation. After three days her headaches were only a minor annoyance, she was joyous, and this positive change continued.

Mrs. Jones'anecdote illustrates one case where medical treatment was symptomatic and ineffective. Simple practical application of biblical principles was effective. That is not to say that physical causes should not be sought or that biblical application is always necessary. This example serves to illustrate that the availability of counseling is essential to a Christian physician's practice.

Pneumosomatic is a more desirable word than "holistic" (Greek: *holos*, whole), because of the association of "holistic" with Eastern religious practices.[28] To reiterate, pneumosomatic represents the unity of man's spirit and body: *pneuma* and *soma*. Even though pneumosomatic health is not equivalent to perfect health, it does represent the optimal state of health achievable by believers and involves a thorough application of biblical principles.

Four characteristics and seven activities describe a balanced Christian life.[29]

Perfect balance is unachievable in earthly life but definitive progress can be made to promote health.

The first characteristic is *salvation*; a definitve understanding and trust in the Lord Jesus Christ as the substitutionary sacrifice for original sin as inherited from Adam as well as personal sins (Rom. 5:12-21). Man's greatest need, far beyond any other, is reconciliation with God through Christ.

The second characteristic, *obedience*, flows from this substantial faith. Obedience is specified because Scripture clearly describes the behavior of a believer as distinct from that of the unbeliever; "walk no longer as the Gentiles walk" (Ephesians 4:17).

The third characteristic, *a right attitude*, or motive, involves a consistent *internal attitude and outward action*. The Pharisees were not repeatedly criticized by Jesus Christ because of their righteous behavior, but for their attitude or heart (Matthew 6:1-6, 15:8-20; Luke 11:37-46). Inner attitude and outward activity must *both* be directed to God's glory (1 Corinthians 10:31).

The fourth characteristic, *perseverance*, emphasizes that the Christian life is not just a profession, but involves persistence throughout life. Such perseverance results in one's being "mature and complete, not lacking in anything" (James 1:2-4, NIV). Believers must consciously be aware that it is the enabling and enlightening Holy Spirit "who is at work in you" (Phil. 2:13) and who teaches (John 15:13) works are to be accomplished. Salvation is a precondition for perseverance because the believer must be conscious of God's readiness to forgive His children (Psalms 103:8-14; 1 John 1:9). Without the clear understanding of God's readiness to forgive because of Christ's sufficient atonement, the believer's guilt will limit or prevent his perseverance.

Manifest activities of the balanced Christian life are:

(1) *Prayer.* Christians are called to pray both throughout the day (Ephesians 6:18) and at a designated time each day (Psalms 5:3; Matthew 6:6).

(2) *Bible study.* Many Christians *read* their Bible but do not *study* it (Hebrews 5:12-14).

(3) *Fellowship.* The Greek word, *koinonia* means to share, but it is commonly misunderstood. First, true fellowship is co-participation in an activity that is specifically spiritual such as prayer, hymn singing, and ministry (Col. 2:16-17; Phil. 2:1-2).

(4) *Physical health.* Specifics will be discussed under preventive practices, but it is a spiritual imperative as well (1 Cor. 6:19-20).

(5) *Putting off sin.* A sinless life is commanded (Matthew 5:48) but will not be achieved in this life (1 John 1:8). Two extremes must be avoided: the idea that a state of sinlessness can be achieved in this earthly life (1 John 1:8) and the wrong notion that progression from a sinful attitude or behavior is not necessary in Christian life (1 John 3:3-10; Romans 6:1-23, 8:1-12; 1 Corinthians 3:1-2). The process of sanctification means a movement away from sin toward biblically sound activities and attitudes.

(6) *Ministry.* This activity involves service or love to others. Specific works

vary according to gifts and opportunity, even so there is a biblical hierarchy of responsibility. The mutual obligations of husband and wives have the highest priority in any area of ministry (Ephesians 5:22-33; Col. 3:18-20; I Peter 3:1-7). Often a person makes the mistake of giving work a higher priority than spouse or children. The biblical position reflects the permanence of the marriage as opposed to the temporary presence of the children in the home. The second priority for both husband and wife are their children. Work, careers, recreation, and even other areas of Christian ministry are lesser priorities.

(7) *Daily disciplines.* A balanced Christian life includes daily tasks which are essential, i.e., eating, sleeping, dressing, and bodily care, and require an orderly arrangement. Disciple, discipline, sound mind, and other New Testament words describe the orderliness of the believer's life. If these activities are disorderly, spiritual and physical effectiveness will be severly limited.

The balanced Christian life is well-defined biblically and is achieved only by disciplined effort. Christians are obligated to live so they fully experience pneumosomatic health that results from such commitment.[30]

Achieving Pneumosomatic Health

Pneumosomatic health involves three areas which may be ranked according to their influence. Of greatest importance is salvation through belief in Jesus Christ *and* obedience to His Word. Second is a lifestyle based upon those preventive behaviors which medicine currently demonstrates to be effective or possibly effective. Third is the practice of medicine. If this ranking is accurate, then the efforts of Western medicine even by proponents of so-called wholistic health, are reversed. The conviction that most diseases are a direct result of sinful behaviors, does not mean that disease is always a direct result of sin. It may be, but the direct association is frequently absent. For example, cigarette smoking is definitely a causal factor in coronary heart disease (CHD). In CHD several other risk factors are known, so it would be erroneous to conclude that a heart attack, one manifestation of CHD, in an individual who smokes, resulted only from the effect of the cigarettes. His genetic predispositon for which he has no responsibility may have been more detrimental than the cigarettes.

We will review the general effects of joy and peace as the opposite of stress, both biblically and empirically. Then empirical evidence will demonstrate the association of specific, identifiable sins with the more prevalent diseases of Western society.

Upon initial reflection, the Bible may not appear to say much concerning health. A more thorough investigation reveals a considerable number of texts which are directly or indirectly associated with health. For example, two of the many promises for Israel in their journey from Egypt to Canaan were health and long life (Exodus 15:26, 20:12, 23:25-26). These promises were continued throughout the history of Israel (1 Kings 3:14; Psalms 38; Proverbs 3:7-8, 16, 21-26, 4:10, 9:11, and 10:27). Two characteristics of these promises are pertinent to our discussion: they were *conditional* upon obedience and they were a *designed* pattern for God's people.

Figure 1

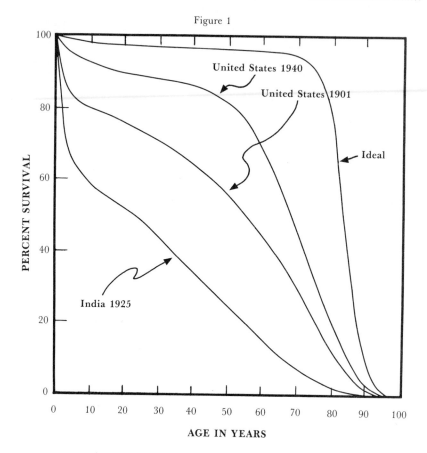

Percentage of survivors of live births for population indicated.

Another example demonstrates the correspondence of biblical teaching and empirical evidence. Without question, longevity is associated with health. Psalm 90:10 states, "As for the days of our life, they contain seventy years, or if due to strength, eighty years." Figure I plots the survival curves of three societies[31] which represent marked contrasts in medical and public health resources.[32] In undeveloped India or the modern United States, the upper limit to longevity is constant, even though the average longevity in the latter has increased from forty-seven years in 1900 to seventy-three years in 1980. Thus, the upper limit of longevity is consistent, biblically and empirically. This limit is likely a major effect of the fall of man and he is unable to extend it beyond God's design.

The New Testament does not have the detailed promises of health found in the Old Testament; even so the New Testament espouses health no less than the Old Testament. Truths from the Old Testament are not abrogated in the New Testament and the unity of truth between the two testaments is fundamental to a biblical faith. Second, it would violate the unity of the body with the spirit for the believer to be directed in a manner inconsistent with the health of the body as the temple of the Holy Spirit. The effect of spiritual directions on physical health is an idea consistent with modern empirical evidence.[33]

The primary benefits of the balanced Christian life are joy and peace. Thus, health produced by life under the New Testament has a similar conditional aspect found under the Old Testament. Some of these "conditional" directives are: John 14:23-27, 15:10-11; Philippians 4:6-9; James 1:2-4; Matthew 25:25, and Galatians 5:22-23, in association with John 15:1-9. Biblical evidence of the fruit of peace and joy that a believer may expect are:

> Peace I leave with you; my please I give to you; *not as the world gives*, do I give to you. Let not your heart be troubled, nor let it be fearful.
> (John 14:27).

> And the peace of God, which surpasses all understanding. . . . (Phil. 4:7)

> A joyful heart is good medicine, but a broken spirit dries up the bones.
> (Prov. 17:22)

> . . . the joy of the Lord is your strength (Neh. 8:10). Additional weight to this verse occurs when it is related to Psalms 90:10: ". . . if due to strength, eighty years. . . .

It seems reasonable to regard joy and peace as the opposite of stress, which, particularly as a result of life changes, is recognized in modern medicine as a very common precursor of disease.[34] One study reported twenty-one percent of arrhythmias (an irregular heartbeat which may precipitate a heart attack or sudden death) occur immediately, within the last twenty-four hours, in association with emotional disturbances.[35] Two-thirds of these experienced the disturbance within the previous sixty minutes! One might wonder whether this phenomenon only represented already present heart disease, but in actuality these patients had less heart disease than the comparison patients in the series. Ventricular tachycardia, a life-threatening arrhythmia, occurred in one patient during marital disputes and in another patient after the hospital visit by his wife because he feared that she might be attacked in the streets. Seventeen of twenty-five episodes involved *anger.*

The potential effect of joy and peace, as well as biblical solutions to situational problems should not be missed. Very possibly, these arrhythmias would not have occurred had these patients been "balanced" Christians. Further, such arrhythmias are commonly the cause of death in coronary heart disease.

Type-A stress behavior, a strong drive, competitivness, the attempt to meet multiple deadlines, and a constant sense of time urgency, has been thoroughly studied in association with coronary heart disease. Where fatty desposits in the walls of the arteries of the heart may occlude, death of the heart muscle itself occurs. One of the manifestations of CHD causes 550,000 deaths each year in the U.S. and seven million people live with health problems caused by CHD.[36] In one study after a follow-up experience of eight and one-half years, it was found that "the type A behavior pattern was strongly related to CHD incidence.[37] In another study two risk factors, those biochemical or behavioral characteristics which have been shown to be closely associated with CHD and many scientists conclude that they are causal of CHD, were found to be associated with Type A behavior: high plasma triglyceride and cholesterol.[38] From these and other such studies, one summary article reported that "it was the consensus of the First National Conference on Emotional Stress and Heart Disease that emotional stress be considered a risk factor equal to other recognized risk factors."[39] Further, it was proposed that the relaxation response was possibly effective to modify this risk factor. One wonders whether Christian "peace" might not be even more effective!

Although heart disease has probably been studied more than any other disease in association with stress, much evidence is available for other disease processes. For example, when stress is measured by "life-change units" a wide variety of illnesses have a higher incidence during periods when these units are increased.[40] Family physicians commonly recognize that more disease is prevalent in those families in whom serious problems exist between family members. A study which supports this observation found "multiple episodes of trauma, infections, and surgery."[41]

A unique study which provides a close look at the psyche-soma relationship began in 1942 with initial and periodic psychological and physical evaluations and continues today. One striking finding was "a relatively weak association of obesity, alcohol use and cigarette smoking with health deteriorations." Similarly, the longevity of parents and grandparents had a weak association. These findings and others caused the author to conclude:

> . . . chronic anxiety, depression, and emotional maladjustments, measured
> in a variety of ways, predicted early aging, defined by irreversible deteriora-
> tion of health. . . . I have speculated that stress does not kill us so much
> as ingenious adaptation to stress (call it good mental health or mature coping
> mechanisms) facilitates our survival.[42]

This study provides evidence that physical health is preceded and can be predicted by "mental health, the presence or absence of stress, since a frequent argument is that physical health is a prerequisite to mental health.

Interestingly, some research has been done on the association between health and religion. A paper which was presented at the First National Conference on Emotional Stress and Heart Disease and was published later concluded: "It is clear that the conceptual and operational clarification of the relevance of religious experience to heart disease is an important issue.[43] In his section on religious behavior and CHD, the author cites several studies which show a positive association:

1. The age-adjusted rate of CHD was significantly lower for "church-goers" than "non-church goers."
2. The same held true for blood pressure.
3. After controlling for certain variables, a sixty percent less risk of CHD

existed for white males (forty-five to sixty-four years of age) who attended church regularly.

4. The incidence of tuberculosis increased as religious attendance decreased in three categories: weekly, once-monthly, and twice-yearly.

5. The five-year CHD rate for white women (ages forty-five to sixty-four) was more than twice the risk among infrequent vs. frequent church goers.

6. Orthodox, traditional, and non-religious Jews had an age-adjusted rate of twenty-nine, thirty-six, and fifty-six, cases of CHD per 1,000 population.

The author discusses methodological and conceptual problems but does not answer the question whether religious factors are causally related to the precipitation, treatment or prevention of CHD. His review of the literature seems comprehensive of that time period and is an excellent resource.

If the hypothesis that stress is the opposite of peace and joy is accepted, then empirical science and the spiritual fruits of joy and peace are compatible; to the extent that unbelievers are able to practice the external principles of the Christian life, for example, an ordered life and a priority for family relationship, they can also experience health "benefits." Can every Christian have joy and peace? As fruits of the Spirit, the New Testament is clear that joy and peace is normative for the Christian. It should not be overlooked, however, that these fruits are based upon the previously described, committed, balanced, and active life of the believer. Modern research provides empirical coherence for the prevention or postponement of disease in the absence of stress and joy and peace may be therapeutic (healing) as well as preventive. Norman Cousins has received publicity, including wide acceptance by the medical profession, for his self-imposed treatment of laughter and vitamin C for his diagnosis of ankylosing spondylitis, a severe, rapidly progressive arthritis of the backbone.[44] He was given one chance in five hundred for full recovery, but today is virtually cured *without* conventional medical treatment. Obviously, one anecdotal case does not establish a universal principle; but it is consistent with biblical and empirical evidence.

To be fully biblical, God's design for individuality must be emphasized. God calls some to unhealthy circumstances and many Christians with a committed, active faith have severe physical disease or handicaps. These variations reflect the biblical emphasis of spiritual values over temporal values. Nevertheless, in general the physical benefits for the believer are real. Jesus Christ promised abundant life (John 10:10), a certainty for all believers. There is a state of health significantly greater for *any* Christian in his *particular* circumstances because of the committed life. Biblical and empirical evidence cohere.

"What is the specific mechanism and site of interaction between the physical and spiritual components of man?" The answer must remain entirely speculative because the spiritual dimension is metaphysical and by definition is not demonstrable *empirically*. However, God has revealed that interaction of the material and immaterial does occur and it is clear from empirical evidence that the physical site of thought and behavior is the brain. Logically, the brain is the site of interaction. The conclusive answer, however, resides in the mystery of man's being as created and designed by his Creator.

Specific Preventive Behaviors

". . . the diseases which attack men are now under control."[45] Thus, the prevalence of health problems may be quantitatively summarized. This prevalence has direct biblical correlation and further underscores the health-producing effect of a biblical lifestyle. In fact, the Bible goes beyond preventive medicine in its directions for health.

TABLE I
CAUSES OF DEATH—ALL AGES—1976

Cause of Death	Males	Females
Heart Disease[a]	400,536	323,193 (1)
Cerebrovascular Disease[b]	80,597	108,026 (2)
Accidents[c]	70,277	30,484 (4)
Cancer of Lung	65,910	20,502 (5)
Pneumonia, Influenza	32,513	29,353 (7)
Cancer of Colon and Rectum	24,544	
Cirrhosis of Liver	20,688	
Cancer of Prostate	20,352	
Suicide	19,493	
Homicide	15,142	
Cancer of Breast	----	33,119 (3)
Diabetes	----	20,483 (6)
Arteriosclerosis[d]	----	17,553 (8)
Cancer of Uterus		11,289 (9)
Cancer of Ovary		10,870 (10)
Cirrhosis		10,785 (11)

Total Number of Deaths from all Causes: 1,909,440

a. Coronary heart disease (see previous discussion this chapter) comprises greater than 90 percent of heart diseases).
b. This term predominately refers to "strokes," i.e., clotting of a blood vessel of the brain or bleeding into the brain which results in the death of brain tissue.
c. Approximately two-thirds of these are automobile accidents.
d. Arteriosclerosis involves the same process which is present in CHD and cerebrovascular disease but this usage refers to the occlusion of vessels to organs other than the heart and brain.

e. Since the ranking for females differs from males, the numbers in (   ) refer
to the ranking of that disease.

TABLE II
CAUSES OF DEATH—AGES 35-54—1976

Cause of Death	Males	Females
Heart Diseases	45,278	13,613 (1)
Accidents	13,446	4,519 (4)
Cancer of Lung	10,080	4,276 (5)
Cirrhosis of Liver	8,040	4,109 (6)
Suicide	5,547	2,753 (7)
Cerebrovascular Disease	5,075	4,988 (3)
Homicide	4,548	
Cancer of Colon and Rectum	2,445	2,414 (8)
Pneumonia, Influenza	2,446	
Diabetes	1,654	
Cancer of Breast		8,269 (2)
Cancer of Uterus		2,302 (9)
Cancer of Ovary		2,278 (10)

TABLE III
LIFESTYLE RISK FACTORS OF SPECIFIC DISEASES[46]

Coronary Heart Disease (Cerebrovascular Disease and Arteriosclerosis)
1. Cigarette Smoking
2. High Blood Pressure
3. Elevated Serum Cholesterol
4. Elevated Serus Triglyceride
5. Decreased Serum High Density Lipoprotein
6. Lack of Exercise
7. Diabetes
8. Obesity

Cancer of Lung
Cigarettes

Accidents[a]
Alcohol[b]
Carelessness and emotional
states (anger, depression, etc.)
Driving too fast
Tranquilizers, sedatives, and
other drugs
Failure to use seat belts

Cancer of Colon and Rectum
Dietary Fiber

Suicide/Homicide
Situational Problems[c]
Alcohol[b]
Personal guns and weapons

Pneumonia	**Cirrhosis of Liver**
Alcohol	Alcohol
Cigarettes	
	Diabetic Control
Homicide	Obesity
Situational Problems[c]	Imprudent Diet
Alcohol[b]	Lack of Exercise

a.   Approximately two-thirds of all accidental deaths involve automobiles.
b.   Alcohol is involved in one-half of all fatal automobile accidents and one-
     third of those which involve the death of a pedestrian. Alcohol is signifi-
     cantly involved in other types of accidents: poisoning, falls, burns, and
     drowning. Homicides and suicides are commonly associated with substan-
     tial concentrations of alcohol.[47]
c.   Situational problems or problems of life are listed here rather than the usual
     terms, e.g., depression, anxiety, and failure to cope. Chapter 10 will explain
     the personal preference for the terminology.

First, we will look at those diseases which are most prevalent and to which
the large majority of medical care is directed. The ten most common causes
of death in the United States are listed in Tables 1 and 2.[48] Those risk factors
which are related causally, with variance as to degree, are listed in Table 3.
These tables clearly identify the extent to which individuals need to assume
responsibility for their health. Biblically, these behaviors are sin. Thus, sin
is directly and specifically related to most causes of disease and death.

The devastation is even more apparent if one considers that many of these
behaviors cause premature morbidity of mortality.[49] For example, accidents
cause twenty-seven percent of the ten million "estimated annual total of potential years lost before age sixty-five"; but only accounts for 3.7 percent of the
total number of deaths each year (risk factors for accidents are listed in note
b of Table III). Another example combines suicide and homicide. These deaths
account for two percent of the total number of deaths annually but fourteen
percent of "potential years lost" (risk factors for suicide and homicide appear
in note *b* Table III, also). "The wages of sin is death" is literal, as well as
spiritual.

Alcohol and cigarette smoking stand out as the most harmful behaviors
because of their prevalence and they produce devastating disease and social
problems. Biblically, alcohol and cigarettes are considered differently.
Alcoholism is mentioned specifically as a sin (Ephesians 5:18; 1 Peter 4:4; Proverbs 20:1, 23:29-35, 23:20, 31:4-6). The biblical standard proscribing cigarettes
is implicit, but nonetheless clear. The body is the temple of the Holy Spirit
(1 Corinthians 3:16-17, 6:19-20); all behaviors are to glorify to God (1 Cor.
10:31); and self-control requires restriction of those things which are harmful
to the body (1 Cor. 3:25). Both alcoholism and smoking are a violation of God's
design for man. Empirically, through physical diseases and social consequences,
the correspondence is apparent.

Many dietary instructions in the Pentateuch have been shown empirically to promote health. These laws are primarily moral/spiritual, but their impact on physical health is consistent with the principle that spiritual health promotes physical health. Excellent dietary instructions allow fruits and vegetables, designated meats were generally low in fats and cholesterol (Lev. 11:1-12, 29-31), and old food was not to be eaten (Lev. 19:5-8).[50] Proper (even though the instructions were written almost 4,000 years ago) nutrition is another example of health produced by a biblical lifestyle.[51]

Exercise is generally considered to be a healthful practice but its specific biblical reference states: "bodily discipline is only of a little profit, but godliness is profitable for all things, since it holds promise for the present life and also for the life to come" (1 Tim. 4:8). Three interpretations are logically possible: "prof-it" refers either to physical life, to the spiritual life in the temporal realm, or to eternal life. The latter part of the verse explicitly states the eternal aspect and thus rules out that interpretation. Then, whether the reference is to the temporal body or to the spirit does not matter, because of the aforementioned incompatibility of spiritual health resulting in physical harm.[52]

A large body of literature provides empirical support for preventive behaviors. In a study of 28,000 white, Protestant clergy from 1950 to 1960, the death rate from all causes and in all ages was seventy-two percent of the rate in the general population.[53] Between the ages of twenty and sixty-four the death rate was fifty-six percent of the expected! Even though many variables were present, the study probably represents a composite effect of both the spiritual dimension and preventive behaviors (i.e., fewer clergy are likely to smoke).

Some studies support preventive measures without regard to spiritual dimensions. Nonsmoking populations show a significant decrease in the mortality rate from virtually all types of cancer, not just those which are directly related to smoking.[54] Seventh Day Adventists and Mormons[55] have been studied many times because of their strict health practices, and the cancer mortality in Mormons was twenty-two percent less than that of the United States population.[56] The lowest death rate from coronary heart disease in the United States is found in Seventh Day Adventists.[57]

The effect of specific lifestyle practices is reflected in a study of residents in Alameda County, California.[58] The mortality rate in the adult population, for men and women whose life had seven specific characteristics was studied for almost ten years. The seven characteristics were:

1. Duration of sleep: men—8 hours, women—7 hours
2. Habitual breakfast-eaters (that is, it was not omitted)
3. Regular and active exercise
4. Three meals per day with no in-between meal snacks
5. Alcohol in moderation (1-2 beverages per day)
6. Average weight (that is, their weight averaged only slightly above the standard
7. No cigarette smoking

These people experienced only fifty-two percent of the total mortality rate of a comparative sample of other Alameda County adults!

Simple biblical directions promote health in ways which are overlooked. In God's plan for sexuality, the only approved context for sexual intercourse is heterosexual marriage (Exodus 20:14). If everyone practiced this plan, all venereal disease, such as gonorrhea, syphillis, and herpes genitalis, would almost totally be wiped out within one generation because very rarely is a venereal disease transmitted by any means other than immoral sex. Billions of dollars are spent by local, state, and national governments and other organizations to prevent and treat these diseases, yet they remain epidemic. Fidelity in marriage removes the possibility that these very prevalent diseases would be contracted.

Another health benefit of biblical marriage is companionship (Gen. 2:18). *The Broken Heart* by James Lynch demonstrates the devastating effect of loneliness.[59] In ten different tables, four categories (married, single, widowed, and divorced) are related to the death rates of a wide variety of diseases (such as high blood pressure, coronary heart disease, specific types of cancer, and strokes) and mental health. Consistently, death rates increase through the four categories in this order: married, single, widowed, and divorced (the last two rates alternate being the highest but almost always follow the first two). As loneliness increases in our society one wonders what future impact these changes will have upon health.

Other biblical patterns which are related to health but have little or no empirical documentation can be found: (a) Work in its proper priority results in a sense of satisfaction and rest: [Ecclesiastes 2:24 (NIV), 3:13 (NIV), 5:12; Col. 3:23-24]. (b) Sufficient rest, both daily and weekly, is necessary (Exodus 20:8-11; Psalms 127:2). (c) The orderliness of both the mind and the life is described throughout the New Testament, as discipline (1 Timothy 4:7; 2 Timothy 1:7), sound judgment (Romans 12:3) and self-control (Galatians 5:23). (d) Gluttony may be an archaic word, but its application includes any behavior which is excessive (1 Corinthians 9:25).

Finally, there is personal and professional dental care—daily flossing, brushing, and regular dental visits. The Bible does not mention dental hygiene, but dental research seems to indicate that decay and gum disease can be prevented by these practices.

In considering medical ethics, it is crucial to understand that health and biblical teaching are not antithetical, but many current medical practices are antithetical to scriptural truth. The ethical choice is not between the health that medicine can provide and the biblically-governed life.

In Summary

Certain distinctives are essential for a biblical concept of health. Biblical anthropology states that man is composed of body and spirit. Man is not "whole" until he is rightly related to God through the Atonement of Jesus

Christ. Any wholistic approach without the centrality of salvation is antithetical to biblical wholism. Following salvation, wholistic health is dependent upon the balanced Christian life which consists of four characteristics (certainty of salvation, obedience, right attitude or motive, and perseverance) and seven activities (prayer, Bible study, fellowship, physical health, putting off of sin, ministry, and management of daily essentials). The joy and peace which result from these characteristics and activities are the most important ingredients for pneumosomatic health. Preventive measures are second in importance. Correlations between the health benefits associated with the balanced Christian life and preventive practices has been demonstrated biblically and empirically. The practice of medicine is third.

In an attempt to make such distinctives clear, the discussion can be formulated into succint statements:

1. Man is composed of two distinct substances, the body and the spirit, yet these exist and function as a unit.
2. Biblical and empirical evidence correlate that health is positively affected by the balanced Christian life, preventive practices and modern medicine.
3. Pneumosomatic health is not possible for the unbeliever; although preventive and medical practices will improve and/or maintain health.
4. Pneumosomatic health is possible for all believers; but its implementation in an individual's life is dependent upon God's sovereign will for that life.
5. Perfect pneumosomatic health existed in the Garden of Eden and will exist in heaven.
6. Since unbelievers are not aware of man's spirit or the necessity of biblical concepts only physicians who are Christians are able to practice pneumosomatic medicine.
7. No final conflict exists between pneumosomatic health and empirical evidence when the latter is controlled by biblical principle.
8. The most common health problems in the United States are a result of personal sin.
9. Sickness and death are not "normal" according to the biblical account of creation.
10. Many specific sins result in specific diseases. For example, syphillis is contracted through extramarital sex.
11. Physical health primarily involves individual responsibility and only secondarily is a responsibility of the medical profession (except for the education of the patient).
12. Many diseases cannot effectively be treated without simultaneous application of biblical principles. Sometimes, these will be more important than the medical treatment.
13. The effect of sin is to program man's body to age and die with an upper limit to its longevity.[60]

14. Biblical principles may not be violated for medical reasons. For example, a divorce designed to relieve stress in a heart disease patient is a violation of the sanctity of marriage.

15. Health resource allocation in the United States is reversed according to the effectiveness of pneumosomatic, preventive, and medical practices.

The biblical ethic for health is distinct from the ethic of naturalistic science and its ethical principles will never be inconsistent at any point when a thorough biblical approach is realized.

NOTES

1. D. Martyn Lloyd-Jones, *The Doctor Himself and the Human Condition* (London:Christian Medical Fellowship Publications, 1982), pp. 99, 102.

2. Ibid., p. 51.

3. Helmut Thielicke, "Ethics in Modern Medicine," in *Who Shall Live?*, ed. Kenneth Vaux (New York: Harper and Row, 1964), p. 159.

4. Louis Berkhof, *Systematic Theology* (1938; reprint ed., Grand Rapids: Eerdmans Pub. Co., 1969), p. 191.

5. Ibid, p. 192.

6. Gordon H. Clark, *Behaviorism and Christianity*, (Jefferson, Maryland: The Trinity Foundation, 1982).

7. W. E. Vine, *An Expository Dictionary of New Testament Words*, (Old Tappan, N. J.: Fleming H. Revell Company, 1966), pp. 54-55.

8. Jay E. Adams, *More Than Redemption*, (Phillipsburg, N.J.: Presbyterian and Reformed Pub. Co., 1979), p. 115.

9. Ibid., p. 116.

10. Joseph H. Thayer, *Thayer's Greek-English Lexicon of the New Testament* (Grand Rapids: Baker Book House, 1977), p. 571.

11. Jay E. Adams, *More Than Redemption*, p. 117.

12. Robert H. Gundry, *Soma in Biblical Theology* (London: Cambridge University Press, 1976), p. 40.

13. Ibid., p. 50.

14. Ibid., p. 50.

15. Ibid., p. 160.

16. Ibid., p. 154.

17. Edmund D. Pellegrino and David C. Thomasma, *A Philosophical Basis of Medical Practice* (New York: Oxford University Press, 1981), p. 58.

18. D. W. Clark and B. MacMahon, *Preventive and Community Medicine* (Boston: Little, Brown, and Co., 1981), pp. 3, 5.

19. This concept alone destroys any pretense that "quality of life" is any criteria for medical action. None are healthy. Any choice of quality becomes entirely arbitrary.

20. Pellegrino and Thomasma, *A Philosophical Basis of Medical Practice*, p. 149.

21. D. W. Clark and B. MacMahon, *Preventive and Community Medicine*, p. 4.

22. Abraham Kuyper, *Principles of Sacred Theology* (1898; reprint ed., Grand Rapids: Baker Book House, 1980), p. 200.

23. James I. Packer, "Poor Health May Be the Best Remedy," *Christianity Today* (May 21, 1982), pp. 14-16.

24. Ibid., p. 15.

25. Karl Menninger, *Whatever Became of Sin* (New York: Hawthorn Books, Inc., 1973).

26. James F. Jekel, "A Biblical Basis for Whole-Person Health Care," in *Whole-Person Medicine*, eds. David E. Allen, Lewis P. Bird, and Robert Herrmann (Downers Grove: InterVarsity Press, 1980), p. 144.

27. James I. Packer, "Poor Health May Be the Best Remedy," p. 16.

28. A perspective on the involvement of Eastern religious practices into modern medicine is presented in the SCP Journal, August, 1978, "Holistic Health Issue." (Spiritual Counterfeits Project, P. O. Box 2418, Berkley, California, 94702.) Another author has predicted the "end of the age of science" (Walter Thorson, "The Spiritual Dimensions of Science" in *Horizons of Science* (San Francisco: Harper & Row Pub. 1978).

29. It is recognized that various terms can be used to define these areas of the Christian life. Those terms chosen here are not meant to be the only biblical possibilities, nor to be completely detailed. As summarized, however, the areas present are considered to be mimimal to a balanced, and therefore, health-producing spiritual life.

30. Bruce Larson has written a book which discusses the relationship of health and Christian living. It is particularly good in its presentation of how wrong attitudes and behavior in life and personal relationships results in bad health and disease. For example, he discusses the principle, "Do you want to be right or well?" One desires that his biblical solutions be more thorough and direct, but he does expose these issues very well. (*There's a Lot More to Health Than Not Being Sick*. Waco: Word Books, 1981).

31. The curve from India, 1925 did not appear in the cited reference. It was adapted from a similar figure from another source (H. J. Curtis, *Biological Mechanisms of Aging*. Springfield: C. C. Thomas, 1966).

32. James F. Fries, "Aging, Natural Death and the Compression of Morbidity," *New England Journal of Medicine* 303 (July 17, 1980): 130-135.

33. Biblical truth *never* requires empirical evidence for its validation, but the latter should have coherence (a test of truth) to biblical truth if it is correctly performed.

34. Stress is not necessarily harmful. Indeed, some stress is necessary for the development of optimal health. For example, exercises for the heart and the muscles generate a stress that results in increased performance. Further, most people recognize that they work better under some pressure. Education and mental development involve cognitive stress. Stress, unless otherwise stated, will refer to a situational stimulus which is beyond the ability of the individual to recover. Such stimuli may seem outwardly positive (for example, a job promotion) or outwardly negative (for example, a job loss). (It is interesting that spiritual stress produces increased spiritual ability as well, James 1:2-4).
The association of stress and disease is more thoroughly present in these large volumes: (a) G. S. Everly and R. Rosenfeld. *The Nature and Treatment of Stress Response* (New York: Plenum Press, 1981) and (b) Hans Selye. *Stress in Health and Disease* (Reading: Butterworth, 1976).

35. P. Reich and Regis A. DeSilva, "Acute Psychological Disturbances Preceding Life-Threatening Venticular Arrythmias," *Journal of the American Medical Association* 233 (July 17, 1981): 233-235.

36. D. W. Clark and B. MacMahon, *Preventive and Community Medicine*, p. 194.

37. R. H. Roseman and R. J. Brand, "Coronary Heart Disease in the Western Collaborative Group Study," *Journal of the American Medical Association* 233 (August 25, 1975): 872-877.

38. M. Friedman and S.O. Byers, et al, "Coronary-Prone Individuals (Type-A Behavior Pattern)," *Journal of the American Medical Association* 212 (May 11, 1970): 1030-1037.

39. R. S. Eliot and Alan D. Forker, "Emotional Stress and Cardiac Disease," *Journal of the American Medical Association* 236 (November 15, 1976): 2325-2326.

40. R. H. Rahe and Ransom J. Arthur, "Life-Change Patterns Surrounding Illness Experience," *Journal of Psychosomatic Research* 11 (1968): 341-345.

41. G. L. Rainsford and Stanley H. Schuman, "The Family in Crisis: A Case of Overwhelming Illness and Stress," *Journal of the American Medical Association* 246 (July 3, 1981): 60-63.

42. George E. Vaillant, "Natural History of Male Psychologic Health: Effects of Mental Health on Physical Health," *New England Journal of Medicine* 301 (Dec. 6, 1979): 1249-1254.

43. Berton H. Kaplan, "A Note on Religious Beliefs and Coronary Heart Disease," *Journal of the South Carolina Medical Association* (February Supplement): 60-64.

44. Norman Cousins, "Anatomy of An Illness (As Perceived by the Patient)," *New England Journal of Medicine* 295 (Dec. 23, 1976): 1458-1463.

45. D. Martyn Lloyd-Jones, *The Doctor Himself and the Human Condition*, p. 16.

46. The tables are summaries of data in which one table listed cancer as a single cause of death and another table listed types of cancer as a cause of death. These tables were combined to demonstrate the ranking of specific types of cancer to other causes of death, rather than all cancers being considered together. This method allowed separation in the basis of probable causes. *Cancer Journal of Clinicians.* (January-February 1979), pp. 2-21.

47. D. W. Clark and B. MacMahon, *Preventive and Community Medicine*, p. 116.

48. The associations of risk factors and diseases are somewhat simplified when the complexity of these relationships are fully considered. Currently, however, it represents our understanding of these diseases. Further, the preventive behaviors advocated have substantial agreement within the medical profession. The risk factors are adapted from: J. H. Hall, M.D., and J. D. Zwemer, D.D.S., Ph.Dl, *Prespective Medicine* (Indianapolis: Methodist Hospital of Indiana, 1979), pp. 75-86. A few modifications were made based on data which was not included there, and on the context of this chapter.

49. "Monthly Mortality, and Monthly Physician Contracts—United States," *Morbidity and Mortality Weekly Report* 31 (March 12, 1982): 109-110.

50. James F. Jekel, "A Biblical Basis for Whole-Person Health Care," p. 135.

51. The Pentateuch instructed many other health practices that included personal cleanliness (Lev. 15:5), pure water (Lev. 11:32-36) and isolation of disease (Lev. 13, 15:1-3).

52. For a thorough discussion and practical plan concerning exercise, the following reference is recommended: Kenneth Cooper, *The Aerobics Way* (New York: Bantam, 1978).

53. Haltung King and Frances B. Locke, "American White Protestant Clergy as a Low-Risk Population for Mortality Research," *Journal of the National Cancer Institute* 65 (5) 1980:1115-1124.

54. James E. Enstrom, "Cancer Mortality Among Low-Risk Populations," CA- *A Cancer Journal for Clinicians* 29 (6) 1979:352-361.

55. These comments no way refers to religious or theological comparisons. Our focus only concerns the preventive health practices of Mormons.

56. Joseph L. Lyone and M. R. Klauber, et al, "Cancer Incidence in Mormons and Non-Mormons in Utah, 1966-1970," *New England Journal of Medicine* 294 (Jan. 15, 1976): 129-133.

57. R. S. Johnson, "Can You Alter Your Heart Disease Risk," *Journal of the American Medical Association* 245 (May 15, 1981): 1903-1907.

58. James E. Enstrom, "Cancer Mortality Among Low-Risk Populations," pp. 352-361.

59. James J. Lynch, *The Broken Heart: The Medical Consequences of Loneliness* (New York: Basic Books, Inc., 1977).

60. If people were to practice preventive medicine fully, this distinctive would replace number 8. It is interesting to speculate how the practice of medicine and the frequency of specific diseases might change. This achievement of prevention, however, is extremely unlikely to occur.

REFERENCES

Belloc, N. B. "Relationship of Health Practices and Preventive Medicine." *Preventive Medicine* 2:67-81.

Centers of Disease Control. Introduction to Table V: Premature Deaths, Monthly Mortality, and Monthly Physician Contracts—United States. *Morbidity and Mortality Weekly Report* 31 (Mar. 12, 1982): 109-110, 117.

Cousins, Norman. "Anatomy of An Illness (As Perceived by the Patient)." *New England Journal of Medicine* 295 (Dec. 23, 1976): 1458-1463.

Dorland's *Illustrated Medical Dictionary*. 25th ed. Philadelphia: W. B. Saunders, 1974.

Eliot, R. S. and Alan D. Forker. "Emotional Stress and Cardiac Disease." *Journal of the American Medical Association* 236 (Nov. 15, 1976): 2325-2326.

Enstrom, James E. "Cancer Mortality Among Low-Risk Populations." *CA—A Cancer Journal for Clinicians* 29 (6): 352-361.

Friedman, M., S. O. Byers, et al. "Coronary-Prone Individuals (Type-A Behavior Pattern)." *Journal of the American Medical Association* 212 (May 11, 1970): 1030-1037.

Fries, James F. "Aging, Natural Death and the Compression of Morbidity." *New England Journal of Medicine* 303 (July 17, 1980): 130-135.

Gundry, Robert H. *Soma in Biblical Theology*. London: Cambridge University Press: 1976.

Hindson, Ed. "Biblical View of Man." *Journal of Pastoral Practice* 3 (1): 33-58.

Johnson, R. S. "Can You Alter Your Heart Disease Risk." *Journal of the American Medical Association* 245 (May 15, 1981): 1903-1907.

Kaplan, Berton H. "A Note on Religious Beliefs and Coronory Heart Disease." *Journal of the South Carolina Medical Association* February (Supplement), 1976, pp. 60-64.

King, Haltung and Frances B. Locke. "American White Protestant Clergy as a Low-Risk Population for Mortality Research." *Journal of the National Cancer Institute* 65 (5) 1980: 1115-1124.

Lyone, Joseph L., M. R. Klauber, et al. "Cancer Incidence in Mormons and Non-Mormons in Utah, 1966-1970." *New England Journal of Medicine* 294 (Jan. 15, 1976): 129-133.

Menninger, Karl. *Whatever Became of Sin*. New York: Hawthorne Books, Inc., 1973.

Packer, James I. "Poor Health May Be the Best Remedy." *Christianity Today*, May 21, 1982, pp. 14-16.

Pellegrino, Edmund D. and David C. Thomasma. *A Philosophical Basis of Medical Practice*. New York: Oxford University Press, 1981.

Rahe, R. H. and Ransom J. Arthur. "Life-Change Patterns Surrounding Illness Experience." *Journal of Psychosomatic Research* 11:341-345, 1968.

Rainsford, G. L. and Stanley H. Schuman. "The Family in Crisis: A Case of

Overwhelming Illness and Stress." *Journal of the American Medical Association* 246 (July 3, 1981): 60-63.

Reich, P., Regis A. DeSilva, et al. "Acute Psychological Disturbances Preceding Life-Threatening Ventricular Arrythmias." *Journal of the American Medical Association* 246 (July 17,1981): 233-235.

Roseman, R. H., R. J. Brand, et al. "Coronary Heart Disease in the Western Collaborative Group Study." *Journal of the American Medical Association* 233 (Aug. 25, 1975): 872-877.

Stott, John R. W. *Christian Counter-Culture: The Message of the Sermon on the Mount.* Downers Grove: InterVarsity, 1978.

Thayer, Joseph H. *Thayer's Greek-English Lexicon of the New Testament.* T. and T. Clark, 1901. Reprint. Grand Rapids: Baker Book House, 1977.

Vaillant, George E. "Natural History of Male Psychologic Health: Effects of Mental Health on Physical Health." *New England Journal of Medicine* 301 (Dec. 6, 1979): 1249-1254.

Vine, W. E. *An Expository Dictionary of New Testament Works.* 1940. Reprint. Old Tappan, N.J.: Fleming H. Revell Company, 1966.

Webster's New Collegiate Dictionary. Springfield, Mass. G. and C. Merriam Company, 1977.

7 | Toward a Theology of Medicine

Attention can now be turned to particular biblical references related to physicians, healing, sickness and patients. The presentation will be based almost wholly upon the New Testament[1] because: 1) the New Testament is generally more clearly explicit than the Old Testament in its directions for Christian practice and 2) some Old Testament principles of health fall under the ceremonial law which no longer has direct application today.[2] Principles will be developed which will provide for a practical application of our findings.

Since the selected words are used in New Testament contexts where the indicated healing may be spiritual, physical, both, or unidentified, those contexts which clearly reveal the healing to be of a physical nature are referenced more frequently than the others.[3] I continue to use healing, health, etc. only to refer to man's physical nature. For example, when Jesus healed (*hugaino*) the man with the withered hand, and made it "like the other (hand)"—an explicit physical restoration occurred.

The Physician in the New Testament[4]

Physician. The Greek word for physician (*iatros*) appears seven times, six of which are used by Jesus. In Matthew 9:12, Mark 2:17, and Luke 5:32, he is speaking to scribes and Pharisees during a banquet in the home of Levi. These Jewish leaders have criticized His association with publicans and sinners. He responds, "It is not those who are healthy (*ischus*—Matt., *hugies*- Mark and Luke) who need a physician but those who are ill" (*kakos*). His statement might be used to justify those who are ill to see a physician but clearly Jesus is making a spiritual analogy since the next verse states that He came "to call the righteous, not sinners." Thus, the spiritual instruction of this context where "physician" is used gives no direction for the moral practice of the Christian in his relationship to physicians.

In Mark 5:25 and Luke 8:43 the account of a woman with a "flow of blood" is given. Over a twelve year period this woman had suffered at the hands of physicians, had spent all that she had and had gotten worse. She was hoping to be healed (*sozo*), and was cured (*iaomai*) by touching Jesus' garment. Then, Jesus pronounced her healed (*sozo*) and whole (*hugies*). *Iatros* is used only historically, not didactically, from which a principle cannot be derived concerning the Christian's relationship to a physician.

In Luke 4:23 Jesus quotes a colloquial proverb, "Physician, heal (*therapeia*) yourself." John Calvin comments upon the context and the application:

> A physician ought to begin with himself, and those immediately connected with him, before he exhibits his skill in healing others. . . . (Christ) acts improperly (from their point of view) in paying no respect to his own country (Nazareth), while he renders cities of Galilee illustrious by his miracles.[5]

Since the saying is quoted by way of colloquial analogy, the context does not allow for a principle to be established for physicians and patients.

Finally, in Colossians 4:4 Paul calls Luke, the "beloved physician." Several passages in Acts (16:11-18, 20:5-16, 21:1-19, and 27:1-28:16) use the first person plural pronoun, indicating Luke's travels with Paul. Further, Luke was probably with Paul when he died (2 Tim. 4:11). No passage states that Luke either did or did not function as Paul's physician. However, "it cannot well be regarded as an improbable or arbitrary assumption that one at least of the apostle's objects in this visit to Philippi was to have the benefit of the beloved physician's advice for the state of his health."[6] This probability seems more certain when one considers that Paul was beaten, shipwrecked, imprisoned, and hungry (2 Cor. 6:4-5), and had a physical ailment which God chose not to heal (2 Cor. 12:7-10). Even so, these passages are historical in nature, and lack explicit reference to Luke's medical skills and knowledge of Paul's ailments. Such supposition, no matter how likely, cannot be extrapolated into a general principle.

In the Old Testament the word "physician" appears four times. King Asa is chastised for seeking help from physicians rather than the Lord (2 Chron. 16:12); Egyptian physicians embalmed Jacob (Gen. 50:2); Job calls his accusers "worthless physicians" (Job 13:4); and Jeremiah calls for the spiritual healing of the wounds which have been produced by the sins of Israel (Jer. 8:22). These references are also historical in nature and thus cannot be used as the basis for a principle for all believers.

In summary, the occurrences of the word, physician, in both the Old Testament and the New Testament do not allow for the derivation of an ethic for a Christian's relationship to physicians. It is worthwhile to note that there is neither an explicit command for any Israelite or believer to seek the services of physicians *nor* is there an explicit command not to do so.

Heal, Healing. All instances of healing in the Old Testament and the New Testament are miraculous with no recorded healing from treatment by a physician. The following validate the fact that a correct biblical use of the word *healing* has reference to healing of the spirit, as well as healing of the body. In some instances it is difficult, if not impossible, to decide which is indicated by the context. Today, the practice of medicine frequently cannot distinguish between the two since many patients have problems that are not clearly physical or spiritual (in secular terms, emotional or psychosomatic). It is erroneous, however, to conclude that all instances of healing in the New Testament are spiritual because many contexts provide sufficient detail to leave no other conclusion except that a true healing of a physical disorder occurred. Finally, only Christ and His apostles are recorded to have performed these healings.

Therapon. This word occurs forty-nine times in the New Testament, thirty-eight times as verbs (*therapeuo*). All but three instances (Matt. 8:7, 17:18; John 5:10) refer to acts of generic healing (e.g. Matt. 4:23, 8:16; Mark. 6:5; Luke 9:6; Acts 28:9). In Matthew 15:30 a variety of problems are listed: the lame, crippled, blind and dumb. Etiologies (causes) are not always specified, but a demonic cause is specific in some (Matt. 12:22; Luke 6:18, 8:2). The primary use of *therapon, therapeuo,* is to designate generic acts of healing, that is, there is no specific reference as to whether it is spiritual or physical. It is sometimes used of persons with problems that are clearly demonic in origin. It does refer explicitly to physical healing in some instances.

Iaomai (noun). This stem is the same as that from which the word physician (*iatros*) is derived. It contrasts with *therapon*, first in its frequent use to refer to individuals with identifiable physical problems: paralysis (Matt. 8:8), hemorrhage (Matt. 13:15), demonic fits (Luke 9:42), dropsy (Luke 14:4), leprosy (Luke 17:15), a severed ear (Luke 22:51), fever (John 4:47), lameness (John 5:13; Acts 3:11), and dysentery (Acts 28:8). Second, this word is distinctively used to denote spiritual healing. (Luke 4:18; Heb. 12:13; 1 Peter 2:24). The same quote from the Old Testament appears three times (Matt. 13:15; John 12:40; Acts 28:27). In comparison to *therapon* it is also used generically (Luke 5:17, 9:2; Acts 10:38). Total New Testament occurrences are thirty-three; twenty-four are clearly physical (including demonic cause); three are spiritual; three are generic; and three (1 Cor. 12:9, 28, 30) designate gifts of healing.[7]

Sozo (verb). The primary use of this word, which occurs 101 times in the New Testament, denotes salvation (root of soteriology, the study of salvation). In other instances it refers to salvation of the body (e.g. Matt. 8:25, 14:30). When it is translated "healing," the context often identifies a physical problem: the woman with the flow of blood (Matt. 9:21, 22; Mark 5:28, 34; Luke 8:48, 50), the blind Bartimaeus (Mark 10:52; Luke 18:42), the lepers (Luke 17:19), and the man lame from his mother's womb (Acts 4:9). The contexts do not allow that salvation of the souls as well as physical restoration occurred. It is clear, however, that *sozo* does refer to healing of physical problems seventeen times.

Diasozo (verb). Derivations of this stem occur eight times; two *may* refer to physical healing (Matt. 14:36; Luke 7:3), but the context does not explicitly identify a physical problem. It more commonly refers to being safely brought through some threatening circumstance (Acts 23:24, 28:1).

Hugies. From this root comes the English word, hygiene, but biblically *hugies* may designate spiritual health (Luke 5:31, 15:27) or physical healing: a man with the withered hand (Matt. 12:13; Mark 3:5), a woman with the flow of blood (Mark 5:34), and a lame man (Acts 4:10). It is interesting that seven of eighteen occurrences in the New Testament concern the paralyzed man at the Bethesda pool (John 5:4, 6, 9, 11, 14, 15, 7:23). The reason for its frequency in this context is uncertain. The context, "Do you wish to get well," suggests a pneumatic (spiritual) etiology, i.e. of the will to get well, but that conclusion could not be stated dogmatically. Other uses are sound doctrine (1 Tim. 1:10, and Titus 1:9) and sound speech (Titus 2:8).

These five words have a contextual use to denote the miraculous healing of physical problems, yet there are distinctives among them. *Therapon, iaomai,* and *sozo* include healing in instances of demonic possession.[8] Only *iaomai* has contexts unrelated to healing. *None are ever used of healing accomplished apart from God's miraculous intervention or have association with physical agents or physicians.*

Dramatically, a decrease in the frequency of the word "healing" occurs after the Gospels and Acts. This fact seems to support the conservative position that the primary and overriding purpose of all the miracles of the New Testament was to validate God's presence and action through His Son and His apostles.

Another observation recorded by New Testament authors is that physical healing and spiritual healing may occur separately or together. Thus, these records identify the distinct components of man that may be healed separately or together.

Disease and Sickness in the New Testament

Asthenes. Derivations of this stem occur eighty-two times in the New Testament but they are rarely used with an identifiable physical problem (John 5:5; 2 Cor. 12:5, 9; Gal. 4:13). In all but two instances associated with disease (John 5:5, 7; Acts 4:9), the word designates such a severe state that it approaches or results in death: Lazarus (John 11:1, 2 , 3, 4, 6), Epaphroditus (Phil, 2:20, 27), a boy with fever (John 4:47) and Tabitha (Acts 9:37). Most contexts where this root occurs involves healing in a generic sense (Matt.10:8; Luke 10:9; and Acts 5:15, 16). Thus, its primary use with reference to disease connotes a life-threatening severity or generic acts of healing.

Most uses reflect various types of weaknesses, e.g., of the conscience (1 Cor. 8:7, 9, 10, 11, 12), of the flesh (Matt. 26:41; Mark 14:38), of physical appearance (2 Cor. 10:10; 1 Cor. 2:3), of the ability of the commandments to save (Heb. 7:18), and of the wife as the weaker vessel (1 Peter 3:7). Further, it is contrasted to strength, e.g., between God and men (1 Cor. 1:25), between the earthly and the resurrected body (1 Cor. 15:43), and between believers (1 Cor. 4:10, 12:22; 2 Cor, 13:3; 1 Thess. 5:14). Its diverse uses are apparent.

To summarize, *asthenes* primarily describes various weakness and states of weaknesses, often contrasted to strength. Some passages, however, clearly indicate its association with physical disability of a physical state which threatens life. It would seem reasonable to conclude that this word also reflects the association between the physical and spiritual components of man.

Nosos. Derivations of this stem are used fourteen times in the New Testament. In every instance except two, it is used of generic healing: Matt. 4:24; Mark 1:34; Luke 6:17; and Acts 19:12. One exception may be the healing performed by an angel at the Bethesda pool. In another exception *nosos* indicates an excessive interest in controversy and disputes (NASV—morbid). Thus, this word from which *nosology*, the classification of diseases, is derived, never refers to identifiable physical problems.

Arrhostos. Five occurrences are found in the New Testament, but it does not specifically refer to identifiable disease, either. Two passages are noteworthy. In 1 Corinthians 11:30 *arrhostos* ("sick") is the result, even to death, of judgment for participation in the Lord's Supper in an "unworthy manner." In Mark 6:13 the twelve were sent out to anoint people who were *arrostos.*

Kakos. The derivations of this stem in the New Testament predominantly refer to that which is evil or destructive. For our concern, it is used of physical injury in Acts 16:28 and 28:5. Its compound form, *kapopatheo*, relates to suffering and hardship (John 5:10, 13; 2 Tim. 4:5, and 2 Tim. 2:9). Paired with *echo* (to have), it mostly connotes generic healing as in Matt. 14:35 and Mark 1:32, 34. It does denote, however, the specific problem of the centurion's servant (Luke 7:2). Further, Christ made the analogy that He came to those who were "sick" (Matt. 9:12; Mark 2:17; Luke 5:31).

Kamno. Only three times does this word appear in the New Testament. In Hebrews 12:13 and Revelation 2:3 it is opposite to endurance and perserverance. In James 5:15 it designates those upon whom the prayer of faith is effectual.

Malakia. All three occurrences are used to name those who were healed generically.

Adunatos, "inability," contrasts with *dunatos* (power or ability—Matt. 6:13, and miracle— John 6:14). In Acts 14:8 the lame man was "without strength" in his feet.

Miscellaneous. The Greek words which refer to specific physical disorders, e.g. *cholos* (lame) or *paralutikos* (paralysis), are not considered. Such specific entities are necessary only to demonstrate that healings were physical (organic) in nature. The purpose of this review is to examine the *means* by which healing occurred.

Naos, hieron. These words are both translated *temple.* The former, however, is used to denote a particular part of the temple, the Holy of Holies, where the priest only entered once each year (Heb. 9:1-7). The latter refers to the entire building or its parts, as distinct from the inner sanctuary. Further, *naos* refers to the fleshly body of Christ (John 2:19, 20, 21) and the body of the believer (1 Corinthians 3:16, 17, 6:19; 2 Corinthians 6:16. Thus, the physical body, at it is indwelt by God the Holy Spirit is identified with the Holy of Holies.

Oinos. Wine was suggested to Timothy (1 Tim 5:23) to use for his stomach and frequent illnesses (*asthenes*) and was used by the Good Samaritan (Luke 10:34). Thus, in the New Testament this one substance (wine) is used medicinally both internally and externally. In the first instance its medical value is not clear, although Paul may have suggested wine to Timothy for its appetite-stimulation or the quieting of his anxieties since Timothy was young and reserved yet faced many responsiblilities. A possible physical manifestation of such anxiety is a poor appetite. The wine could have been used for both these reasons causing Timothy to relax enough to eat and overcome his weakened condition (*asthenes*). Of course, even this explanation is conjectural, and its recommendation came, not from a physician, but an apostle! Since the Bible warns repeatedly of the dangers of alcohol (Eph. 5:18; Prov. 23: 20-21, 29-35), Timothy was specifically instructed to use a *little* (*oligos*) wine! In the case of the Samaritan, alcohol does have antiseptic (germ-killing) properties which make its use appropriate in an open wound.

These two situations demonstrate recommended (Timothy) and applied (Good Samaritan) uses of wine which are consistent with some known medical properties. Although physicians were not involved, these passages record the moral use of wine (a drug) for physical symptoms and injury.

Elaion. Twice oil was used to anoint the sick: *asthenes* (James 5:14) and *arrhostos* (Mark 6:13), although an identifiable physical problem was not named. The Good Samaritan applied oil, as well as wine, to the beaten man's wounds, but in this instance medical knowledge is not helpful. Olive and other oils may be used to soften and prevent skin from drying, but are currently thought to be contraindicated where the skin is broken, particularly burned, and likely to increase the incidence of infection. Of course, medical science changes and remains incomplete. It is inconceivable that Christ would have told a parable that included an injurious mode of treatment.

Conclusion. Can any principles, relative to physicians and their practices, be derived from this overview of New Testament terminology? Definitively, the texts which involve oil and wine seem to allow for the use of both internal and external applications of medications. It is interesting that neither are applied or directed by a physician. Further, no explicit or implicit didactic or historical passage in the entire Bible refers to a specifc example of healing by a physician. The only explicit direction to believers concerning sickness is James 5:13-18. From this passage some theologians have concluded that anointing with oil (a medicine) may be interpreted to allow for the various treatments of physicians. In a personal review of conservative references on these passages in James, interpretations were varied, inconsistent, and even contradictory. Without consistent agreement it would seem tenuous and unreasonable to vary from a literal interpretation, i.e., a simple application by elders in conjunction with possible confession and repentance. Thus, an ethic for the relationship of physicians and believers must be established from other biblical principles since no texts offer explicit or clearly implicit instruction.

Freedom and Principle in Medical Care

Adiaphora "denotes acts or church rites which in themselves are neither morally right nor wrong, but matters of Christian liberty."[9] The concept is applicable to our biblical review because the Bible does not have clear directive concerning the relationship of Christians to physicians and their medical treatments. Some writers substitute "nonmoral," but whether *adiaphora* or nonmoral is used, one must be careful not to ignore the following biblical characteristics of this concept which do prescribe the principle necessary to the physician-patient relationship.

First, a principle must consider all other scriptural principles. Even though options exist in one area, other biblical directions must not be violated. For example, a Christian man is free to marry any Christian woman (2 Cor. 6:14), but he should give priority to the important characteristics of her inward beauty (1 Peter 3:1-8). It would be sin for him to marry a woman who professed Christ, yet who was more concerned about physical beauty than her relationship to Jesus Christ.

A second characteristic of "nonmoral" concerns motive. God is concerned about both inward motive *and* outward action since the Word is "able to judge the thoughts and intentions of the heart" (Heb. 4:12). Continuing with the example of Christian marriage, a man who gave priority to a woman's physical appearance, would have the wrong motive. His action would be sinful because his priority was personal preference. If he sought women who were serious in their Christian committment, however, and found two who were essentially equal in this respect, then he could freely choose according to his personal preferences. If motive is not carefully weighed (Ps. 139:23-24), nonmoral choices may involve sin.

A third characteristic of nonmoral is the clear position of Scripture that nothing which a human thinks or does, is nonmoral. "For we must all appear before the judgment seat of Christ, that each one may be recompensed for his deeds in the body, according to what he has done, whether good or bad (2 Cor. 5:10). That every thought, word, and deed is either "good or bad," i.e., moral, evokes an appropriate seriousness to any decision making.

A fourth characteristic of nonmoral is the avoidance of legalism. The Bible states clearly that certain persistent lifestyles are incompatible with salvation (1 Cor. 6:9-10; Rev. 21:8). On the other hand, some organizations of believers may determine a person's spiritual maturity, even his salvation, according to nonbiblical criteria, such as the avoidance of dancing, card playing and cigarette smoking. These activites in themselves are not explicitly prescribed or proscribed by Scripture. Their morality is decided on other factors, like motive, time commitment, desire, and physical health, not merely the presence or absence of the activity itself. To consider such activities as a basis for or against fellowship or salvation would be legalism.

Further, other characteristics, e.g., one's defiling of conscience (Rom. 14:23), one's becoming a stumbling block to weaker believers (1 Cor. 8:9) or to unbelievers (1 Peter 3:15), and one's being bound with unbelievers (2 Cor. 6:14), demonstrate that nonmoral issues must not be approached lightly. Based upon these characteristics, the following principles for the relationship of physicians and believers are proposed. It will be apparent that many current practices within the physician-patient relationship must be at least questioned, if not changed. The reader is reminded that immediate agreement or implementation is not expected. What must be established initially, however, are those biblical principles that should govern our practice.

Believers have indiscriminately accepted the role of physicians in their lives. Empirical and biblical evidence has been presented to demonstrate the close link between sin and sickness. Therefore, if almost all medical care is practiced without consideration of, or is opposed to spiritual realities, the most important dimension in believers' lives has been neglected (2 Cor. 4:16-18; Rom. 8:18; 1 Tim. 4:7-8). Most Christians, both lay and professional, are consciously unaware of this neglect, even opposition. Therefore, in order to assure the possibility of spiritual, as well as physical ministrations, *the first biblical principle to be established is that Christians be cared for by Christian physicians primarily.*

Sally went to a Christian counselor because of severe headaches. She had called her private physician who had prescribed successively three different medications (analgesics or antidepressants), but none of these had helped. She knew, as did her physician, that the headaches were caused by her intense worry over a family situation. From close acquaintance the counselor knew that she was committed to spiritual growth and as she responded consistent with that commitment, only one thirty-minute session was necessary. Three simple instructions were given her: irregular devotions must become regular and be conducted in the morning rather than the evening (to insure that nothing would interfere); when she became aware of her thinking about the family situation, she was to apply biblical thought-control, that is, change her thoughts to a "right" object (Phil. 4:8); and she was to pray for the problem only once weekly, instead of daily to decrease the frequency that she thought about the situation with its accompanying worry. No counsel was given for the family problem because it involved relatives and as far as the counselor could determine, Sally was not responsible in any way for its development or current difficulties. Within twenty-four hours the headaches were no longer a problem and within a few days they were gone completely. Sally had been almost incapacitated by a physical symptom which could not be treated with drugs.

There are four substantive reasons why Christians should see only Christian physicians. First, a physician is the best trained person to distinguish between a problem that is physical, spiritual or a combination of both. In many instances the patient could make these distinctions, but he would have to have been trained how to do so. If he could make such an evaluation, he could seek biblical counseling, preferably from his pastor or someone else at his local church, instead of seeking a physician. Frequently, however, neither the patient nor his counselor would be able to distinguish between the two areas *and* a physical condition may coexist with the spiritual problem. Second, seeing a Christian physician would be the most efficient approach for the patient, the counselor, and the physician. The major portion of a medical office practice involves minor or routine problems for which the physician is trained. Temporally, it would be impossible for a biblical counselor to be involved in all these conditions, yet each one is potentially related to a spiritual problem. For example, a simple cold may be secondary to stress which has been inappropriately handled and has caused a decrease in the patient's immunity to infection. Appropriate waiting room material (which to my knowledge is not yet available) and appropriate instruction in the church situation could contribute to the patient's education in such self-diagnosis. A physician, however, learns a great deal about patients and their habit patterns over years of observation. Frequently, from this knowledge-base he would recognize spiritual problems where the patient was unable to do so.

Third, the unity of both sides of man's nature means that a physical problem will affect one's spiritual life. Obviously, physical problems will have extreme variations in their relationship to the spiritual. On the one hand a cut finger for which stitches are needed may be almost entirely a physical problem, but on the other hand psychosomatic symptoms from depression may be entirely spiritual if the depression results from the patient's failure to act responsibly. Further, the spiritual side should have dominion over the physical, at least as a present fruit of the Spirit (self-control, temperance, etc.). Joni Eareckson is an example: as a teenager she became paralyzed from the neck down, yet she has overcome this handicap to the extent that she is a compentent artist who ministers to others through her testimony, counsel, and books. Physical problems should only bring about a spiritual *effect* because of the weakness (through ignorance, immaturity, or intention) of one's spirit. Although this attitude is never achieved perfectly (Paul in Romans 7), it is available to the maturing believer (Paul in 1 Cor. 9:27). The discerning Christian physician, from his knowledge and experience with both physical and spiritual problems, frequently will be able to determine the necessary effect of each upon the other. Nonmedical counselors would have difficulty obtaining the expertise to make such evaluations. At times it is difficult even for the experienced counselor-physician to determine the extent of influence of the spiritual on the physical and vice versa.

Fourth, a probability exists that a patient who sees a non-Christian physician is "unequally yoked" (2 Cor. 6:14-18). True intimacy exists between the patient and his/her physician. The physical body is exposed in a manner that usually is not allowed by any other person. Similarly, intimate details of the patient's life are revealed. Should an unbeliever be privileged to such exposure of the believer, especially with the known frequency of a cause-effect relationship between sin and physical illness? Further, should the unbeliever be allowed entrance into the Holy of Holies (see *naos*, above), even to prescribe treatment and to give direction to the method of its use (moral direction)? The answer to these questions seems unavoidable: the unholy physician may not enter and rearrange the utensils of worship, and *absolutely* he may not prescribe the method worship, i.e., "to present your bodies a living and holy sacrifice, acceptable to God, which is your spiritual service of *worship*" (Rom 12:1).[10]

This first principle requires that the physician have biblical counseling available to his patients. The counselor may be himself, one of the staff in his office, a pastor or someone else. Ideally, the counselor should be the patient's pastor.[11] The situation today, however, is not ideal so biblical counseling may not be available. Even so, the Christian physician is obligated to seek its availability. The best approach would be to persuade a biblically conservative local pastor to seek training in biblical counseling. Many centers are beginning to provide this training.[12] If such a pastor is not available, the physician may choose to study counseling himself or one of his male office personnel may be trained.[13] In this instance women may not have authority over, teach, or counsel men (1 Tim. 2:12). How can a medical practice be Christian without biblical counseling? Many physicians are evangelistic, but counseling is needed also. From personal experience the provision of both counseling and medical care by the same person is an arduous and time-consuming task.

Apart from the physician, pastors are obligated to locate a Christian physician with whom they can interact on counseling cases which are not clearly physical or spiritual and to whom he can direct his members since his provision of spiritual oversight includes the physical care of the body as it is united with the spiritual. The paucity of biblical counselors and biblically-discerning physicians creates a distressing situation, but God never leaves one of His adopted children to his own resources. Here, the Christian patient and physician's dilemma is mostly one of disordered priorities: to find a community where complete spiritual oversight of both body and soul are practiced.[14] Rarely, however, are places of residence chosen with that spiritual necessity as a conscious, high priority.

The other side of the believer's freedom to choose medical care is the second principle of the believer-physician relationship; the freedom not to choose medical care or to choose an alternative. Many examples are being presented where medical treatment must be avoided for ethical reasons, e.g., abortion, treatment of children who are still at home without the knowledge and consent of the parents, and active euthanasia. Other reasons not to choose medical care are the possibilities of complications or adverse outcome (chapter 4). Informative decision making is needed since these issues may abbreviate or extend life and alleviate or cause physical disability. Some medical treatments are clearly efficacious and necessary: the treatment of car accident victims, the delivery of a baby whose mother has pregnancy complications, and the repair of congenital heart defects in children. Other situations are less clear: the prolongation of life for a short time at great expense in some cases of terminal illness, surgery which is not clearly necessary, and experimental methods of treatment.

Recently, a Christian friend told me this account of her back problem. She had been managed by an orthopedic physician (a Christian) for several months but she became steadily worse. Her physician advised, and she was scheduled for, surgery. Two days prior to the surgery, she decided as a last resort to see a chiropractor. At that time she was unable to get into a sitting position because of the inflexibility and pain in her back. Following the adjustment by the chiropractor (a Christian), she was able to sit, as the pain and spasm was reduced markedly. She cancelled the surgery and with continued visits to the chiropractor, obtained complete relief. Although she has occasional recurrences, they have never been as severe as they were previously and have continued to respond to occasional chiropractic adjustments. This anecdote illustrates the fact that the provision of medical care is not restricted to physicians. This principle is consistent with those areas of freedom for the believer: the absence of explicit direction to seek any particular therapist. Indeed, earlier in the chapter it was pointed out that Paul who prescribed for Timothy, and the Good Samaritan who applied oil and wine, were not physicians!

Admittedly, dangers are present in this position. Many persons are duped, harmed and deprived of their money by unscrupulous charlatans. Five guidelines should prevent these adverse possibilities: (1) The most soundly-based therapies are those of formally trained physicians and their traditional helpers: nurses, physical therapists, etc. No other healing discipline is as well-researched, and the onus is on other disciplines to begin to develop their research base. At the same time flexibility must be allowed because traditional medicine has serious problems of its own. (2) There should be little danger from the therapy. An example would be the use of chiropractic for problems which are limited to muscle spasm of the spinal column without a bony deformity which could be aggravated by adjustments. Unfortunately, many drugs and therapies used by nonmedical practitioners are extremely harmful. With a reasonable openness Christian physicians could assist fellow believers to evaluate the potential of these therapies for harm *and* benefit. Certainly, scriptural freedom allows the nonphysician to treat physical problems. (3) A formal training program has been developed by the nonmedical discipline and the therapist himself has had that training. (4) The cost should be reasonable. If someone is not going to make a large profit, he is not as likely to promote a false treatment. (5) As with a physician, the therapist should be a believer to whom all the aforementioned discussion applies.[15]

A third biblical principle is the possible etiology of disease as a result of satanic influence. (Examples have already been given in the biblical references.) In addition, a wayward believer who is involved in gross sin may be delivered "to Satan for the destruction of his flesh" (1 Cor. 5:5). Paul had a thorn in his flesh which was a "messenger of Satan" (2 Cor. 12:7).[16] The practical value of this truth in the Western world, however, is uncertain. What seems certain, is that demon possession does occurs. Diagnostically, I have not read of any account where a physical illness was due to demonic influence *in the absence of* symptoms other than those of the physical problem itself. On this basis the current approach to focus on the common etiologies of sin-engendered disease and injury which is a result of the fall of Adam is appropriate. The attention to these will likely be effective against, or at least expose, a demonic etiology when it is present. One must be careful not to search for demons where they are not, but the Scripture is clear concerning the reality of their presence and possible influence to cause disease.

In conclusion, the New Testament does not give explicit directions to believers concerning their involvement with physicians. Thus, Christians are free to choose or not choose medical care. With all areas of freedom, however, other clear principles should be brought to bear. On this basis three principles have been presented: (1) Christians should ideally be treated by other Christians with the realization that expedients are currently necessary because of the current paucity of trained people. (2) Christians may choose not to accept medical care and to seek help from other healers if they give strict attention to certain guidelines. It would be morally wrong to reject medical care where the result of its rejection was almost certainly to be worse than its acceptance. To the contrary, it could be morally right to reject medical care where the result was equivocal or likely to be worse than the disease. Biblical counselors and physicians, particularly, need to be aware of this freedom. Often, their counsel will be the deciding factor in the decisions of their counselees. (3) Satanic deception is a rare, but nevertheless real, cause of disease.

Healing, Patient Responsibility, Truthfulness and the Family
Biblical Principles of Healing

> On a rainy afternoon in the early summer of 1972 about fifteen people gathered together in a tiny oak church not far from my home. . . . We began by reading aloud from various Scriptures. . . . I left the church parking lot in exactly the same frame of mind that I had entered it—fully expecting God to heal me. . . . A week went by . . . then another . . . then another. . . . Fingers and toes still didn't respond to the mental command, "Move". . . . Three weeks became a month, and one month became two . . . Is there some sin in my life? Had we done things right? Did I have enough faith? Since that time I have had years in a wheelchair to ponder this question, "Why wasn't I healed?" I still don't have all the answers about healing. But I do have some of them—answers that come from the Bible.[17]

A treatment of medical ethics is incomplete without developing biblical principles of healing, especially since this topic is one manifestation of Christians' renewed interest in the miraculous.[18] Despite divergence of opinion, it is possible to develop sound biblical principles which may be applied to particular situations. Broadly, healing may be divided into two general categories: that which is of God and that which is of Satan. God may use various means, but all healing is dependent upon His created design whether natural or supernatural.[19]

Since the principle has already been developed that all illness, disease, suffer-ing, and death is attributable directly or indirectly to sin, scriptural clarity dic-tates that only God is able to remove the effects of sin through Christ's Atone-ment. Any healing is only temporary in the sense that all people eventually die physically.

Satan's healing is not true healing because he is a deceiver (Gen. 3:1; 2 Cor. 11:13-14; Rev. 20:8). His healing occurs by the delusion that sickness is present when it is not, or that he caused it in the first place and then removed his influence. He intervenes into God's natural and spiritual design *only* by God's permission (Job 1:10, 2:4-6). Since men are not able to perceive the invisible spiritual world, it is difficult, if not impossible to discern these decep-tions. It is doubtful, however, that Satan ever heals, even as a delusion, except through such means as occult practices, e.g., mediums, spiritual healers, and black magic. Since Christians are forbidden to become involved with the oc-cult, strict avoidance of such practices cannot be overemphasized.

God's healing may be subdivided into two types. First, God heals by physical means such as medications, physical therapy, radiation, or surgery. This is performed by physicians, through self-treatment, or by nonmedical practi-tioners. The action of these agents may be direct or indirect. Direct methods are those where there is a known biochemical or physiological effect. For ex-ample, antibiotics kill bacteria; surgeons remove appendices; digitalis increases the pump-ing ability of the heart. The indirect method is the placebo effect in which a biochemical effect is unknown. Nevertheless, the physical response is real and can be documented objectively. Both actions, however, involve God's created design. No surgeon can cause skin or other organs to grow together, he only approximates their edges. Orthopedists align bones, but fusion is in-herent within their cellular and organic structure. Antibiotics kill bacteria, but white blood cells and other tissues must clean out the debris and then the organ must repair itself. Thus, physicians never heal the body by their practices alone, they assist an extremely complex design that is "fearfully and wonderfully made" (Ps. 139:14).

Second, healing may result from the application of biblical (spiritual or super-natural) principles or God's miraculous intervention. Biblical principles are the normative pattern for every Christian life and their influence upon the physical body extends to all bodily processes. God both prevents and heals disease.

Also God may heal miraculously through supernatural means; in other words, he acts apart from both His natural and supernatural design. In the case of the woman with a flow of blood, natural means, the healing mechanisms within the body and the practice of physicians, were inadequate; but God healed apart from these means. Objectively, a miracle can only be recognized if it is distinguishable from the ordinary means, even though God works miraculously in association with mundane physical means. A surgeon may operate to remove a cancer, but overlook some cancerous tissue. God may choose to destroy all the remaining cancer, but from all appearances the surgeon cured the patient. In this instance God intervened, but the result could not be known objectively to be a miracle because God's special action could not be distinguished from the usual means of surgery.

How a miracle may be recognized needs to be explored further. Unless a physical problem has been established by objective evidence, a miracle cannot be known to have occurred.[20] For example, a person may announce that he has been healed of cancer in the abdomen that was self-diagnosed. By contrast a patient may be operated upon, found to have inoperable cancer and closed without an attempt at curative surgery. If that patient then claimed to have been healed at a later date with no evidence of tumor on x-rays or other tests, and his health continued without evidence of any further occurrence of the cancer, then a miracle was more likely to have occurred.

Without documentation the claim of a miracle should not be made. Even with documentation a miracle may not have occurred since natural processes occur in ways we do not yet understand. Spontaneous cures of cancer that occur quite apart from religious influences are known.[21] Thus, healing that is based upon objective evidence in a believer or an unbeliever may be a miracle but it cannot be absolutely known to have occurred. A miracle is more likely to have occurred where spiritual ministrations, anointing and prayer, etc., are in very close proximity to a healing.

An exception where doubt could not exist would be the presence of objective evidence of a physical problem for which recorded cures were otherwise unknown. For example, a withered hand restored to health (Matt. 12:13); a man blind since birth could see (John 9:1-7); and a lifelong cripple who could walk (Acts 3:1-10). In such cases the Scripture does not leave room for doubt that a miracle took place. Any modern claims to the miraculous should have similar objective data. If these criteria are applied, almost all claims of a miraculous nature could be dismissed. If these criteria are present, the occurrence of a miracle would be virtually certain. Further, it should be noted that healings in the Bible were instantaneous.

Did miracles cease with the end of the apostolic age? If they did, no miraculous healing could take place today. Highly respected theologians differ. B. B. Warfield, expressing the predominate thought within Presbyterian and Reformed denominations, believes miraculous healings did cease, although he does concede that God heals supernaturally through prayer and other revealed designs.[22] On the opposite side is D. Martyn Lloyd-Jones, "We must not exclude dogmatically, as we have often tended to do so, the manifestation and demonstration of the power of God to heal diseases, or to do anything that He wills and chooses to do."[23] More recently, J. I. Packer agrees that, ". . . does Jesus still heal miraculously? Yes, I think on occasion he does. . . . There is much contemporary evidence of healing events in faith contexts that have baffled the doctors."[24]

I agree with Lloyd-Jones and Packer. Experience and/or phenomena never invalidates or validates Scripture; but the Bible does not explicitly state that miraculous healing ceased with Christ and the apostles. Extrabiblically, missionaries and others have given accounts of healings which are sometimes documented or otherwise seem to have objective reliability. Objective criteria for a miracle would exclude most claims, and apart from these, any specific case of claimed healing is purely subjective.[25]

Writing with reference to the gift of healing, Lloyd-Jones has instructed:

> I believe that the 'faith' referred to by our Lord and by James as 'the prayer of faith,' is . . . 'given' faith. I put it into the same category as 'commission' that was given to the Apostles and others, who in my opinion, have worked miracles since the days of the Apostles. Not experimentation, not an announcement on Sunday that there is going to be a healing meeting on Thursday next. They cannot truly say that because they do not know. All true divinely wrought miracle is 'given'; and 'the prayer of faith' is given. No one can work it up; either he has it or he does not have such faith. It partly depends upon a man's general spirituality and his general faith in God, and still more upon His sovereign will.[26]

Few men can lay claim to more adherence to the faith than the apostle Paul, yet he could not heal whenever he desired: himself (2 Cor. 12:7-8); Timothy, (1 Tim. 5:23); or Epaphroditus (Phil. 2:27). No one has objectively substantiated the gift of healing apart from the biblical record in an individual. As D. Martyn Lloyd-Jones said, an individual cannot create faith from within to be healed; neither can an individual claim to heal whenever he personally wills; it is God's choice and His time.

The Bible records more accounts of healing by Jesus Christ than any other person. His healings were primarily to validate that He was the Son of God and the Messiah (Matt. 11:1-6; Luke 4:16-21; John 10:22-42; Heb. 2:3-4). The New Testament gives no evidence that physical healing has ever become a primary concern of God the Father, nor the predominant manifestation of Christ's miraculous power—the Resurrection established the priority of the supernatural over the physical. A focus on healing by medical, spiritual, or miraculous, should always be of secondary importance. The more important spiritual dimension should never be neglected (Heb. 2:3).

Believers should always consider spiritual factors in association with physical illness as a possible cause and effect. Close self-examination is necessary to determine whether or not sin is a contributing factor. Questions to consider include: Have I been under more stress lately? Are my devotional times observed daily, unhurried and meaningful? Do I get along with my spouse? Am I getting enough restful sleep each night? Am I truly resting one day per week (Ex. 20:8-11)? Do I have an aerobic exercise program? Am I considerably overweight? Do I worry? If one is not sure whether illness is a result of lifestyle, then one's physician should be consulted. Believers will be amazed at the correlation between spiritual problems and physical problems. Even if the physical problem is entirely unrelated to anything spiritual, a time of illness can be advantageously used for a spiritual "checkup"—a period of hospitalization allows timely personal reflection.

Christians have the understanding, ability, and motivation with which to understand a balanced, healthy Christian life. Unfortunately, even among Christians, there has been an increasing dependency upon physicians for health. *Self-responsibility through preventive effort cannot be overemphasized.* Although Christians have greater resources than non-Christians, the ability of non-Christians to be responsible and change should not be underestimated. Many have been able to stop smoking or make other healthy behavioral changes. If they are not open to eternal benefits which also maximize temporal benefits, then Christians must do all that is possible to demonstrate the love of God. Behavorial, pyschological and medical directions may be a part of this demonstration.

If a person has a chronic illness that persists for months and years without hope for a cure and for which only palliative treatment is possible, he should read extensively on that disease. Too many individual variations exist for physicians to consider every one with every patient. In addition, the physician may overlook something that the patient can do to help himself in the management of his problem. Today, many self-education materials as well as organizations are available to maximize one's understanding of the patient's role, the physician's role, and the roles of others. A personal health record may be helpful. A brief account of a problem and its time of occurrence may indicate a previously overlooked pattern.

Since our bodies are temples of the Holy Spirit, Christians cannot neglect personal responsibility for their health. The evidence is conclusive that the patient can better maintain his own health and prevent disease if he does not totally rely on his physician. Often pastors, physicians and other committed Christians discover that schedules are their worst health enemy; primarily because of resulting conflicts in their relationships with God, spouse, children, and Christian brothers and sisters. Such patterns are sin (Ps. 48:10; Isa. 40:31; Matt. 11:28-30).

The Importance of Truthfulness in Medical Care

The patient stared into her physician's eyes as if trying to see into his soul. His thorough examination, including laboratory studies, revealed an initial diagnosis of gastritis (irritation of the stomach). All results were conclusive, but he assured her that simple treatment would resolve the condition. After a momentary pause, she responded, "Well, thank you, I was sure it was cancer. I had to hear the diagnosis from somebody I could trust, and I think that I can trust you." The intensity of her gaze became apparent as she told her story. When her mother had asked another physician whether she was dying, that physician had said, ". . . You'll feel better before you know it. Don't worry. Just trust me." A few minutes later in the hallway that physician had nformed the family that she had terminal cancer. Her mother died the same night.

This patient, now a middle-aged lady, had seen her mother's physician for her stomach pains. He again responded. "Don't worry . . . you'll be feeling fine very soon." In tears she hurriedly had left his office and sought the second physician for advice.[27]

Doctors should not lie, it is a sin. "You shall not bear false witness against thy neighbor" was God's command from Mt. Sinai (Ex 20:16). God's very nature is truth (1 John 5:6; John 14:17, 15:26, 16:13). His Word is truth (Hos. 10:13; Amos 2:4; 1 John 2:4, 22). This realization prompted John Murray to conclude:

> When we speak, therefore of the sanctity of truth, we must recognize that what underlies this concept is the sanctity of the being of God as the living and true God. He is the God of truth and all truth derives its sanctity from Him. That is why all untruth or falsehood is wrong, it is a contradiction of that which God is.[28]

The biblical position and goal for the Christian is truthfulness in thought, word, and deed in every area of life—including the practice of medicine. Traditionally, lying to patients has been considered a prerogative of the physician for the good of his patient. Plato, in *The Republic* wrote that the physician should embrace skillful deception as a means of medical treatment.[29] The Hippocratic Corpus (of which the Hippocratic Oath is a part) instructs the physician to reveal "nothing of the patients' future or present condition."[30] Alexander Dumas was explicit in his *Camille*: "When God said that lying was a sin, he made an exception for doctors and gave them permission to lie as many times a day, as they saw patients."[31] A trend toward candor is occurring, but regardless of the current non-Christian thought, Christians should tell the truth because the Bible is explicit in its command.

The manner in which truth is presented must be guided by the "fruits of the spirit." One would think that gentleness and kindness are obvious, but too many physicians seem to be ignorant or insensitive to patients. Instead of informing the patient of a serious problem in a clinical and curt fashion, the physician should set aside proper time to answer questions. Later, follow-up would allow further questions and concerns to be voiced by the patient. Insensitivity to the confusion and mystery of medical terminology and medical milieu are frequent errors by physicians. The patient's concerns need to be anticipated, even actively sought, because strong emotions may prevent his ability to verbalize these concerns.

A second factor in truth-telling is its timing. Drugs, physical traumas, procedures, and other events may markedly reduce the patient's ability to concentrate and to remember. These circumstances are commonplace to the physician, but emotionally overwhelming to patients. The best time to inform a mother that one of her children has been killed in an auto accident is not in the emergency room as she is being stabilized for blood loss and injuries which she herself has sustained in the same accident. In another situation, a patient will probably recall nothing, if told the results of his surgery as he is awakening from anesthesia. Ideal situations are difficult to plan, but every consideration should be given the patient who receives bad news. An instance in which unnecessary delay should not occur is terminal illness and the spiritual urgency of such situations should not be overlooked.

After a lengthy discussion of several Bible instances, John Murray concludes that "the Scripture confronts us with difficulties" but it necessarily establishes the biblical concept of truthfulness.[32]

> . . . the upshot of our examination has been that no instance demonstrates the propriety of untruthfulness under any exigency. We would require far more than the Scripture provides to be able to take the position that under certain exigencies we may speak untruth with our neighbor . . . but the Scripture warrants *concealment of truth from those who have no claim upon it . . .* and concealment is often an obligation which truth itself requires (our emphasis).[33]

Two principles emerge. First, partial disclosure of truth may be appropriate, rather than untruth (Samuel at Bethlehem). Second, a concealment of truth is warranted from those who have no claim upon it (Joshua's deception of Ai).[34]

These principles are essential to the truthfulness which may be complicated in medical practice. Partial truth is only permissible because of practical necessity and medical facts exist as probablities rather than unchanging truth. In any particular situation all contingencies are too numerous to cover or even to predict! Thus, the physician must decide what he will tell the patients. Great lattitude, in both the content of the information and its emphasized points, is possible for the physician. This complexity is illustrated by a study in which the method of presentation determined whether a patient would choose surgery or radiation as treatment for lung cancer.[35] Another study on the avoidance of laryngectomy has show that patients would choose a lessened chance of survival in order to preserve their speaking ability.[36]

As early as 1903, a physician provided evidence that the truth did not harm the patient.[37] In addition real benefits have been found to occur: "pain is tolerated more easily, recovery from surgery is facilitated and compliance with therapy is markedly improved."[38] Thus empirical, medical evidence and Scripture agree that truthfulness is both influential in the patient's decision and that it positively affects his prognosis. A physician's concern ought to be, if medical disclosure is impossible, a partial presentation of truth which would most honor the God of truth.

The second principle, concealment of truth, has no application in medical practice. In Scripture each situation involves concealment from an enemy. Clearly the physician is not the enemy, rather he is the patient's advocate. The patient is responsible for his body and should seek knowledge of his health. Physicians are wrong to withhold information. The patient should know at least as much as any family member. Although pragmatic value is not necessary to validate biblical truth, a benefit of this principle is that no family member need be concerned about information that the patient might hear inadvertently.

A method which would facilitate patient and family understanding would be to assemble all concerned. The patient would have to give permission since only the spouse or parents have access to medical information. Much time could also be saved by the physician.

The Christian physician may face difficult tests when dealing truthfully with patients in the variety of situations which constitute the doctor-patient-family relationship. The above principles should assist the doctor to be truthful. The traditional relationship of medical practice to the the family has been one of support and strength. However, the character of this relationship is changing as the practice of medicine has an increasing, even destructive, power over the family.[39] Consider these facts:

> Teenagers may abort their unborn children without parental consent. An older woman can abort without the consent of her husband, or the biological father of the child if she is unmarried.
>
> Teenagers may be treated for venereal disease, pregnancy (and drugs prescribed for contraception), and drug abuse without parental consent.[40]
>
> Physicians-in-training are taught that the confidentiality of the patient-physician relationship has priority over the marriage or family commitments. The courts uphold this confidentiality.[41]
>
> Parents or spouses are limited or prevented from being with their hospitalized loved ones; especially in Intensive Care Units.
>
> On the testimony of physicians, children can be removed from homes for child abuse or for medical treatment for which the parents will not grant permission.
>
> The family is being redefined to include homosexual ''couples'' which physicians are taught to accept ''unconditionally.''
>
> In some states single women may receive artificial insemination. Denial of this service is said to involve ''discrimination.''
>
> Psychiatrists are becoming the primary resource to the needs and problems of children. Pediatricians and other physicians are effectively influenced by their theories and practices.
>
> Eighty-two percent of families who institutionalize their retarded children do so on the advice of a physician.[42]
>
> Behavioral problems at school and at home are diagnosed and treated, primarily if not entirely as hyperactivity—a medical problem.
>
> Elderly people are placed in nursing homes for chronic management and terminal illness, often when their condition could be managed at home.

Admittedly, some individual instances of these general developments are helpful to the family. The list demonstrates the influence and power physicians have over the family. Perhaps, the most destructive situations involve those physicians who depend exclusively upon psychiatrists and psychologists in these and other situations.

In general Christian physicians have remained ignorant that in many such instances transgressions of biblical norms have occurred. The concept that medical care takes precedence over intrafamily responsibilities is so ingrained that a proposed policy change by the federal government has been met with "outrage." This policy would require that family planning clinics notify the parents of any girl under eighteen who receives a prescription for a means of birth control.[43]

Biblically, the father is the head of the marriage and the home (1 Cor. 11:3-4; Eph. 5:23-24; 1 Tim. 3:4.) The husband-wife relationship is the most intimate and permanent of human relationships since children are only temporarily in the home. The goal of their being in the family is to be trained in the way that they should go (Prov. 22:7), as the God-given authority of the parents is transferred gradually to God's authority with their developing maturity. The husband and wife, however, were designed to become "one flesh," even prior to the Fall (Gen. 2:24), with a severence of parental authority and primary responsibility to each other. Communication between them should be open and frequent (preferably daily). Even their bodies no longer belong to themselves (1 Cor. 7:4-5).

Given this biblical structure for the home, how can physicians withhold information about a child from a parent? To do so is to intrude the physician's authority into the biblical unity and dependency of the family. Children are to obey their parents (Eph. 6:1-3), but the physician who withholds information from parents may aid disobedience. No biblical text validates an agent outside the family to be privileged to information which is not available to parents.

Husbands and wives may be in situations where the doctor needs to exhort one spouse to communicate with the other spouse. A communicable disease, such as tuberculosis, is a risk to spouse and the family. The presence of a venereal disease needs to be communicated for both the medical threat of the disease and the marital problems inherent with extramarital sex. Life-dominating problems such as alcoholism and drug abuse impact severely upon the family. Finally, a request for an abortion may not be the sole choice of the wife.

Physicians must realize medical practice often breaches biblical responsibilities designated to family members. He must research and weigh applicable biblical principles and not assume that orthodox medicine has taught him correctly how to manage these situations.[44]

Perhaps, the following principles will provide some focus for reflection and direction:

1. The non-Christian patient cannot be expected to understand or follow biblical responsibility within the family. He must first believe in Christ. Therefore, evangelism remains primary.
2. The Christian patient should be informed of his biblical responsibility to communicate to his spouse and family members.
3. The physician cannot assist any patient in immorality (sin) even if he hopes

to achieve good later. It is "pernicious logic that we may do evil that good may come".[45]

4. The Christian physician must strive to conduct his practice in such a manner that the unity of his patient's marriage, the headship of the father over the family, and the parent's responsibility for their children, is not compromised.

NOTES

1. The Old Testament is cited for the word, "physician" because of its explicit relationship to the study here. An extensive reference to the physician and the value of his work does appear in the Apocrypha (Ecclesiasticus 38:1-15). Among Protestants the Bible excludes the Apocrypha as Holy Scripture. Even the Roman Catholics, who accept the Apocrypha as Holy Scripture, did not do so traditionally, e.g., Jerome's translation into Latin did not include it.

2. Even though the believer under grace is no longer bound by the ceremonial law, current empirical evidence defines what could not be otherwise: what is spiritually healthy through the ceremonial law is physically healthy, as well, since man is a physical and spiritual unity.

3. This study was fascinating because the Holy Spirit has written many passages in such a manner as to define both the process of healing and the specific physical problems by context without the dependence of the interpretation upon lexical definitions.

4. *Young's Analytical Concordance* and *Vine's Expository Dictionary of New Testament Words* were used to locate the pertinent words which follow. These two resources are referenced to the King James Version of the Bible, but quotations continue to be taken from the New American Standard Version. The Greek stems (in parenthesis) were referenced in Young's to locate the various Bible passages where they occurred. This procedure prevents an inadvertant ommission of a Greek word which has an unexpected English translation.

5. John Calvin, *Commentary on a Harmony of the Evangelists* (reprint ed., Grand Rapids: Baker Book House, 1979), pp. 231-232..

6. W. H. Hobart, *The Medical Language of St. Luke* (Dublin: Hodges, Figgis and Co., 1882), p. 295.

7. The uses of *iaomai* in a spiritual sense would allow the gift of healing to be applied to a person who is gifted by the Holy Spirit to heal spiritually. Such healing would consist of the practical application of biblical teaching which redirects a person in such a way that sin is put off and right living is put on: thus, spiritual change and growth are enhanced. By this translation many believers would have this gift today. It becomes doubtful that anyone in recent times has had the gift of physical healings (pp. 112-115) when his or her ministry has been examined carefully.

8. The cited passages clearly indicate that demonic possession is one etiology of a variety of physical problems. Thus, three etiologies of physical problems exist: physical (with no other etiology), demonic, and spiritual (a sinful lifestyle).

9. Robert D. Preus, "Adiaphora," in *Baker's Dictionary of Christian Ethics*, ed. Carl F. Henry (Grand Rapids: Baker Book House, 1973), p. 89.

10. Carl F. H. Henry, *Christian Personal Ethics* (1957; reprint ed., Grand Rapids: Baker Book House, 1977), p. 433.

11. Jay E. Adams, *Competent to Counsel* (Nutley, N. J.: Presbyterian and Reformed Pub. Co., 1970), pp. 65-78.

12. For Information write: National Association of Nouthetic Counselors, Box 889, Bryn Mawr, PA 19010.

13. If such a pastor is not available, particularly in the physician's own church, why is the physician in such a community? The neglect of regular exposure to biblical preaching and teaching is almost certain to result in spiritual neglect (Heb. 2:3). The necessity of a vital, dynamic fellowship cannot be emphasized enough! In a day where many believers search intently for God's will, this principle is clearly His revealed will. Many true believers choose a lukewarm church with a detrimental effect upon their souls (Rev. 3:16). Also, see following note.

14. Such a proposal seems to concentrate believers into communities and neglect the commands to "go" (Matt. 28:19) and to be "salt" and "light" (Matt. 5:13-16). Certainly, I am not advocating that these be neglected for those Christians who are *gifted* and with deliberation discern that God would have them to follow these commands. My concern, however, is a very common overestimation of one's ability to affect, or grow spiritually in a church where both the leaders and a significant number of believers are not committed to a life similar to the "balanced" life. I am convinced that Christians would have a greater impact on the above commands if first they spent several years where they could learn and participate in what a serious committment to Jesus Christ practically means.

15. Brief reviews of many nonmedical therapies are provided in these books:

(a) J. Weldon and C. Wilson, *Occult Shock and Psychic Forces* (San Diego: Master Books, 1980), pp. 149-246.

(b) P. C. Reisser, T. K. Reisser and J. Weldon, *The Holistic Healers* (Downers Grove: InterVarsity Press, 1983).

16. The particular diesase has been the subject of much discussion among physicians and theologians. For a full discussion, see *The New International Commentary of the New Testament*, (2 Cor.), pp. 442-448.

17. Joni Eareckson, *A Step Further* (Grand Rapids: Zondervan, 1978), pp. 122-134. Miss Eareckson's testimony is used to demonstrate the effectiveness of biblical truth to answer sufficiently the difficult problems of the Christian's life in which one may still experience God's blessings in ministry, productiveness, joy, and peace. Readers are encouraged to read this chapter in her book for her personal testimony to a biblical balance that covers more fully my brief presentation here.

18. Only physical healing is being considered here. Bibically, healing of the mind and spirit (entities which are not necessarily distinct) apart from an obvious physical effect may occur. In this chapter, however, spiritual healing without a physical effect is not my subject. First, my continuing distinction between the spiritual and the physical is maintained. Second, claims to spiritual and mental healing are too nebulous in their assoction with objective evidence to ascertain whether healing occurred or even the existence of a definite problem was present in the first place.

19. On the one hand, it is artificial to distinguish between natural (physical) and supernatural (spiritual). Ultimately, God is the first cause of all events since He is Omnipotent. On the other hand, humans are limited to the observation of the physical side of events. We are not able to separate the independent effects of the natural and the supernatural.

20. We would not say in a particular instance that a miracle did not occur, but that such a claim has no validity. Indeed, many such miracles may occur, but without objective documentation they should not be claimed publicly to be miracles. The objective testimony of the visible church must be a vital concern to God's people (Matt. 18:15-18; 1 Cor. 5:1-13; Eph. 4:17-19; 1 Thess. 3:14).

21. Tilden Everson and Warren Cole, *Spontaneous Regression of Cancer* (Philadelphia: Saunders, 1966).

22. B. B. Warfield, *Counterfeit Miracles* (Carlisle, Pennsylvania: Banner of Truth Trust, 1976).

23. D. Martyn Lloyd-Jones, *The Supernatural in Medicine* (London: Christian Fellowship Publication, 1971), p. 24.

24. James I. Packer, "Poor Health May Be the Best Remedy," *Christianity Today* (May 21, 1982), pp. 14-16.

25. I must admit that I have never encountered personally an instance which meets these criteria, although I have heard first-hand reports from others.

26. D. Martyn Lloyd-Jones, *The Supernatural in Medicine*, p. 22.

27. Paul Brand, *Fearfully and Wonderfully Made* (Grand Rapids: Zondervan Publishing Co., 1980), pp. 78-79.

28. John Murray, *Principles of Conduct* (1957; reprint ed., Grand Rapids: Eerdmans Pub. Co., 1978), p. 125.

29. Steve Holve, "Truth Telling in Medicine: A Historical Perspective," Society for Health and Human Values, 925 Chestnut Street, Philadephia, PA 19107.

30. Ibid.

31. Ibid., p. 6.

32. Rahab in Joshua 2:1-24; Samuel in 1 Sam. 16:1-13; the Israelite midwives in Ex. 1:15-21; and Joshua in Joshua 8:1-29.

33. John Murray, *Principles of Conduct*, pp. 146-147.

34. The reader is referred to Murray's detailed discussion of these concepts. Space does not allow the detail which would be necessary to examine such biblical instances of lying or conceal-ment. His biblical research is thorough and his conclusions are sound. They supply a practical approach which would minimize possibilities of sin in medicine or any other endeavor.

    Although Murray does not comment specifically, his (biblical) position would seem to necessitate a biblical definition of lying which is distinct from the usual definition of "intent to deceive". In his analysis of Joshua's deception of the people of Ai (pp. 143-145), he concludes, ". . . we are at a loss to find untruth." Joshua did intentionally deceive the people of Ai and "the Lord himself was part of the strategem" (Josh. 8:18), but the "deception arose from their failure to discover its (the retreat's) real purpose." No untruth was involved, but concealment of the reason for the Israelites' action was. Thus, a biblical definition of lying would have to in-clude intentional deception or concealment of the true purpose of an action against a recognized enemy. This deception would not include circumstances where mutual understanding is a "rele-vant or requisite" consideration. Certainly, this qualification is extremely limited and cannot be extended to "our right to speak untruth" in any situation.

35. B. J. McNeil and S. C. Pauker, "On the Elicitation of Preferences for Alternative Therapies," *New England Journal of Medicine* 306 (May 27, 1982): 1259-1262.

36, Ibid.

37. Steve Holve, "Truth Telling in Medicine," Society for Health and Human Values.

38. Ibid.

39. These laws and practices vary among states but these listed are prevalent throughout the United States.

40. Richard M. Martin, "Law and the Minor Patient," *Southern Medical Journal* 75 (1982): 1245-1248.

41. "Doctors Business: Disclosure to Patient's Wife Ruled Actionable," *Medical World News* (June 21, 1982), pp. 69-70.

42. M. H. Apell and W. J. Tisdall, "Factors Differentiating Institutionalized from Noninstitu-tionalized Referred Retardates, *American Journal of Mental Deficiency* 73 (1968): 424.

43. *Medical World News* (March 15, 1982), pp. 17, 24.

44. Larry Spalink, "Confidentiality and Biblical Counseling," *Journal of Pastoral Practice* 3 (3) 1979: 56-62.

45. John Murray, *Principles of Conduct*, p. 146.

REFERENCES

Apell, M. H., W. J. Tisdall. "Factors Differentiating Institutionalized from Noninstitutionalized Referred Retardates." *American Journal of Mental Deficiency* 73 (1968):424.

Benson, H., and M. D. Epstein. "The Placebo Effect. A Neglected Aspect in the Care of Patients." *Journal of the American Medical Association* 232 (June 23, 1975):1225-1227.

Brand Paul. *Fearfully and Wonderfully Made*. Grand Rapids: Zondervan Publishing Co., 1980.

Clark, Gordon H. *What Do Presbyterians Believe?* Phillipsburg, PA: Presbyterian and Reformed Publishing Co., 1979, pp. 12-13.

"Doctor's Business: Disclosure to Patient's Wife Ruled Actionable." *Medical World News* (June 21, 1982):69-70.

Eareckson, Joni, *A Step Further*. Grand Rapids: Zondervan, 1978. Everson, Tilden and Warren Cole. *Spontaneous Regression of Cancer*. Philadelphia, Saunders, 1966.

Hobart, W. H. *The Medical Language of St. Luke*. Dublin: Hodges, Figgis and Co., 1882.

Holve, Steve, "Truth Telling in Medicine: A Historical Perspective." Society for Health and Human Values, 925 Chestnut Street, Philadelphia, PA (19107).

Lloyd-Jones, D. Martyn. "The Supernatural in Medicine." London: Christian Medical Fellowship Publication, 1971.

Martin, Richard M. "Law and the Minor Patient." *Southern Medical Journal* 75 (1982):1245-1248.

McNeil, B. J., S. C. Pauker, et al. "On the Elicitation of Preferences for Alternative Therapies." *New England Journal of Medicine* 306 (May 27, 1982):1259-1262.

McNeil, B. J., R. Weichselbaum, S. G. Pauker. "Speech and Survival. Tradeoffs between Quality and Quantity of Life in Laryngeal Cancer." *New England Journal of Medicine* 305 (Oct. 22, 1981):982-987.

Packer, James I. "Poor Health May Be the Best Remedy." *Christianity Today*, May 21, 1982, pp. 14-16.

President's Commission for the Study of Ethical Problems in Medicine and Biomedical and Behaviorial Research. Making Health Care Decisions: A Report on the Ethical and Legal Implications of Informed Consent in the Patient-Practitioner Relationship. Washington, D.C., October 1982.

Spalink, Larry. "Confidentiality and Biblical Counseling." *Journal of Pastoral Practice* 3 (3):56-62.

Vine, W. E. *An Expository Dictionary of New Testament Words*. 1940. Reprint. Old Tappan, NJ:Fleming H. Revell Company, 1966.

Young, Robert. *Analytical Concordance to the Bible*. 1964. Reprint. Grand Rapids: Wm. B. Eerdmans Publishing Company, 1978.

FURTHER STUDY: Healing

B. B. Warfield. *Counterfeit Miracles*. 1918. Carlisle, PA: Banner of Truth Trust, 1976.

Henry W. Frost. *Miraculous Healing*. Overseas Missionary Fellowship, 1972. Reprint. Grand Rapids: Zondervan Publishing House, 1979.

James I. Packer. "The Theology of Healing." (Cassette Tapes). Dallas: Christian Medical Society, 1983.

William A. Nolen. *Healing: A Doctor in Search of a Miracle*. New York: Random House, 1974.

Linda Coleman. "Christian Healing: Is It Real." *Spiritual Counterfeits Project Journal* 2 (1):42-51.

Paul C. and Teri K. Reisser and John Weldon. *The Holistic Healers*. Downers Grove: InterVarsity Press, 1983.

8 | The Role of the Church in Health Care

The World Health Organization has defined health as "a state of complete physical, mental, and social well-being and not merely the absence of disease or infirmity." Paul Ramsey's comment on their definition is worth quoting at length:

> The broad definition of health will either have to be withdrawn or else consistently applied. The latter would mean that professional medical judgments assume the responsibility for the full range of human moral considerations. . . .This, I rather think is an alarming suggestion from which the medical profession should draw back in the direction of a stricter construction of medical judgments as such. . . .(There should be) a continuing distinction between the medical meaning and the theological-moral or humanistic meaning of imperative and elective procedures . . . he (the physician) should make room for the primacy of the human moral judgment on the part of the men who are his patients, the relatives of his patients, and their spiritual counselors.[1]

By the nature of what they do, physicians make pronouncements, personally and professionally, about what people may or may not do. For the Christian the "full range of human moral responsibilities" is the prerogative of the church to define principle and implement practice. A dialogue between physicians and theologians who are solidly convinced that the Bible is the ultimate source of truth, is imperative if we are to arrive at biblical principles and practice. Until that occurs, the following discussion will act as a catalyst.

The unity of the body and spirit and the relationship between sin and illness commands that the church play a central role in and outside the church. Generally conceptualizations of the church are either missing or incomplete in systematic theology, personal Christian ethics, and Christian medical ethics.[2]

Since the doctrine of the church is central to the Christian life, this neglect is being remedied. A ramification is that the church is a central doctrine in the development of biblical/medical ethics.

Historically, "there is no doubt that hospitals received their greatest impetus from the church in the centuries after Christ."[3] However, most church-initiated hospitals in the United States are now functionally indistinguishable from secular hospitals. The reality and daily existence of man's spiritual component is conspicuously absent within the hospital. Local churches need to re-establish an emphasis on the spiritual, as well as the physical; an emphasis that is both biblical and historical. Perhaps, the church's ministry to both believers and unbelievers will exceed the effectiveness of any present and historical applications.

One warning is necessary. There is a general tendency of the church, both individually and corporately, to become preoccupied with secondary matters, e.g., its buildings, its comfort, and its social programs. Physical health can become such a preoccupation. The primary purposes of the church are evangelism and edification of the saints. In some churches a preoccupation with health, for example, jogging clubs, weight loss programs, and miraculous healing, already exists. These pursuits in themselves are not necessarily wrong, but unless they contribute to the church's outreach and/or spiritual edification they are misdirected. These two purposes produce the best environment for health. The principles that follow will involve these primary and secondary issues. Each local church must set priorities for their development and implementation.

Counseling and Psychotherapy

Believers are primarily to be counseled within the church because Scripture contains the only principles which truthfully govern life (Rom. 12:2).[4] Unbelieving psychotherapists and their theories represent "conformity" to the "foolishness" of the world (1 Cor. 1:20). As such they cannot perceive the obvious, elemental truths of Christianity: it is necessary to be "born again" (John 3:5-8) and given a new heart (Ps. 51:10); only the Spirit can illumine the mind (John 16:12-15; 1 Cor. 2:12-14); the believer is able to live a transformed life only because of the indwelling Spirit (Phil. 2:12); and the Scriptures contain all that is needed to be "thoroughly furnished unto all good works" (2 Tim. 3:16-17). The unbelieving counselor cannot pray for or with his client, nor can he use the spiritual and physical resources of the church.

Although Christians should not take counseling lightly, all believers are to counsel in various ways (Rom. 15:14). Counseling on a regular basis requires certain spiritual gifts, life experience, and a thorough knowledge of Scripture. God's organizational structure for the church has officers for this function. The elders or bishops are given oversight of, and responsibility for, the spiritual welfare of the local assembly of believers (Acts 6:1-6; 1 Tim. 3:1-7, 5:17; Titus 1:5-10; 1 Peter 5:1-4). These officers have largely turned over counseling to secular professionals, but this does not lessen their biblical responsibilities. Secular theory and practice have taught that such "psychotherapy" is possible only for "professionals."

Is the Bible a textbook for counseling? Since non-Christian psychotherapists are guided by non-Biblical principles, the believer should not have his thoughts and actions directed by attitudes derived from any metaphysical basis other than the Bible; otherwise it would be a violation of the First Commandment.

What about the Christian psychologist or psychiatrist? As spiritual leaders of a local church they could counsel. But the counseling they do would be a function of their church affiliation *not* their psychological training. The serious danger is the false integration of biblical truth with the theory and practice of secular training.

> No Christian sets out to pervert and to deny God's truth; the process is gradual. It happens in stages, not all at once. This is the warning of Psalm 1 . . . One of Satan's ruses (as an angel of light) is to convince those who claim theological sophistication to accept error under the slogan "All truth is God's truth." Under that banner nearly every error in the book has been blamed on God!. . . . You can be sure that it is not the result of common grace that rival ways of counseling exist side by side. God cannot be charged with such contradiction. . . . Only those who ruminate upon God's Word, day and night, will resist such temptations to compromise.[5]

There are exceptions where biblical counseling is unavailable at certain times. Included in this exception is the believer who has neglected his walk with God to such an extreme that a nervous breakdown suddenly occurs.[6] In this instance, hospitalization may be necessary for a few days and a psychiatrist may have to be utilized in the absence of a Christian physician to admit and manage the patient. While the patient is hospitalized and immediately upon discharge, the pastor or elder should supervise his care; and the psychiatrist's role should be primarily limited to management of medications.

These thoughts are radical to most Christians today, but God's full provisions for the growth of belivers are encompassed within the church, primarily the local body. Counseling has been surrendered to secular professionals, yet it is crucial to the spiritual health and the physical health of the church. Counseling by God's design falls within the domain of the church and the personal dynamic of the indwelling Holy Spirit. A biblical-medical ethic is needed to recover spiritual counseling and place it under the God-intended authority of the church.

Prayer For Healing

The sign read, "NO ADMITTANCE, HEALING IN PROGRESS."[7] Betty Farmer was scheduled for surgery the next morning, but in her hospital room were several elders who had come to anoint her with oil and pray for her. Only a short time had passed since the x-rays of her colon (barium enema) had shown the pathognomonic "apple core" configuration of cancer. Betty and her husband, Ray, had decided to "call for the elders of the church," as well as to utilize modern surgical technique. Surgery was performed as scheduled, but the presence of cancer or any other abnormality could not be found anywhere in her abdominal cavity. For completeness, a colonscope (lighted tube) was passed twice to the midtransverse colon, but it also revealed no lesions. The sign on her door following surgery read, "HEALING COMPLETE. PRAISE THE LORD." This anecdote illustrates a case of probable miraculous healing which fulfills our healing criteria.

Adam and Eve were created with perfect health and thus would have lived forever. Following their sin, however, they became susceptible to physical disease and faced certain physical death. On this basis all sickness immediately bears a cause and effect relationship to sin; even though the relationship of sinful thoughts and behaviors to disease may or may not be clear. Disease may even be planned by God (John 9:2-3; John 11:4), or sent by Satan (2 Cor. 12:7; Job 2:5-6) without personal sin as the direct etiologic agent. Most illness results from sinful choices (lifestyle). The position of Scripture is equally clear that sin is not *always* causal. These distinctions of cause and effect are necessary because much harm may occur even with biblical balance.

James 5:13-17 is a unique passage in the New Testament because it places the church squarely responsible for the care of the sick, but every pastor and lay person should do a sound exegesis of these verses to decide what they should do in practical application.

> Is anyone among you suffering? Let him pray. Is anyone cheerful? Let him sing praises. Is anyone among you sick? Let him call for the elders of the church, and let them pray over him, anointing him with oil in the name of the Lord; and the prayer offered in faith will restore the one who is sick, and the Lord will raise him up, and if he has committed sins, they will be forgiven him. Therefore, confess your sins to one another, and pray for one another, so that you may be healed. The effective prayer of a righteous man can accomplish much.
>
> (James 5:13-16, NASB)

It would be unwise to neglect this passage which is explicit concerning the church and the care of its sick. Some might think that the following application would place elders and pastors in the uncertain and precarious position of evaluating and providing medical care. However our goal is to define the church's role in medical care and not allow it to be blocked by medical personnel and their treatment. Under current practice, it is not uncommon for the patient to become isolated from family, fellowship, and spiritual care.

Several conclusions may be drawn from these verses. First, the sick person is to "call for the elders of the church" (v. 14). The question then becomes which sicknesses and what degree of sickness; since no disease is specified, the believer can determine his need and initiate the action. The degree of sickness is a consideration because colds and other minor illnesses are so frequent they could create an unnecessary burden for the elders. The emphasis of the Greek verb, *astheneo*, is extreme physical or spiritual weakness and lack of strength. Perhaps the illness has so weakened the believer that he is unable to pray and must ask others to pray for him. In the practical application of this text, serious illnesses would qualify but would not necessarily have to be incapacitating. For example, the elders might be called prior to major surgery when the patient feels no ill effects. Major surgery is a life threatening state of health for anyone! In any situation it would seem appropriate that the elders respond when called.

Secondly, the elders are explicitly expected to: (a) pray over the person and (b) anoint (*aleipho*) him with oil. (v. 14) The first action is self-explanatory. There is disagreement about the second action. Oil is frequently a biblical analogy to the Holy Spirit. Thus, the anointing could be symbolic of the involvement of the Holy Spirit: to attribute the work of the Holy Spirit to the oil itself is "trite and common."[8] Since oil was frequently used as a medicine in biblical days, some commentators have concluded that the oil is representative of all ministrations of the physician. Further, *aleipho* (anoint) may be used for the application of oils and ointments. There are difficulties, however, with this interpretation. First, the context is clear that the elders anoint. If the elder was the sick person's physician, the interpretation might include what the physician does. Rarely, however, is that the case. Second, the oil is applied externally ("anoint"). The inclusion of internal medication and surgical procedures is a considerable departure from the external application of an innocuous substance (oil). Neither of these reasons, however, excludes the use of medical treatments. My contention is that this passage does not direct Christians to use physicians in general. The simple act of anointing with oil followed by prayer is the literal interpretation. How can the church neglect such a simple instruction?

Thirdly, the elders are to determine whether the sick person has sin which needs confession and repentance (vv. 15-16). The literal interpretation of the entire passage is fully consistent with our idea of sin as the frequent etiologic factor in illness. Others have recognized this relationship.[9] Confession leading to healing is a literal interpretation (v. 16). This passage, then, involves more than the simple call and response of the elders. First, every person who has a significant illness should be interviewed by an elder to determine whether sin exists that might be directly or indirectly related to the illness. This interview must be without an accusative attitude or manner (Gal. 6:1), but it should be done. Common evidence which bears out this association is seen by family physicians who find that members of stressed families are frequently in their offices with a variety of illnesses. Second, the causal relationship may be suggested in preaching or teaching. If any in the congregation are frequently ill they should examine their lives for unrepented sin. As above, it should be explained clearly that all illness does not have sin as a direct cause, but sin's significant contribution should result in a *spiritual* examination as well as a *physical* examination. The Holy Spirit will convict and disclose sin in these instances when it is present (Ps. 139:23-24).

Fourthly, several variables must be taken into account. (a) Although these biblical instructions should be carried out; healing is not automatic. Any effect or lack of it resides in God's sovereign will. The fact that God will work in these situations to heal or restore is verified by the literal context. On the other hand, the work of the Holy Spirit in a particular circumstance is unpredictable (John 3:8). A rite, even a sacrament, is not of itself efficacious. Many who are baptized never demonstrate any outward evidence of inward regeneration by the Holy Spirit. Further, participation in communion may result in the opposite of its intended effect (1 Cor. 11:30). (b) Literally, this passage in James states that the righteousness (v. 16) of the elders who are called is a factor in the result and certainly spirituality will vary among groups of elders. (c) The righteousness of the believer is an unstated but likely factor. For example, if the anointed person has conscious sin in his life and has no intention of confession and repentant change, God is unlikely to heal that person and allow him to continue in rebellion. Such healing would be inconsistent with God's plan for believers to increase in holiness. (d) The manner of healing is another factor. The anointed believer may be restored to complete health or may be healed of a particular crisis. (e) The ultimate factor against the occurrence of healing in every instance is death. No one would die if prayer for healing could be administered prior to death in each instance. To summarize these points, this practice may be efficacious at times but is not an automatic means of healing because God retains His sovereignty and purposes which are far beyond the understanding of man (Isa. 55:8-11; Rom 11:33-34), and variable factors which may inhibit or enhance healing are present in both the person and the elders involved.

In conclusion of this section, sin significantly contributes directly to illness, but not always as an etiologic factor. Evidence for personal sin should be sought by church officers but they must be gentle in their attitude and manner without trying to prove what is not readily confessed. James 5:13-18 should be exegeted and practiced by individual churches and/or denominations. Elders have these God-given responsibilities in the physical and spiritual health of their sheep. These responsibilities should not be neglected because of the attempted interference of hospital staff or physicians who might see these actions as unnecessary and detrimental. That is to say that elders should be sensitive and reasonable to accommodate medical personnel and their treatments. This passage directs church leaders to be involved with their sick and diligent to implement this instruction.

Balancing Hospital Policy and Spiritual Care

Jane Smith, a patient in her mid-fifties, had a type of cancer which was intermittent in its effect; that is, it would get better then worse over the course of months and years. One sudden exacerbation resulted in her hospitalization in an intensive care unit. She was an active member of a local church, but her parents were unbelievers. Because of hospital policy she was allowed only visits by her family with an occasional visit by her pastor. Prayer and Bible reading were quite noticeably uplifting for her, but this opportunity was only possible for a few minutes each day because of hospital restrictions to people outside the family. Her disease worsened and she died after several weeks.

Many details are omitted from this patient's complex medical problems, but those presented illustrate her suffering with only brief infrequent opportunities for spiritual ministry. Though the course of her illness would not have been any different, obvious comforts and sources of strength were available because many people were on hand to help. Yet, she was isolated from them for "health" reasons. Churches should realize that spiritual needs exceed routine visits by the pastor and plan means by which both the physical and spiritual needs of the hospitalized person may be administered. Christian physicians on hospital boards should propose flexible regulations that will permit such spiritual care. Usually, such care would not interfere with the best medical care, particularly with open communication between the hospital, medical personnel, patient, family and church officers.

The needs and desires of patients will vary with personality, the illness, the medical treatment and spiritual maturity. Some patients will want few or no visitors, others will desire more. Because of their illness, patients are usually unable to direct traffic themselves. Thus, one person may be designated as a patient advocate. This person may be a family member or another person close to the patient, but he must be a believer. The patient advocate could direct visitors, inform inquirers, answer the phone, and in other ways assist the patient. Also, he may inquire if any of the hospital staff are believers. Their presence will likely be an additional comfort and help to the patient. People who have been severely ill know the comfort of having someone constantly present who provides quiet but attentive companionship. Since patient advocacy requires twenty-four-hour coverage, others should be sought to help the advocate. He can instruct those who relieve him, but one person should retain responsibility for oversight. The advocate can be invaluable in the medical care of the patient.

With sensitivity to the provision of necessary medical care, church councils should challenge the isolation that results in intensive or coronary care units. Medical evidence exists that such isolation may be detrimental to the patient! Most units would not be inhibited in their function by the quiet presence of someone around-the-clock. The spiritual welfare of patients should be integrated with their physical care. A spiritual ministry will actually contribute to physical healing. This point is mentioned only in passing and is not central because the spiritual welfare of patients alone is sufficient indication to reconsider current practice and policy.

A pastor makes this plea to hospital staff:[10]

1. Please do not expect me to see one of my sheep during visiting hours only.
2. Please do not accuse me of bad timing.
3. Please do not deny me information I must have about the patient.

4. Please do not treat me as an enemy or an intruder.
5. Please do not think of yourself as the only one who is caring for the patient at this time.
6. Please do not assume that I am ignorant and untrained.
7. Please feel welcome to talk to me about these matters.

His experience validates the need for the church to be seen as an integral part of the medical team. From the perspective of the church, it should see itself as responsible for the spiritual care of its members in every situation.

Evaluating the Need for Hospitalization

The hospitalized person who is not seriously ill can use this time to reflect seriously upon his life and spiritual condition. In the fast pace of modern life, the inactivity of hospitalization may be a rare opportunity to have an extended time for meditation. Such reflection should include problems or patterns of living which may have contributed to the need for hospitalization. Often a fast pace and overscheduling results in stress and, subsequently, physical symptoms and/or disease. I have personally known many people, including knowledgeable and experienced Christians, in whom a chaotic lifestyle resulted in hospitalization. These symptoms may be psychosomatic but eventually real disease may develop.

Can hospitalization be avoided? The patient's physician can present the probabilities of real disease being present or absent and the possibility that a workup or treatment may be carried out on an outpatient basis. Also hospitals are dangerous. Although uncommon, some severe diseases may be acquired in the hospital setting. These problems result from immobilization, exposure to unusual infectious agents, medications, and other things which are unnatural and uncommon to the patient. Of course, hospitals should not be feared unnecessarily and they are essential to diagnosis and treatment care, but avoidance is desirable where there is a reasonable alternative. If appropriate questions are asked, patients will find that admission may be avoided frequently. Reflection upon one's lifestyle is essential to the possible avoidance of hospitalization. Self-corrections can be accomplished. Such lifestyle changes may preclude hospitalization.

Both medical and nonmedical Christians need to assess accurately the biblical morality and the true efficacy of common medical practices. The awe and overconfidence with which modern medicine is viewed has allowed it to encroach upon many areas not in its proper domain. Physicians and their practices need to be questioned, especially if the patient's family or elders do not understand the full implications of what is to be done. It is apparent that the general morality of physicians has declined with our cultural morality. Many medical procedures are not straightforward, as many patients who have seen two physicians and had two different alternatives suggested, are aware. The imprecision of medical choice and the current moral tenor of medicine mandates that the Christian, his family, and his church be active participants in medical decisions.

Two situations where alternatives to hospitalization should be sought are chronic and terminal illness. Nursing homes are one alternative; personal homes are another. Although each situation is distinctive, frequently day-to-day management of these patients is simple and straightforward. Most nonmedical people could be trained easily to provide necessary care for patients at home. Medical people within a congregation may consider such help as an area of ministry. One circumstance I know involves a family of two older women, neither of whom is able to walk, yet who are able to live together in a home of their own with the help of other members of their family and Christians who minister to them. It is a joy to see that they are able to live outside a nursing home where their intimate relationship would be seriously limited.

Health Education and the Church

To give some direction for sermons may result in an epithet—usually directed toward pastors as meddlers. The following comments point to health as a subject for sermons. The body is a temple of the Holy Spirit (1 Cor. 3:16-17,6:18-20) but some Christians teach that the body is intrinsically evil. The sinless perfection of Jesus Christ precludes His inhabiting sinful substance (John 1:14). In the Old Testament the temple had meticulous rules and regulations to govern its conduct and care. Likewise, the believer should care meticulously for the physical body, maintain it properly, and not abuse it.

The most definite causes of disease and death which could be called in are cigarettes and alcohol. Alcohol has been covered as a specific biblical prohibition, but cigarettes are causally linked to many types of cancer, heart attacks, lung disease, atheriosclerosis, restriction of growth of unborn babies and other disease. Smoking should be proscribed by the church, and counsel provided to assist in its cessation. Obesity is not as clearly linked to disease, but usually involves gluttony.

The health benefits from exercise are highly probable, but a difference of opinion remains among medical authorities. First Timothy 4:7 is a stronger exhortation toward exercise than the biological data. The latter provides guidelines concerning frequency, intensity, duration, and type of exercise.

Many Christians advocate certain health practices, such as natural foods and vitamins, but the data on which they depend is conflicting and uncertain. The results of a relatively new treatment, biofeedback, are best provided through the joy and peace of the obedient, repentant Christian. The few areas which have been covered indicate that simple health practices can have a profound effect upon health. Both spiritual and physical health are primarily to glorify God and only secondarily for the believer's benefit (1 Cor. 10:31).

Finally, pastors should seek to disciple Christian physicians. A great need exists for physicians to be evangelical, that is to be completely committed to Jesus Christ and the inerrant Scriptures and also be willing to consider that the best approach to health and ethics may not be that which is traditional or common to the medical profession. As the pastor exhorts the physician to examine himself spiritually, and the physician shows a growing responsiveness, the physician could be directed to additional reading sources—those which are suggested at the end of each chapter. Those books which question medical practice from the biblical and nontraditional viewpoint are especially indicated. The extensive growth of medicine dictates that a growing number of these physicians discern those practices which are or are not scriptural and from that discernment to direct the universal church. The anti-Christian milieu of modern medicine with its political authority may lead the church to break off involvement with an unbelieving medical system. Let us pray that that day never comes, but such an eventuality is possible and should be watched for. It may even be a blessing in disguise if it increases the biblical and spiritual framework within which medicine is practiced!

NOTES

1. Paul Ramsey, *The Patient as Person* (1970; reprint ed., New Haven: Yale University Press, 1979), pp. 123-124.

2. Louis Berkhof, *Systematic Theology* (1938; reprint ed., Grand Rapids: Eerdmans Pub. Co., 1969), pp. 553-40.

3. John E. Woods, "Hospitals," in *Baker's Dictionary of Christian Ethics*, ed. Carl F. Henry (Grand Rapids: Baker Book House, 1973), pp. 299-300.

4. "Psychotherapy" is used here, as previously, to refer to the activity of all professionals who regularly counsel people concerning solutions or direction to problems and dilemmas of life. Psychotherapy connotes the "professional" concept and represents a primarily secular process, so "counseling" is the preferred word for what is essentially the same process.

5. Jay E. Adams, *More Than Redemption* (Phillipsburg, N.J.: Presbyterian and Reformed Pub. Co., 1979), pp. 8-9.

6. Although a nervous breakdown occurs suddenly, it is the result of weeks, months, or years of sinful practices. It is usually a physiological overload, similar to an electrical circuit overload, not a breakdown. The overload occurs because of improperly managed choices. For a thorough review of the process, see *You Can Avoid or Overcome a Nervous Breakdown*, a booklet written by Louis O. Caldwell and published by Baker House, 1971.

7. *Guideposts* (June, 1982); pp. 11-14.

8. John Calvin, *Institutes of the Christian Religion*, vol. II (Grand Rapids: William B. Eerdmans Pub. Co., 1979), p. 636.

9. The Report of the Committee on the Relation of Christian Faith to Health (Adopted by the 172nd General Assembly, May, 1960). The United Presbyterian Church in the United States of America, Philadelphia, PA, p. 320. Darryl McNabb, "The Biblical View of Ill Health," *Journal of Pastoral Practice* 3 (1) 1979: 67-73.

10. Donald R. Miller, "A Shepherd's Plea to Hospital Staffs," *Journal of Pastoral Practice* 1 (1) 1977: 23-24.

REFERENCES

Calvin, John. *Institutes of the Christian Religion* Translated by Henry
    Beveridge. vol. II. Grand Rapids: Wm B. Eerdmans Publishing
    Company, 1979.
McNabb, Darryl. "The Biblical View of Ill Health." *Journal of Pastoral Prac-*
    tice 3 (1) 1979:67-73.
McQuilkin, J. Robertson. "The Church." Class Notes: Christian Ethics.
    Theology 509 and 401. Columbia Bible College, Columbia, S.C.
Miller, Donald R. "A Shepherd's Plea to Hospital Staffs." *Journal of Pastoral*
    Practice 1 (1) 1977:23-24.
The Report of the Committee on the Relation of Christian Faith to Health
    (Adopted by the 172nd General Assemply, May 1960. The Relation of
    Christian Faith to Health. The United Presbyterian Church in the United
    States of America, Philadelphia, PA.

9 | Abortion: Historical and Legal Aspects

(Coauthored with Harold O. J. Brown)

> To kill the child in the womb by abortion is only anticipated murder.
> Tertullian. (Third Century)

With the number of abortions in the United States currently running at 1.5 million per year—or about one abortion to every two live births—abortion presently constitutes the first compelling life-and-death issue that most Americans are likely to encounter, especially in a situation which demands they can make a clear-cut ethical decision.

Abortion is a problem that thrusts itself with inescapable urgency on many sectors of American society. Unmarried young girls—and fellows—are lured, cajoled, or pushed into sexual intimacy not only before marriage, but often before attaining even a moderate level of psychological and emotional maturity. Many girls become pregnant and are totally unprepared to handle the situation. Friends, classmates, and sometimes (but not by any means always) parents are consulted. When children would prefer to conceal a pregnancy from their parents, sex educators and civil libertarians help them do so—although almost inevitably the parents will have to deal with the problems that result, even if the pregnancy is terminated by an abortion performed without the parents' knowledge.

Physicians are seldom involved in abortion against their will, although young interns and residents in obstetrics and gynecology are frequently compelled to assist in abortions or even to perform them in order not to lose their positions and possibilities of advancement. Nurses, operating room attendants, and other health-care personnel are less privileged than the doctors. Despite U.S.

government regulations permitting them to refuse to participate in operations they oppose, they may simply be discharged for refusal to cooperate and securing redress is long and difficult. Many personnel not directly involved in the abortion procedure have to participate in one way or another, taking medical histories, performing laboratory work, preparing the patient for the procedure, and the like. One of the grislier abortion-related tasks includes disposal of the "products of conception," a technical term referring to the placenta, the amniotic sac, the umbilical cord—and the baby.

Conscience clauses supposedly protect health care personnel from being obliged to work on abortion cases. On the other hand, both federal and state court decisions as well as many individual laws and regulations oblige hospitals to provide all "medical services," including abortion procedures. Groups such as the American Civil Liberties Union and the National Abortion Rights Action League have been at the forefront of successful efforts to force hospitals, including religious ones, to provide abortions, regardless of their convictions. Every year, six to ten million individuals are confronted with the problem of abortion, some of them—physicians, nurses, social workers, and other health care personnel—over and over again.

The Grim Statistics

Since 1973, the year of the infamous abortion decision known as *Roe* v. *Wade*, abortion has touched, directly and indirectly, more people than the Vietnam War and the draft ever did. And this leaves out of account the 1.5 million tiny victims who are, in John Calvin's prophetic words, "robbed of the life they had not yet begun to enjoy."[1] Abortion, beyond a doubt, is a situation where more Americans face an ethical dilemma than in any other life and death issue. What about the theoretical reason for the importance of abortion? The German Supreme Court gave it with precision in the preamble to its abortion decision of 1975; which prohibited abortion on demand, even in the first trimester, as a violation of the fundamental human right to life.[2]

The German court squarely and explicitly acknowledged that it was dealing not with the question of whether or not a certain right may be derived from a constitutional document, but rather with "problems in the area of biology, especially human genetics, anthropology, but also of medicine, psychology, sociology, and political sociology, and not least of ethics and moral theology. "The import and seriousness of this question of constitutional rights becomes apparent when we consider that we have here to do with protection of human life, a central value of every legal order.[3] It is no accident that Francis Schaeffer and C. Everett Koop devoted the first episode in their film series, *Whatever Happened to the Human Race?* to abortion. What will ultimately become of the human race certainly depends to a large extent on how it deals with abortion; because abortion, and the way we deal with it, will be symptomatic of what we think about human life and how we value it.

Abortion is taken directly from the Latin *abortio*, originally meaning premature birth or miscarriage. Since ancient times, premature births often resulted in the death of the infant.[4] Etymologically the old Latin term abortion means "untimely appearing" and does not necessarily involve the death of an untimely fetus—it could be a premature birth and did not necessarily imply a deliberately provoked miscarriage involving the death of the fetus, contrary to the modern German term *abtreibung* which is literally "driving away" or "driving off."

Less than two years ago in English and American medical parlance, abortion referred to a spontaneous, accidental, or provoked incident that resulted in the death of a relatively premature fetus. If the fetus was full term or close to it, the incident was not called a spontaneous abortion but a stillbirth. The deliberate abortion of a full term fetus was unheard of and would have been called infanticide. Today, such fetuses can legally be aborted in the United States and thousands are killed annually.

In most countries that allow abortions, second trimester abortions are allowed only for grave medical reasons and third trimester abortions, which are considered the equivalent of infanticide, are not allowed at all. Caesarian sections are performed instead. *The United States must be recognized as the only country where abortion in the third trimester, right up to birth, can legally be obtained if a physician can be located who is willing to affirm that it is "medically necessary."* The judge of the "medical necessity" of a late abortion is in almost every case the physician who performs it.

Prior to the late 1900s, the vast majority of the incidents referred to as abortions were medical accidents caused by disease, fetal deformity, or injury. In other words, they were called "miscarriages" in common parlance and "spontaneous abortions" in medical language. In addition to unintentional miscarriages, a very small number of abortions were induced for medical reasons. These were called therapeutic because they were held to be necessary to heal, i.e. prevent death or serious injury to the pregnant woman. Abortions induced for nontherapeutic reasons were not unknown, but were almost universally regarded as immoral as well as illegal, and hence were called criminal abortions. The concept of the criminal abortion made the term "abortionist" a bad word, morally on the same level as "terrorist" or "extortioner" until recent years. Today, "spontaneous abortion" has more or less been dropped from medical parlance. Abortion now generally means deliberately induced abortion and is divided into two categories: therapeutic, involving the relatively small number of procedures thought to be medically necessary for the sake of the pregnant woman's life or health; and elective, close to 1.5 million per year, which are performed in deference to "freedom of choice" apart from any therapeutic goal or significant medical indication.

The reality of abortion on demand in the United States has made the older terms "spontaneous abortion" and "therapeutic abortion" all but obsolete. The vast majority of abortions can be designated "elective" i.e., performed on the basis of "freedom of choice" without any necessity of a medical nature. Today abortion may be defined as the extraction or expulsion of the immature fetus from the uterus, resulting in its death.

The History of Abortion

In antiquity, abortion was available but seldom practiced. Ancient techniques, and indeed all abortion techniques until recent times, were very dangerous for the woman. Consequently women would only seek abortions when they felt themselves to be under tremendous pressure to conceal a pregnancy. In addition, infanticide, or the killing of newborn infants, was widely practiced and in some cases even had the complete sanction of law. Inasmuch as it was not illegal to kill an unwanted child after birth, practical Greeks and Romans usually waited until the child was delivered before deciding whether it was wanted or not. Moral codes and civil laws that permitted abortion also permitted killing newborn babies and the killing of newborns was completely without danger to the mother.

Ancient medicine was familiar with situations in which it was not possible to give birth to a baby without endangering the mother or even costing her her life. The most common situation was one in which the baby's head was too large for the birth canal and a normal birth became impossible. Once the child's head was wedged, it was impossible to save its life with the medical skills of the ancient world. The condition, if allowed to persist, would soon take the life of the mother as well. Today such problems can be anticipated and forestalled by Caesarian section, but back then it was impossible to do major abdominal surgery without anesthesia and antiseptics. Caesarian takes its name from Julius Caesar who was delivered by such a method, but this was immediately following his mother's death. Had she still been alive, she could not have survived the operation. Ancient authorities, such as Hippocrates, the "father of medicine," (460-375 B.C.) and Soranus of Ephesus, the "father of gynecology," explain how a woman can be saved when the child is wedged in the birth canal; its head can be crushed with forceps, permitting the physician to extract it dead, but saving the life of the mother.

The only modern parallel that is at all common is the case of ectopic pregnancy, or tubal pregnancy, in which the newly-conceived zygote implants itself and begins to grow *ek-topou*, literally, "out of place," usually in the Fallopian tube. If allowed to develop, the fetus will soon rupture the tube, almost certainly causing the mother's death as well as its own. Fallopian tube pregnancies are normally ended by excision of the fetus. Under current medical conditions, it has not yet become possible to save the life of a fetus growing in a Fallopian tube. Nevertheless, the removal of a tubal pregnancy is not normally called an abortion. Perhaps a major reason lies in the intent of the pregnant woman and her physician. The death of the fetus is not desired, but is accepted as an unavoidable and tragic necessity. Most women with tubal pregnancies desperately want to save the child. If and when it becomes possible to save the baby in ectopic pregnancy, it will mean that the gestational age at which infants can be saved has been pushed back so far that it will no longer make sense to speak of abortions, even quite early in pregnancy, as involving "nonviable" fetuses.

The birth of Louise Brown, the first "test-tube baby," in the summer of 1978 clearly demonstrated that conception can take place outside the. womb. After being conceived *in vitro*, outside the womb, or literally, "in glass," the embryonic Louise Brown was carefully implanted in her mother's womb. It is not yet possible to replace the uterus as the place where a baby can live through the early months of its prenatal life, and thus Fallopian-tube embryos, although several weeks older and many times larger than Louise at implantation, cannot yet be saved by any readily available techniques.[5]

Ancient medicine was familiar with other techniques and rationalizations for destroying the developing child by abortion before birth. Even though both pagan Greeks and Romans traditionally practiced the exposure of unwanted infants, leaving them to be killed by wild animals or to die of starvation and inattention, their leading physicians discouraged abortion. In his oath, Hippocrates included the pledge not to provide or even counsel abortions, and for over two thousand years physicians have sworn to have nothing to do with abortion. Prior to the advent of Christianity, the Hippocratic Oath and the medical standards it inculcated were followed only by a minority of physicians. It was intended to raise the standards of medicine, but it did not find universal acceptance in the ancient world until Christianity combined both the biblical and Hippocratic view that man is made in the image of God. With the advent of abortion on demand as a widespread and lucrative medical procedure, most medical societies in the English-speaking world have dropped their opposition to abortion and abortionists, and a number of medical schools have formalized their disregard for the Hippocratic Oath by replacing it with pledges such as the one to "do nothing illegal."[6]

In the early centuries of Christendom, abortion, like infanticide, all but disappeared. It was sporadically practiced in medieval Europe, usually by Jewish physicians, some of whom salved their consciences by interpreting Genesis 2:7 to mean that human life does not begin until the baby takes its first breath. Nevertheless, because all techniques were dangerous to the pregnant woman and because the universal Christian conviction that abortion was tantamount to infanticide, deliberate abortion remained a relatively rare occurrence.

Legal History of Abortion

The legal history of abortion takes place almost entirely in the past 150 years; or since the time when medical science first understood exactly how human life originates. The union of sperm and egg to produce a new, individual zygote was first observed in 1875, but postulated somewhat earlier. Thereafter medical societies in all of the scientifically advanced countries worked to outlaw abortion, which was also becoming medically practical for the first time with the introduction of anesthesia and antiseptics. Even so, abortion was generally condemned by Christian doctrine and church law but was not often the object of direct legislation.

Two of our most ancient legal documents, the Code of Hammurabi and the

Middle Assyrian Code do contain explicit prohibitions of abortion.[7] Pagan Roman emperors, in an effort to stimulate and protect family life during the decadence of the empire, also legislated against abortion, but such efforts were sporadic and apparently had little impact. After the conversion of the Emperor Constantine to Christianity, the Empire was rapidly Christianized and abortion all but disappeared. It is probable that the virtual disappearance of abortion as a practice is the explanation for the fact that there was little specific anti-abortion legislation even on the part of Christian emperors.

Abortion was a crime at common law in the English-speaking world, although prior to "quickening," the old term for the imprecisely-determined point at which the mother begins to feel the baby's movements, it was widely regarded as less serious than afterward. The concept of quickening refers to the beginning of life as the expression "the quick and the dead" in the old form of the Apostles' Creed. Life was incorrectly thought to begin when the mother could first feel the child's movements. Because all scientists and health care personnel know that the child is in fact alive long before the mother feels it, in fact from the moment of conception, the term quickening has largely been replaced by viability. The concept of viability refers to the ability to survive without extraordinary aid outside the womb. Like quickening, it is a very imprecise concept and does not refer to any actual change in the developing fetus, but rather to the ability of modern medical science to sustain its life. From the beginning of the third trimester onward, fetuses are increasingly viable even with techniques available in ordinary hospitals, and in a few cases viability has been pushed back to the twentieth week of pregnancy. The concept of viability, like the earlier concept of quickening, is a rough-and-ready term with no clear-cut medical significance. Unfortunately viability has been adopted by the United States Supreme Court as a criterion for the permissibility of abortion. In *Roe* v. *Wade*, the Court held that fetuses before viability may be aborted on demand and are not to be protected in any way by law. *Roe* v. *Wade* seemed on superficial reading to allow the possibility that states might restrict or even prohibit abortion after viability. For this reason *Roe* v. *Wade* is often incorrectly described as "permitting abortion early in pregnancy," or "permitting abortion during the first trimester." In fact, however, *Roe* v. *Wade* explicitly permits abortion *without restriction up to the beginning of the third trimester*, and allows it *during the third trimester* whenever there is any question of the woman's health being adversely affected by the pregnancy—in other words, even in the third trimester *Roe* v. *Wade* provides for virtual abortion on demand.

The question of ensoulment derives from the assumption that man is essentially dichotomous and that the soul is "an immortal, yet created, essence".[8] If the soul is separately created by God while the body results from the union of sperm and egg, it is relevant to ask when the newly created soul is joined to the body: at conception, or several weeks later. The Bible uses the dichotomous language of soul and body, but on occasion it also uses trichotomous language, speaking of body, soul, and spirit. The Court took an interest in this issue only because it wanted to use the uncertainty this issue raises to justify taking the life of a fetus as if it had not yet received·its soul and thus was not yet truly human. Jesus told his hearers not to fear those who can destroy the body, but not the soul (Matthew 10:28). If the Supreme Court was consistent, it should have no objection to murder or capital punishment because they also destroy the body.

Even if one adopts the dichotomous view of man, the concept of the time of ensoulment is not really relevant to the issue of abortion and certainly not for the civil law because the soul is always present in human life. Many Protestants, particularly those influenced by Luther, hold what is called traducianist view of the origin of the soul. The soul is an offshoot of the parents' souls, just as the body is an offshoot of their bodies and it is in harmony with our fundamentally wholistic view of human beings. Although the traducianist viewpoint is gaining followers, the majority tend to follow the Calvinistic and Roman Catholic tradition of "creationism," the view that God specially creates a new immortal soul to go with each new human being conceived.[9]

Most Christians who are "creationists" simply hold that God creates a soul and ensouls the developing child as soon as human life begins. Indeed, the Latin word for soul is *anima*, used to designate a sentient being as opposed to vegetables and minerals. Because they were not sure that the fetus was alive until the woman could feel its "quickening," it was possible for medieval Christians to suppose that it had not yet received its *anima*, its soul. Nevertheless, many authorities assumed that the soul was present from conception. Today, scientific evidence confirms that the fetus is animate from conception.

The problem—or pretext—of ensoulment arises because one very important medieval theologian, Thomas Aquinas (1225-1274) followed the classical Greek philosopher Aristotle in assuming that ensoulment occurs forty days after pregnancy has begun in the case of a male baby, and eighty days afterward in the case of a female. For centuries Thomas Aquinas' teaching has been the foundation of Roman Catholic theology. It is strange to observe our modern Supreme Court following Aquinas and Aristotle on a scientific question. In any event, even the arguments of Aquinas would not permit abortions after forty or eighty days—which E.R.A. advocates would have to reduce to forty for every fetus. Finally, we should note that Aquinas was not considering the permissibility of abortion when he brought up the topic of ensoulment, but rather the question of whether a baby that miscarried should be baptized.[10]

Ensoulment was irrelevant to the permissibility of abortion because it was consistently forbidden. Since the justices of the United States Supreme Court permitted abortion throughout the entire period of pregnancy, it is apparent they cited Aristotle and Aquinas in *Roe* v. *Wade* to show that ancient and medieval authorities did not offer valid information on the supposed time of ensoulment. They did not deal seriously with the self-evident implication of the question—namely that every abortion after ensoulment would take a human life.

If one adopts a dichotomous view of human nature and a creationist view of the origin of the individual soul—and probably the majority of orthodox Christians adopt both—what is one then to say about the time of ensoulment? There are three different events when something of decisive significance occurs in the life of the fetus. Christians, in various historical periods, have proposed each of these events as the occasion on which ensoulment occurs. We have already mentioned "viability." It is not an event in the life of the fetus, for it is active and alive from the earliest stages following conception. Viability is a reflection of the development of medical technology at the present time; just as "quickening" refers to the perceptions of the mother-to-be and not to any event in the life of the fetus. If we disregard quickening or viability there remains only conception and live birth.[11]

A few professing Christians allege—contrary to all medical and biological knowledge—that human life begins with live birth. Some simply base this on a naive interpretation of Genesis 2:7: "Then the LORD God formed man of dust from the ground, and breathed into his nostrils the breath of life; and man became a living being." While it is true that Adam did not become fully human until God breathed life into him, it certainly does not follow that Adam's descendants are not human until they draw the first breath. Adam had no human ancestors. His humanness was a direct endowment by God, who made him in his own image and put the breath of life into his nostrils. In other words, it is impossible to generalize from Adam, just as it is from Eve. Each of them was formed in a unique way. But since Adam and Eve, except for the virgin-born Saviour, all human beings have been formed by the union of gametes from two human parents. Hence, it is correct to say that Adam *became* human because he was once less than human ("dust of the earth"). This cannot be said of any of Adam's decendants, who are never anything other than human from the very first.

A somewhat more sophisticated argument is used by some Christians—not necessarily in connection with the issue of abortion—who take a mystical view of breath and the process of breathing. Identifying "breath" with "spirit" and connecting "spirit" with the Holy Spirit, they then argue that man is not truly human until he breathes.[12] We should note that this theory is purely speculative and lacks substantial biblical foundation. In addition it is without any scientific warrant. While science cannot disprove such an unverifiable contention, it would be unfortunate to burden the Christian doctrine of man with an assertion that makes no biological or scientific sense and that appears to ignore God's relationship to man before birth.

Some attempts to justify abortion on the basis of the time of ensoulment involve several questionable assumptions: the human being is fundamentally dichotomous, and the soul can be joined to the body at some specific time during bodily development; the time of ensoulment is either late enough to permit early abortions, or sufficiently indeterminate so that abortions can be performed without being absolutely certain that they are destroying human beings; the concept of ensoulment is the determining factor as far as Christian opposition to abortion is concerned; the state, in determining abortion law, may accept the opinion of some Christians concerning ensoulment as justification for its own refusal to accord legal protection to developing human lives before birth.

Nothing scientifically discernible happens to the fetus at birth to make it anything different from what it was just before birth, i.e. a developing human child. Normal physical birth is common to all human beings and is a natural process. It can readily be observed by natural science. A human being, if he exists at all, is always a human being.[13] We certainly cannot deny *a priori* that a change can take place in us that is indetectable by the tools of natural science. But if such a change were to take place, i.e. if one "became human" in a mysterious way at the end of gestation, then how would we expect to know about it, since according to the hypothesis it would be scientifically indiscernible? It would have to be taught in Scripture—but "humanization" is not taught in the Bible. Even if Genesis 2:7 applied to the whole human race since Adam, to make this eccentric theory the basis for allowing the destruction of a child before it draws it first breath, is certainly inconsistent for a Court and a government that usually prides itself on operating only on wholly secular principles. One wonders why the Supreme Court took up this line of thought in the first place. From the Christian persective, we should note that there is not biblical support for the position that *human* life begins with the first independent breath, *except in the case of Adam himself.*[14]

As we now recognize, the concept of "quickening" is purely subjective and does not refer to any change in the life of the fetus at the time of birth. The fetus goes through no transformation or change of nature perceptible to science, and Scripture does not suggest that it at that time "becomes" anything that it was not already. That leaves the possible time of ensoulment as occurring at conception, when the new human being comes into existence. Since the pioneering work of Oscar Hertwig in 1875, the medical and scientific world has known beyond doubt that a new human life begins at conception.[15] It was not until 1981 that some noted medical figures, in an attempt to support what they consider the "socially necessary" freedom of abortion on demand, have denied that they know when life begins. One noted proabortionist, Leon Rosenberg, M.D., of Yale University Medical School, went so far as to testify before a United States Senate Subcommittee that "science has no criteria for determining humanness.[16] If Dr. Rosenberg was correct—and his argument is a question of definition, for he defines "humanness" as a "value," and then says that science has nothing to say about values—there is no scientific evidence that he himself is human and hence no "scientific" reason for the government to protect him from being killed.

There is, in fact, no biological or medical doubt that at fertilization, a new, individual human life has begun. The only plausible way to deny this is to say that humanness is a matter of philosophical or theological definition, for that which has begun at fertilization is life, it is human, and it is a distinct individual. It possesses all the characteristics of the fully-developed adult. Professor Jerome Lejeune of the Université René Descartes in Paris says, "Science has turned the fairy tale of Tom Thumb into a true story, the one each of us has lived in the womb of his mother. . . . To accept the fact that, after fertilization has taken place, a new human has come into being is no longer a matter of taste or of opinion. The human nature of the human being from conception to old age is not a metaphysical contention, it is a plainly evident experimental fact."[17] From the perspective of science, if ensoulment is necessary for an individual to be a human being, then it must take place at conception, for there is no time after that when the being is anything less than or other than human.

From the Christian perspective, Roman Catholics and others who hold the creationist position concerning the origin of the soul have been forced to improve upon the position of Thomas Aquinas and to hold that life takes place at fertilization. As we have already noted, the creationist position itself cannot be demonstrated from Scripture, but if one wished to postulate a creationist origin for the soul, then the only point at which Scripture permits us to think that ensoulment takes place is the point at which the human being comes into existence, namely, at fertilization. To the extent that Scripture makes reference to babies in the womb, it attributes to them individuality, personhood, humanness and God's direct, personal interest in them.[18]

"Monster," perhaps surprisingly to nonmedical readers, is a medical term that defines "a fetus or infant with such pronounced developmental anomalies as to be grotesque and usually nonviable."[19] Traditionally, the Roman Catholic Church baptizes these conditionally, not knowing whether they have souls or not. Some Protestants have raised this question as well.[20] This position is not consistent with the inevitable conclusion of our prior discussions.

The argument might be presented: all humans have eternal souls; the only nonarbitrary point of ensoulment is conception; therefore, all conceptions are humans.[21] In reference to monsters, this conclusion jars our rationality, but it also presents us with the grotesque and devastating effect of sin. Still, is no other conclusion possible?

We have defined "human" as life which has an eternal soul, yet have proceeded to a biological argument. Is this reasoning inconsistent? No, it is not because we are limited in our analyses to empirical data. One's definition must be theological, but practically, two limitations require biological criteria for this definition. First, beyond the concept that a human is a unity of body and spirit, the Bible gives no criteria by which a soul can be determined to be present or not. Thus, any biological definition that is biblically consistent presumes the presence of a soul. This presumption is crucial and awareness of it must not be lost. Second, beyond biblical criteria, the metaphysical nature of the soul prevents any empirical analysis. Thus, no biblical or empirical criteria exist by which the presence or absence of a soul may be determined. Any measurable criterion of ability, whether physical or mental, destroys the whole argument upon which pro-life Christians stand. For example, an anencephalic (a baby without a brain) could be said to be nonhuman because it does not have a brain. That argument seems simple until one asks how much brain constitutes a human. Immediately, we are back to the quality-of-life ethic.

Most people have heard the argument that we are all imperfect in one way or another. Let's take a closer look. ". . . every person is a carrier of between five and eight recessive, nondominate, deleterious genes that would cause serious disorders if properly paired."[22] In other words the pairing of those genes from each of our parents could have resulted in each of us being a monster! That realization should make us both humble and thankful for the degree of wholeness that God has given us.

Arguments by Christians for or against abortion on the basis of personhood are fallacious. To define personhood in such a way as to exclude some human beings, necessarily involves some set of physical, mental, or moral criteria. These will necessarily be entirely arbitrary. Such arbitrariness is out of place within the biblical world view, particularly with reference to a definition of human personhood.

> Any product of human conception is, by definition, human. Tracing the development of human personhood is appropriate in the areas of morality, cognition , and psychosexuality; such an effort is inappropriate in the field of medicine; it can only lead to the slippery slope of Nuremberg"[23]

In Conclusion

To summarize the above, that which has an eternal soul is human, biblically. Because no biblical or empirical criteria for the presence or absence of a soul exists, we are left with the necessity of a biological identification of humans. Any definition other than a conceptus is entirely arbitrary. Personhood is a deceptive, but eventually lethal, thin edge of the wedge. Arguments that monsters are not human are similarly deceptive and lethal. In all honesty some monsters, gross deformities that they are, may not have been given souls by God. Both consistency of argument and avoidance of a lethal weakness, however, require that every conceptus be considered fully human. The argument of both traducianism and creationism from Christian theological tradition add further soundness to this conclusion.

Some final points are important. First, the abortion issue is a crucial one and abortion principles are much easier to clarify than infanticide and euthanasia. Therefore, abortion more accurately reflects the individual and societal value of human life. If abortion does not become strictly regulated by law and personal morality, human life will become valueless and the evolutionary principle, "survival of the fittest," will prevail. I grieve that my profession not only performs abortions, but fights to defend them as moral medical procedures. Second, there is some correspondence between a Christian's position on abortion and his faith. The Scripture is clear that God is intimately and personally involved in the creation of each human life. Scripture even teaches that God forms us in His mind prior to the existence of time, in eternity past (Ps. 139:16; Jer. l:5). Abortion is a violation of the Sixth Commandment. Certainly, one's position against abortion cannot be equated with one's being a Christian since immaturity as a Christian and lack of good teaching are limiting factors. Nevertheless, for a well-informed and thinking Christian, to advocate destruction of life is inconsistent with being a child of the Author of life. This chapter gives a logical and biblical foundation to the principle that human life begins at conception—that includes all conceptions regardless of abnormalities.

This latter statement should not be confused with the question of the legal status given to unborn life. In our legal system there are examples where individuals do not have full legal rights. Organic brain disease may result in a person losing his legal status to a guardian, but that does not mean that he can be killed at any time and for any reason. Opponents of legislation that life begins at conception overstate the implications of this law. Jurisprudence already recognizes the gray areas and extenuating circumstances of the existence of life. The physician who makes an unavoidable error is not charged or punished to the same degree as one who is careless or malicious. Under such anti-abortion legislation the accidental death of a fetus from medical or surgical intervention would be totally distinct from intentional killing. The physician would not be charged with murder, as some claim.

Third, granting human status to deformed babies does not mean that all that can be done medically should be done. Many recognize that the moral way to deal with terminally ill people is to withhold or stop treatment. (We will discuss these situations in chapters 11 and 12.) The same principles can be applied to the other end of life, the unborn and the newborn. Judgments have to be made concerning what treatment is moral or immoral based upon the special circumstances of each patient and his prognosis. Allowing a natural process to result in death is totally distinct from active killing. The Sixth Commandment forbids killing except in declared war and capital punishment. Even in the situation where a mother's life is threatened by the continued presence of the baby in her womb, biblical morality requires that every effort be made to save both *at every stage of the process* and that neither should be actively killed.

Fourth, we should be aware of numbers and percentages of abortion. Approximately 1.5 million abortions occur annually in the United States. By comparison there are approximately 3.3 million live births and approximately 1.9 million deaths of all other causes. Thus, we are actively killing almost as many humans as die otherwise. Abortion deaths and all other deaths combine to exceed the number of live births! Turning to percentages, pregnancies from rape are extremely rare. The number of pregnancies from incest is unknown, but certainly are rarely reported. Significant congenital abnormalities comprise one to two percent of pregnancies. Pregnancies which threaten the life of the mother are less than one percent. Mental illness is too imprecise a category to be included as a reason for abortion at all. Thus, these common (but unbiblical) arguments in favor of abortion comprise less than five percent of current abortions. Over ninety-five percent are performed for convenience or preference alone! This staggering number should motivate one to work against abortion. In another place Dr. Brown has challenged Christians:

> If we will not react to the substitution of ancient religion (which was the basis of the Supreme Court decision to liberalize abortion) . . . for biblical values, to being obliged to help fund the extermination of one-quarter of the future generation, then we will probably react to nothing.[24]

A Christian's response to the legalization of abortion does reflect his moral sensitivity and intellectual undertanding of Christian (biblical) values.

Finally, for both the Christian and the non-Christian there are only two positions: pro-life, or pro-abortion. The so-called moderate and pro-choice positions are essentially pro-abortion since they compromise the Sixth Commandment and the principle that life begins at conception. Inactivity in educating others and in working toward legal prohibition of abortion promotes abortion. It may take some time for a Christian to study and think through the abortion issue, but the world desperately needs articulate, well-informed Christians who will defend the sanctity of human life.

NOTES

1. John Calvin, *Commentaries on the Four Last Books of Moses* (reprint ed., Grand Rapids: Baker Book House, 1979), p. 42.

2. Harold O. J. Brown, "Abortion: Rights or Technicalities?," *Human Life Review* 1 (3) 1975: 60-74.

3. Ibid.

4. An example is the difference of opinion regarding the Hebrew words of Exodus 21:22, literally rendered, "and her children go forth." Does this refer to a premature birth, as John Calvin, Keil and Delitzsch, Umberto Cassuto, Walter C. Kaiser, and a host of other commentators, ancient and modern, Christian and Jewish, insist, or can it mean miscarriage and imply the delivery of a dead infant, as Luther's translation implies and a certain number of modern writers, including the translators of the Revised Standard Version and the Living Bible as well as J. Barton Payne and Meredith G. Kline contend? The present writers prefer premature birth. Because this text has been abused to hold that the Scripture teaches that the unborn child is not fully human at this point we will anticipate the fuller discussion to follow in order to note that even if one allows the translation "miscarries," as Bruce Waltke does, we should follow Walkte, Cassuto, and others in refusing to see in Exodus 21:22-25 any reference to deliberate abortion. The text refers to violence in which a pregnant woman is accidentally involved, with possible injury to herself and to the child she is carrying. It says nothing about *abortus provocatus* (deliberate abortion), which is what the word in the modern sense involves.

5. There still remains a period of about twenty weeks at minimum between fertilization and the earliest point at which a developing child can be kept alive outside the womb. Of course, many second trimester abortions and all third trimester ones take place after the fetus has become potentially or definitely viable. Approximately 30,000 abortions after twenty weeks of gestation took place in 1978 (*Human Life Review* 7 (4) 1981: pp. 95-96).

6. Such a pledge would not have kept Hitler's physicians from participating in extermination programs and human experimentation, as in the Third Reich it was all perfectly legal.

7. Harold O. J. Brown, "What the Court Didn't Know," *Human Life Review*, vol. 1:2 (Spring, 1975), pp. 5-21.

8. John Calvin, *Institutes of the Christian Religion*, vol. 1, chap. IV, article 2, trans. Henry Beveridge (Grand Rapids: Eerdmans, 1979), p. 160.

9. This "creationism" is not to be confused with the creationism of the evolution debate, which is about the origin of life.

10. Roman Catholics traditionally baptize infants born dead and unbaptized persons immediately after death on the basis of their conviction that the baptism may be valid if the soul has not yet fled the body. That baptism is a necessity if the soul is ever to enter the presence of God.

11. In recent years the term "conception" has taken on an unfortunate ambiguity. Traditionally it has referred to the union of sperm and egg, out of which a new individual arises. However, in certain rare cases (homozygous or identical twins and so-called mosaics) individualization is not complete until the zygote implants itself in the wall of the uterus several days later. The term "fertilization" in now frequently used instead.

12. See the interesting work of Arthur C. Custance, *Man in Adam and in Christ*: Doorway Papers, vol. 3 (Grand Rapids: Zondervan, 1975).

13. The concept of "humanization" or "hominization" is both slippery and dangerous. To speak of "making man human" in the sense of more humane sounds fine, but it suggests that some or most people are not yet human, and thus implicitly that they are dispensible. It also is double talk. As Dr. Paul Marx is fond of saying, "No one talks about ratification. A rat is always a rat, never anything more or less.

14. Most Bible-believing Christians hold that Adam was specially created by God as described in Genesis 2 (some hold that the "dust of the earth" means a previously existing, highly-evolved subhuman). But most of those who support *Roe* v. *Wade* do not believe in a real Adam made by the breath of God. Hence their use of this argument is deceitful.

15. Oscar Hertwig, *Lehrbuch der Entwicklungsges chichte der Menschen and der Wirbel thiere*, 6, Auflage (Jena: Gustau Fischer, 1898).

16. Published in the *Chicago Tribune* (Tuesday, May 12, 1981).

17. Jerome Lejeune, "In Re New Humans," *Human Life Review* vol. 7, No. 3 (Summer, 1981), p. 64.

18. See familiar texts such as Job 3:3, 9-13; Psalms 51:5, 139:13-16; Jeremiah 1:5; Hosea 12:3 and Luke 1:41, 44.

19. Dorlands *Illustrated Medical Dictionary*, 25th ed. (Philadelphia: W. B. Saunders, 1974).

20. Carl F. Henry, ed., *Horizons of Science* (San Francisco: Harper the Row Pub., 1978), p. 141.

21. Pro-life people must be careful not to state that humans consist of 46 chromosomes because some rare examples do not. For example, Turner's Syndrome has 45 chromosomes and Klinefelter's Syndrome has 47. The latter, in particular, may have normal intelligence and a somewhat normal life.

A hydatidaform mole may mimic pregnancy in its early months. A ridiculous argument is sometimes raised, and might be here because of my position, that a mole is a product of conception, and therefore human. A mole does derive from part (the sac which surrounds the baby) of the conceptus but it is an abnormal growth (tumor) no different from a tumor that develops on any part of the body at any time of life. An embryo may be present, although it never survives, further indicating that a mole is not a product of conception any more than any other tumor is a human.

22. "Genetic Revolution," *M D Magazine* 23 (8) (August 1979):69-79.

23. Carl F. H. Henry, ed., *Horizons of Science*, p. 137.

24. Harold O. J. Brown, *Death Before Birth* (Nashville: Thomas Nelson Publishers, 1977), p. 157.

REFERENCES

Brown, Harold O. J. *Death Before Birth*. Nashville: Thomas Nelson Publishers, 1977.
Dorland's Illustrated Medical Dictionary. 25th ed. Philadelphia: W. B. Saunders, 1974.
"Genetic Revolution." *MD Magazine* 23 (8) (August, 1979):69-79.

10 | Psychotherapy: Friend or Foe?

Psychotherapy, as psychology and psychiatry, needs the most critical and detailed examination by evangelical Christians.[1] Many practices in medicine are not clearly dictated by biblical principles, but this overlaps spiritual areas because the goal of psychotherapy is to counsel people to make changes in their thoughts and behavior. Moreover, since the Bible is the Christians's only infallible rule of faith and practice, a conflict of directions with secular psychotherapy is usually unavoidable. Many Christians are influenced more by the concepts of secular psychotherapists than by the Word of God. Psychologists and psychiatrists in evangelical seminaries often teach psychotherapy under the title, pastoral counseling. Since the training of many of these individuals is predominately or wholly secular with little or no formal theological education, their presence demonstrates the emphasis upon secular theories and methodologies.

It is to the discredit of Christians that this statement appeared in a recent journal: "Compatibility is possible, both theoretically and in practice. Our study revealed that there is no conflict between religion and psychiatry".[2] By contrast the apostle Paul spoke of incompatibility of biblical thought and worldly philosophies (2 Cor. 6:14-7:1). The deception of Christians that has resulted from an eclectic process needs to be reviewed if we shall continue to develop a biblical-medical ethic.

The following argument is directed immediately toward the psychotherapies. Ultimately, however, the argument must be directed toward the church, pastors and laymen alike. The church has allowed psychotherapists to teach and practice in the void that has been vacated by the church because she has not recognized the naturalistic philosophical and ethical principles upon which psychotherapy is based. With very few exceptions both theologians and pastors

have failed to give priority to, or make thorough application of, biblical principles in their theory or practice. For example, anthropology is either neglected
entirely or superficially developed. If one searches among so-called Christian
psychotherapies for a thorough biblical anthropology or reference to a systematic
theology that contains a thoroughly developed biblical anthropology, he searches
in vain. Such neglect or superficiality is deceptive at best, and opposed at worst,
to evangelical Christianity. Thus, judgment, and therefore reformation, must
begin with the household of God (1 Peter 4:17).

One Sunday after the worship service, I was approached by the son in a
family who were members of our church. His mother, Mary Jones, was sixty-
years-old and having a problem with depression. Electro-convulsive therapy
(ECT) or shock treatment was recommended as the only approach for her current episodes. The recommending psychiatrist rarely suggests this alternative
but he saw no hope of change. He concluded that such problems late in life
involve such ingrained thought and behavior patterns that such persons rarely
respond to psychotherapy or drugs. She was already on two kinds of ''nerve''
medications. Because of the son's anxiety over ECT and because they were
members of my church, I hesitantly agreed to meet with her and to try to determine whether I might help.

The situation was overwhelming. Unquestionably, severe depression was
present. The mother was not making simple decisions, such as planning daily
activities or grocery shopping. When she read Old Testament accounts where
families were killed, she would cry. Usually, she refused to go to church or
to visit anyone. She had considered suicide. Overall, she didn't enjoy life. She
talked of her depression as though it were an outside force: ''It just came on
me,'' and ''I don't know how to get it away from me.'' She considered herself
a burden to her family.

As I gathered further history, events in her life during the past ten years
were startling. Her husband had died suddenly of a heart attack. Within a year
she was diagnosed as having ulcerative colitis and abdominal surgery was performed three times. During one surgery she had had a permanent colostomy
(the terminal portion of the large intestine was fixed to the skin of the abdominal
wall with defecation into a plastic bag). She was concerned about her appearance
to others and saw the colostomy as interfering with her self-image. Within the
past few months she had severely fractured her shoulder and her doctor had
told her it might be immobile when it healed. Five brothers and sisters had
developed various chronic diseases. One had committed suicide. Finally, she
doubted whether she was truly saved because she thought that her lack of faith
was the reason she was not completely healed of her physical problems.

How should I respond? It seemed that her depression was an unavoidable
response to her numerous and significant problems. I was a family physician
with two months of limited psychiatric training. This woman had seen three
psychiatrists in the past, and currently a fourth one, who had coincidentally
been one of my instructors. At that point I had had three counseling cases which

involved a total of eighteen hours. An experienced psychiatrist had seen no alternative but ECT. Could she have a endogenous (chemical) depression which would necessitate ECT to restructure the biochemical composition of her brain?

Drugs: Prescription for Depression?

Psychotropic drugs are most commonly prescribed in an attempt to affect thinking, emotion, and behavior.[3] This use is based upon the premise that there is a biochemical alteration which one of these drugs will correct; once more permitting the patient to function efficiently. In addition biochemical abnormalities are sought as explanations of various symptoms and signs which have been labeled "mental illness." Therefore, a place to begin a brief analysis of thought, emotions and behaviors is the current scientific understanding of these processes.

A basic textbook in neurophysiology, the study of the brain and nervous system, provides a representative sample of other texts and literature.[4] The cerebral cortex is considered the highest level of activity of the nervous system but:

> It is ironic that we know least about the mechanisms of the cerebral cortex of almost all parts of the brain, even though it is by far the largest portion of the nervous system (p. 192).

> Our most difficult problem in discussing consciousness, thoughts, memory, and learning is that we do not know the neural mechanism of a thought (p. 198).

> Despite the many advances in neurophysiology during the past half century, we still cannot explain what is, perhaps, the most important functions of the brain: its capability for memory (p. 199).

> Now we need to consider the mechanisms by which the brain performs complex intellectual operations, such as the analysis of sensory information and the establishment of abstract thoughts. About these mechanisms we know almost nothing . . . (p. 202-203).

> We are left with an unanswered question: what is the locus of the initiation of voluntary motor activity? (p. 177)

> The basic mechanisms by which the brain accomplishes its diverse acts of attention are not known (p. 182).

These brief excerpts illustrate the lack of scientific certitude in neurophysiology. However, based upon such speculative research many neurologists, psychologists, and psychiatrists claim competence to make sweeping judgments about mankind. The scant scientific underpinning does not permit such comprehensive judgments.

Depression and its treatment by tricyclic compounds is one example of the application of neurophysiological research. A review article about the use of tricyclic compounds appeared in a leading medical journal recently.[5] Some initial comments concern the biochemical etiology of depression, called the "amine hypothesis:"

> Just how the *postulated* decreased aminergic function is mediated in depressed patients is *not yet clear*, although it is currently *believed* to be a genetically transmitted biochemical defect. The relative importance of serotonin versus norepinephrine has also been *debated*, although present *theories* accommodate both neuro-transmitters. . . .
> Current evidence suggests that these predictions might hold, but much *more work* needs to be done to validate it.[6]

The italics indicate those words which reflect uncertainty and tentativeness. Their conclusions concerning the clinical applications of these drugs are ludicrous for a "scientific" paper. Further,

> Many patients with depression improve *spontaneously* (more, *infra*), which probably accounts for some of the enthusiasm about the benefits from the tricyclic antidepressants. . . . The most compelling evidence for their efficacy is in patients with endogenous depression, a diagnosis that is often *uncertain*.[7]

Other research studies show conflicting evidence concerning the ability of these drugs to alleviate depression. One reason for such inconsistency is the difficulty of evaluating subjective complaints in patients. This difficulty is known by all researchers for it involves relative and thus imprecise judgments. To further confuse this "science," some psychotherapists do not think drugs are indicated for depression at all, and if so, only rarely. In summary, the use of tricyclic drugs in depression is "debated," and is based upon probable "theories" of action, which are themselves based upon "believed theories" of the biochemical cause of depression which "might be true." The statement sounds silly but it is an accurate reflection of the above quotes and the science of the use of psychotropic drugs in depression . Other psychotropic drugs in other "mental illnesses" show similar characteristics.

An example of the evangelical acceptance of such weak evidence appeared in *Moody Monthly* magazine.[8] Although the author makes a brief acknowledgement that "research into the biochemistry of depressive illness has not as yet produced proof of any particular biochemical theory of disease," his professional authorities are psychiatrists who prescribe drugs for 50-80 percent of their depressed patients. In addition, they recommend that these drugs be tried for at least three months followed by a different drug if that one does not work. The article is extremely unbalanced with a strong bias in favor of the use of drugs; it inaccurately represents the available research, an example of which was cited above. Worse, it implies that God's resources for depression are inadequate and that historically since these drugs have only been available in the last twenty years, Christians had no hope of overcoming their depression.

Precautions must not be restricted to psychiatrists. Another article on antidepressants reported that 70 percent of prescriptions are written by non-psychiatrists, mostly physicians in internal medicine or family practice. One class of tranquilizers (benzodiazepines) was reported to be prescribed 82 percent of the time by nonpsychiatrists.[9] A national invitational conference concluded that drug therapy among primary care physicians was often used excessively and indiscriminately.[10] The frequent use of these drugs should cause reflection for the believer in the light of Jesus' command not to worry and His promise of peace (John 14:27) without anti-anxiety medications.

Brief, but thoroughly representative evidence has been presented. The incidence and prevalence of prescriptions for these drugs is without empirical support in the medical literature. With such a base and because of problems connected with research itself, a great deal of precaution, rather than indiscriminate acceptance, should be practiced.

The Uncertain Etiology of Mental Illness

The prevalence of psychosocial problems under the umbrella of biological medicine is reflected by various studies. The number of patients seen, evaluated, and treated by nonpsychiatric physicians exceeds 50 percent of all patients who are classifed as having mental health disorders.[11] Patients with supposed mental disorders use nonpsychiatric medical care twice as much as patients without such diagnoses.[12] Of the patients seen by primary care physicians approximately one-half have problems due to "psychosocial" causes rather than biomedical problems.[13] From these data, one can conclude that a significant proportion, perhaps a majority, of a primary care physician's time and effort directly involves care without evidence of organic disease. It is upon this basis that a heavy emphasis is being placed on the training of family physicians to manage these problems.[14]

These problems present a unique opportunity for the Christian physician, but also a warning to Christian patients that they will probably receive drug treatment, rather than biblical counseling for these problems. Christian physicians are missing the opportunity because most are unaware of biblical counseling methods. All physicians, as well as psychiatrists and psychologists, are intimately involved in situations where biblical counseling is the "treatment" needed, not a biomedical approach. God's rich and powerful resources need to be made available to the believer in every area of medical care.

The historical development of psychiatry points out its underlying assumption:

> Even though evidence was lacking for an organic explanation of some important types of mental disorder, early workers assumed that brain lesions would ultimately be found in all.[15]

The following excerpt indicates that little, if any, progress has been made toward organic explanations, since schizophrenia is the most studied of the mental disorders:

> The cause of schizophrenia remains obscure. . . . Although research trends are promising, the hope of discovering a biochemical origin or marker

. . . remains unfulfilled . . . understanding of the nature of schizophrenic disorders remains crude, and ability to treat them successfully remains limited.[16]

Psychiatric diagnoses are under constant revision. Recently the Third Edition of the *Diagnostic and Statistical Manual of the American Psychiatric Association* was published. This manual gives new definitions and descriptions to psychiatric diagnoses. Such changes raise questions about previous theory and research, since all patients who were diagnosed under the previous criteria would have to be recategorized in many research studies.

Finally, there is research on the latest and most (technically) sophisticated biochemicals, the endorphins:

> For several years psychiatrists and neuroscientists have explored a possible association between mental illness and an imbalance in the brain. . . . This approach is part of the trend toward researching for biochemical, rather than developmental, cause of mental illness. A possible link between psychosis and dysfunction in a brain system that is affected by morphine (an endorphin—like substance) was first advanced by psychoanalysts. Experimental support for this link came in the mid 1970's. . . . Somewhat confusingly, however, there is data to support both an endorphin-*excess* and an endorphin-*deficit* basis for psychiatric symptoms . . . studies based on a simple endorphin theory of psychosis have not been fruitful . . .[17]

If consistent, accurate biochemical defects were known to be the etiology of mental illness, then psychiatrists could treat such patients as a physician treats any patient with medication. Research, however, cannot provide consistent biochemical evidence for any so-called mental illness.

How much less can psychiatry speak authoritatively to a patient's thoughts and behaviors? Upon such uncertainty, common practices that masquerade themselves as medicine have been established. Laymen may not be able to examine this evidence but no word of these uncertainities is heard from Christians who are active in these fields and critical examination of statistical and empirical methods is lacking. Biblical direction and hope for individuals has been substituted with a hopeless etiology—a sickness for which there is only an uncertain cure.

In order to retain balance, some benefits of medication in some disorders seem likely; for example, patients who are uncontrollable and psychotic (dysfunctional in everyday life). Even so, a biblical approach may be successful in lieu of, or in conjunction with, drug treatment. It must be underscored that such situations under the large umbrella of "mental illness" are rare—probably one percent or less. The unusual situation should not dictate the usual approach. Even though the biochemical complexities in psychotherapy are so uncertain, they are less important than the incomplete and erroneous application of biblical principles by psychotherapists who are Christians.

Can Psychiatry and Christianity Be Integrated?

Should I try to help Mary Jones? Our pastor, with ten years of pastoral experience had chosen not to counsel her, referring her to the non-Christian psychiatrist who recommended ECT. In the past her personal physician had also directed her to psychiatrists. Christians in both psychology and psychiatry have spoken and written of the integration of Christian principles in psychotherapy. Pastors have been trained by these and non-Christian professionals. The majority of Christians believe that psychotherapy can help Christians "cope."

I was thoroughly familiar with nouthetic counseling and had counseled my previous three cases on this basis with positive results.[18] The nouthetic approach to depression would require Mrs. Jones to resume her daily responsibilities. Her family had been very carefully instructed by her orthopedic physician to wait on her; otherwise the shoulder might not heal properly or she could fall and reinjure it. To accomplish this, the family had arranged for a lady of similar age to move in with Mrs. Jones. She was not permitted to do many things and was never allowed to do anything without assistance.

To direct her to have daily responsibility for herself, would be going against the advice of both a psychiatrist (recommended by our pastor) and by her orthopedic doctor (a Christian). My advice could potentially aggravate her physical and emotional status. The majority of Christian and professional opinion was contrary to the approach that I believed to be correct.

As if that weren't enough to dissuade me, Mrs. Jones' past history pointed out that well-intentioned Christians could be wrong. About three years previously some enthusiastic Christians were emphatic that she could be healed of all her physical problems, *if* she had enough faith. She did believe God had the power to heal her, so she stopped all medications, was "prayed-over" several times and expected to be healed. Nothing happened. According to their theology it was her lack of faith that prevented God's healing. Although her faith had sustained her through past crises, it was not, according to them, sufficient for healing. At that point she began to doubt her salvation. Fortunately, her son had taken her to a Christian psychologist who helped her through that crisis with a biblical explanation of faith and healing. She had functioned adequately since then, but improper application of biblical principles could cause spiritual doubt once again. There was much in the situation that made me hesitant and apprehensive.

A "successful" integration of psychotherapy and Christianity seems to have occurred among most professionals and laymen. Christian periodicals regularly have articles written by professing Christian psychotherapists; their textbooks are used at all levels of Christian education; referral consultations from pastors are made to *both* believing and nonbelieving psychotherapists. The evident conclusion is that psychiatry is able to provide an essential component to Christianity. If this component is essential, then Christians prior to Freud must have missed out. Psychiatry is supposed to provide insights into the Bible and personality which give new dimensions to the believer's understanding of himself, salvation, and especially sanctification.

Psychiatry will be discussed here and psychology excluded because a critique of psychiatry's role in conjunction with the Christian faith has not yet been published, although several books along these lines have been written by non-Christians. In addition, several books have been written in critique of psychology by Christians containing brief discussions of psychiatry. A critique of psychiatry necessitates an understanding of medicine and no Christian psychiatrist or physician has yet criticized his discipline that way.

A thoroughly biblical critique of psychotherapy is *Competent to Counsel* by theologian, Jay Adams.[19] He demonstrates the power of change which has always been available to the believer but has been obscurred, even denigrated, by psychotherapists. Of particular importance is the God-ordained responsibility of the leaders of the local church to counsel its members. Other books by Dr. Adams have further developed a biblical approach to counseling. One, the *Christian Counselor's Manual*, is thorough in its provision for counselors.[20] As such, it should be read by all Christians because of its practical approach to the Christian life. A more recent book, *More Than Redemption*, is a beginning development of a theology of counseling.[21]

It is crucial in any discussion of psychotherapy to recognize its inherent ethical and metaphysical implications. An understanding of such implications is the only approach which will clearly reveal the incompatibility of both theory and application between secular and biblical presuppositions. Some physicians recognize these relationships:[22]

> . . . one realizes that every psychotherapist sooner or later goes beyond the strictly psychological sphere . . . to the consideration of problems which are no longer psychological but spiritual, problems such as the meaning of life and of the world, of disease and death, of sin and faith, or one's own scale of values . . . as soon as there is any question, in the course of treatment, of the patient's attitude to himself, to others, toward life, and toward God, we have left the technical sphere for that of morality and metaphysics. The doctor at this point is no longer engaged in psychotherapy, but in soul healing.[23]

> The efforts of psychology and psychiatry to divest themselves of philosophy have been recognized as futile, since *every system requires the assumption of premises that cannot be proved.* Moreover, these disciplines have inevitably found themselves, when they set out to help troubled people, working in the *ethical realm, where values cannot be evaded.* . . . In a more direct way than any other medical specialty, *the psychiatrist's philosophy of life becomes involved in the therapeutic relationship.* Psychiatry remains "a practical art with scientific aspirations."[24]

The practice of psychotherapy licenses the therapist to be involved intimately with psychotherapy (literally meaning "soul healing"). Every evangelical believer should know that the soul is the prerogative of the Holy Spirit and

His Word *only*. The best counselor should be the most spiritually mature and biblically knowledgeable person available. Psychiatrists have spent far more time in secular study than biblical study. It is natural that the training which has received the most attention will have the most influence upon their practice.

A common practice which illustrates an incorporation of naturalistic principle concerns man as a trichotomous being: body, soul (or mind) and spirit. Although I believe that man is dichotomous, the focus here is not between trichotomy and dichotomy but who does "soul therapy." Many psychotherapists who are Christians believe that the physician should care for the body, the psychotherapist for the soul, and the pastor for the spirit. Such a belief is totally foreign to the biblical pattern for man. How can believers voluntarily engage in a search for understanding of their problems with instruction that is derived from naturalistic values? Since psychotherapy is inherently an intimate encounter, going to an unbeliever or a believer who practices according to naturalistic principles, is to form an unholy alliance that is forbidden by Scripture (2 Cor. 6:14-16). Such a fundamental error clearly illustrates the failure of most Christian psychotherapists to have an elementary grasp of biblical principles.

One issue of the *Christian Medical Society Journal* is a representative example of Christian psychiatrists' misunderstanding of biblical principles. The Affirmation of Faith of CMS is essentially evangelical. However, the superficial manner in which these Christian psychiatrists handle biblical truths place biblical authority in the background rather than giving it the preeminence it deserves. The issue, "Psychiatry and Christianity" contains no reference to Scripture as the historical rule of faith and practice of orthodox Christianity.[25] For such treatment of the Bible, the reader can only receive the impression that psychiatry has more important things to say than the Bible. The word "integration" is a key theme which is prevalent throughout the article. "Integration" describes the process of merging psychiatry with Christianity. The term is a commmon one used by Christians who are involved in psychotherapy. It will be useful to examine briefly some of the articles in this issue.

Dr. Malcolm Beck states, "Both psychiatry and Christianity seek to release man from the bonds of guilt."[26] He does not, however, distinguish between true guilt which is a state of being (culpability before God due to our inherited nature in Adam, Rom. 5:12-19), and intentional or unintentional personal transgression of God's law, and false guilt which violates tradition, childhood teaching or other authority which provokes a sense of guilt. The gravity of this omission by Dr. Beck is apparent; since forgiveness of biblically-defined true guilt is the essence of the necessity of Christ's Atonement, the central truth of Christianity. False guilt by contrast, can be remedied with biblical counseling.

In another article J. R. Runions, M.D., states, "Only on a biological view of man can we come to an understanding of the substrate of human behavior."[27] The biblical accounts are thorough in their analysis that human behavior is generated from within man's heart or soul not by his biological self. Again, this understanding of man is a central truth of the Christian faith. Only when man's spirit is regenerated by the Holy Spirit, can he and his behavior become acceptable to God. Apart from regeneration man cannot, and will not, live a life which fulfills either of the two great commandments by which Christ summarized the law.

Dr. Mansell Patterson, M.D., discusses various typologies relative to psychotherapy.[28] Early in the article he states that psychotherapy is involved in "the every day problems of every day life of everybody" and that psychotherapy is a "normative enterprise." In his last paragraph, however, he concludes that it is sometimes right to be a Christian therapist and other times a secular therapist. Christianity, not psychiatry, is the *only* "normative enterprise" because it involves the plan of reconciliation between man and God and those directives for life which are acceptable to God. To be a secular therapist is to direct, either actively or passively, the patient in a non-Christian manner which is directly contrary to God's normative plan. Christ says "I am the way, the truth, and the life." His "enterprise" is the only normative one.

These psychiatrists have made errors which strike at central biblical truths concerning justification and sanctification—concepts which determine the eternal destiny of men. Any discipline which blurs or minimizes eternal values is a stumbling block and runs the risk of being an alternative to God's scriptural plan.

Another example of the relative unimportance of Christian principles to psychiatrists is found in a psychiatric textbook that is written by a Christian.[29] A. M. Nicholi has written for several Christian periodicals, yet he ignores Christian truths in this text. For example, Christian references do not appear in the index; no statements direct a person toward Christ or the Bible. Such a total neglect of salvation, holiness, peace, and other eternal values strongly implies that Christianity is not important to one's mental health. Such omission by a Christian, which amounts to a denial of truth is incomprehensible. How can "mental health" exist apart from the salvation offered by Christ?

A frequent slogan in these discussions is: "All truth is God's truth." I agree with that statement. The rub comes in the test for truth. In psychotherapy, which of the nearly three hundred varieties does a person choose? Theories conflict and research has serious methodological flaws. With such disarray, the test for truth must come from outside. For the Christian that test is the Bible. If the Bible is the final test of truth in psychotherapy, why is it necessary to seek theoretical or experimental validation of that which is already known to be true? Why not circumvent such an indirect and laborious methodology with a biblical approach; especially with God's promise that He has "granted to us *all* things pertaining to life and godliness . . . in order that by them you might become partaker of the divine nature" (2 Peter 1:3,4). These promises lead to moral excellence, knowledge, self-control, perserverance, godliness, brotherly kindness, and Christian love (2 Peter 3:5-8). A person with those characteristics is in the epitome of "mental health!" How can the relative and changing "truths" of psychology and psychiatry add to such human achievement? "All truth is God's truth" but biblical revelation is always the starting point as well as the final test.

John White, M.D., formerly a pastor and currently a psychiatrist, has a brief chapter entitled, "Psychology or Religion" in a most recent book. His comments are incisive:

> My point is that what I do as a psychiatrist and what my psychologist colleagues do in their research or their counselling, is of infinitely less value to distressed Christians than what God says in His Word. . . . Christian counselors are influenced more than they realize by such psychology, which besides being shoddy, it is at its roots profoundly anti-Christian. . . . I believe it is essential that psychologies of any brand be subjected to the most rigorous examination in the light of Scripture.[30]

For whatever reasons that psychiatry has been found appealing to Christians, examination of its applied theology shows its serious defects. If psychiatry was objectively scientific, its integration which theology would have validity because all truth is ultimately compatible in a Christian-theistic universe. Biochemically, however, psychiatry has a weak and inconsistent scientific foundation. Such weakness coupled with theological error can only lead people astray. This danger cannot be overemphasized. Most psychiatrists who profess Christianity are a serious hindrance, and even antithetical, to the cause of Christ because of their authoritative, but mistaken, influence in the name of Christ.

Psychotherapy: Science or Art?

Jeff Smith had been treated for several physical problems by a physician at a local hospital. Since one of his problems was atherosclerosis of his heart, his marital problems and his frequent reference to Christian beliefs were thought to be related to mental deterioration caused by a similar process in the arteries of his brain. He was a convinced believer, knowledgeable about the Bible, an active member of a local church, and active in evangelism. His psychiatric and psychological evaluations contained such comments, as these: "religious delusional systems which seem to be organic brain syndrome (the atherosclerosis) caused" and "interprets reality through his religious beliefs." It is apparent what his evaluators thought of Christianity: His "generalized anxiety disorder," "obsessive-compulsive personality traits" and organic brain syndrome had produced his beliefs in a transcendant reality. The scientific diagnosis had been made! In reality, it was presupposed.

Modern economic constraints have forced a review of many programs relative to their cost effectiveness. The federal government, as the largest spender for health-related service, is making such analyses. Morris Parloff, Ph.D., extensively reviewed the psychotherapy literature.[31] His results summarize the "scientific" foundation for psychotherapy; and they confirm earlier reports about the lack of efficacy for psychotherapy—which dates back to the 1950s.

Dr. Parloff describes professionals and their practic⟩   ⟩sing psychotherapy:

> Psychotherapy is not a profession but a varied and sometim⟩   ned
> set of practices engaged in by members of a number of diff   ofes-
> sions. Each profession requires that its members be trained firs   ⟩imar-
> ily to *do something else*: medicine, psychology, social work, nursi⟩   ⟩ligious
> ministering. In short, psychotherapy represents ancillary act⟩   ⟩ngaged
> in by various professionals whose preparation in the area of ⟩   ⟩therapy
> may be (is) *quite variable*.[32]

> In short there is *little agreement* regarding what is to be inclu   ⟩ithin the
> perimeter of psychotherapy and, more important, *little consensus* aʋout what
> is to be excluded from its *progressively elasticized* boundaries.[33] (emphasis
> added)

These statements show that psychotherapy is not a well-defined theory or practice, although common usage by lay and professional people strongly implies
that it is. Since many psychotherapies are similiar, these nonexclusive, all-
inclusive psychotherapies depending on the categorization, number several
hundred.

Dr. Parloff proposed that the field of psychotherapy cannot claim lack of
developmental time for failures to achieve definitive research results. He quotes
Dr. Martin Orne:

> Modern psychotherapy antedates modern physics, biochemistry, molecular
> biology, behavioral genetics, and many other highly developed disciplines.
> We can no longer excuse the lack of hard clinical and scientific data either
> by the newness of the field or by the complexity of its problems.[34]

These statements paint Dr. Parloff's additional conclusions along with the remainder of psychotherapeutic research into an inescapable corner. In essence,
psychotherapists have had ample time and resources to demonstrate their
effectiveness, but have failed to do so.

Dr. Parloff continues with a concern for psychotherapy's harmful results.
He observes that a consensus of clinicians agree that "psychonoxious effects"
may occur if psychotherapy is "improperly or inappropriately conducted."

> It may be *assumed* that most psychotherapists act in a manner consistent
> with what they believe to be the patients' enlightened best interests. . . .
> Witness that anyone, mental health professional or not, is permitted to of-
> fer the public *any* form of psychological treatment that his/her ingenuity
> may devise *without* first having to demonstrate its effectiveness or its safety.[35]

Dr. Parloff does not realize the problem of determining the standard by which
the results will be evaluated. Lacking an objective standard, how can anyone
except Christians, determine whether a therapy is in the "best interests" of
the patient. Some therapists become sexually involved with their patients.
Although most professionals decry such therapy, it still happens. Why? The

answer lies in morality and ethics. They never recognize the underlying moral assumptions which place psychotherapy squarely upon its base—metaphysical *assumptions* from which morals are derived. So they continue in sin and "abnormality" according to God's decree.

Parloff presents summaries of approximately 700 published and unpublished controlled studies in which more than 90 percent demonstrate that the treated group was more improved than the untreated group. However, this effectiveness loses much of its impact once realized that there was no measurement of the "magnitude" of the effect. That is, the degree of effectiveness was not reported. Another summary included 475 controlled studies, 66 percent of which included random, not selective, assignment of patients to the treatment or control group. The latter remained untreated, placed on a waiting list, and then received placebo treatment or a second form of psychotherapy. These 25,000 patients averaged 16 hours of treatment by 78 different forms of psychotherapy. At the end of the treatments, 80 to 85 percent had better outcome measures than the controls. Dr. Parloff concludes:

> The size of the effects of psychotherapy can now be judged to be not merely modest but demonstrably great. . . . These findings . . . give persuasive rebuttal to the widely held view that psychotherapy is simply the beneficiary of spontaneous remission.[36]

He calls these results "good news," but turns to the "puzzling news" that certain characteristics seriously limit this apparent efficacy. Summarized, eleven major findings are:[37]

1. No clinically significant differences among the seventy-eight varieties of psychotherapy were found.
2. Fifty percent of the treatment effect is lost two years after completion of therapy. Since studies rarely go beyond that time, it is unknown how much more of the effect will be lost.
3. The more females in the treatment group, the better the results.
4. Patients did better when their therapists were similar in ethnic group, age, social, and educational status.
5. Patients who were chosen or volunteered, rather than randomized, showed greater effects than those selected at random.
6. Objective criteria, work adjustment, school adjustment, personality traits, and physiological reactions were less demonstrable of therapeutic effects than subjective criterias, global adjustment, self-esteem, personal development, and experiences of fear and anxiety.
7. Comparisons across professions and schools showed no characteristic differences in the effectiveness of treatment.
8. There is no relationship between the length of treatment and effect-size.
9. There is little evidence that level of experience is related to effectiveness.
10. The careful analysis of nearly 500 treatment outcome research studies still does not provide data adequate to answer the question of what kinds of therapy are most useful for what kinds of patients or problems.

11. Placebo effects account for about half the size of the effects which were obtained by "recognized" therapies.

A considerably larger proportion of these patients received treatment for "everyday" problems, for example, depression, anxiety, phobias, compulsions, life crisis, and marriage. Dr. Parloff reflects:

> Research has not yet answered the questions of what kinds of psychotherapy are most efficacious and cost-effective in the treatment of particular kinds of patients or problems. At present the method of psychotherapy, length of therapy, and training and experience of the therapist do not appear to bear any strong relationship to the effectiveness of psychotherapy.[38]

Since God's truth never needs empirical validation and since no method is distinctly valid, why not develop one from the Bible? Since God's valid promises could be available to both the "therapist" and "clients," this approach would be advantageous. Loss of effect would not be a problem because God promises to complete the process (Phil. 1:6). Since no mode of training is correlative, time could be spent in Bible study, prayer, and the other means to God's grace through which He promises effectual individual growth (John 15:5; Gal. 5:22-23), and through him to other people (John 7:38; Acts 1:7-8). Further, identity within a patient's life situation promotes the effectiveness of counseling.

How can any Christian who believes in the inerrancy of Scripture and its promises of temporal and eternal benefits to both the individual believer and those he influences, believe that the fuzzy conclusions of scientific evidence offer anything positively by comparison? Even Dr. Parloff, who has no apparent Christian identity, finds his analysis "puzzling." As a scientist, he leaves the "limits of science" in his final comments when he appeals to a "clinical consensus . . . to determine what is 'reasonable and necessary' treatment." In other words, since "we cannot use scientific evidence, we must use our heads."[39] Since he has presupposed the effectiveness of psychotherapy, he will settle for "consensus" arbitrarily. This method is science by majority vote; which is not science. At least he is clear once again that psychotherapy is not "scientific:"

> The best I can say after years of sniffing about in the morass of outcome research literature is that in my optimistic moods I am confident that there's a pony in there somewhere.[40]

What else convinces him but his faith, or metaphysical presuppositions in psychology!

Determining Biblical Principle and Practice

Masturbation as an exemplary topic demonstrates a common failure by Christian psychotherapists: the extension of the letter of the law to the spirit of the law. Such extension is a recognized principle of sound hermeneutics and a necessary part of a methodology for biblical ethics. Masturbation has also been chosen because it is one dimension of sexual immorality (*porneia*).

James Dobson, Ph.D., is well-known. His books are popular and his movie series, "Focus on the Family" has been seen in many churches. In one of the films and in his book *Preparing for Adolescence*, he states that the Bible is silent on the subject of masturbation.[41] He is mistaken. The letter of the law may not cover masturbation, but the spirit of the law clearly does since thoughts, motives, and actions are considered in light of Scripture. Even though Dobson does not encourage masturbation, he does not do so on biblical grounds but only because he is concerned about the subsequent guilt and habit-forming nature of the practice. Thus, he makes two more mistakes. First, true guilt can be resolved through the process of confession and repentance (1 John 1:8-10; Rom. 12:2). Second, a defeatist, "can't stop" attitude is unbiblical (Phil. 4:13; 1 Cor. 6:11). Both principles involve sanctification—to ignore these truths is to immobilize spiritual growth.

M. O. Vincent, M.D., comes closer to the biblical position on masturbation when he writes that the fantasies are lustful and condemned by Christ in the Sermon on the Mount.[42] Also, excessive masturbation is wrong. Then he states: "The Christian cannot oppose masturbation on the grounds that . . . Scripture specifically mentions or condemns it." From this position he believes that masturbation would be justified morally in certain situations.

Jerry White, an aeronautical engineer, a nonpsychotherapist, is more fully biblical than Dobson, Vincent and many other psychotherapists.[43] Only his lack of familiarity with psychotherapy prevents an unequivocol stance. Dr. White lists these guidelines to determine whether masturbation is sin:

1. Can you practice masturbation without engaging in sensuality or lust? (Galatians 5:19)
2. If you practice masturbation, can your mind remain pure? (Matt. 5:28)
3. Without question masturbation is an attempt to experience the same sensations meant to be experienced in marriage . . . a substitute for the real thing.
4. . . . masturbation is totally self-centered. (Eph. 2:3)
5. Finally, masturbation can put us in bondage. (1 Cor.6:12)

By these guidelines I fail to see how masturbation can be practiced without its being sin.[44]

Three reasons may be stated why psychotherapists do not arrive at a biblical position on masturbation. The most basic reason is ignorance of biblical interpretation. Second, they react against the false predictions of blindness, mental illness, and other dire events which popularly have been said to result from masturbation. Third, they may not know how to counsel the person who practices it. In this latter area again, Dr. White is insightful. He lists twelve practical suggestions for making progress against this sin which includes the biblical solution to guilt and the possiblity of total victory. He is convinced that masturbation is sinful based upon his knowledge and ability to seriously and biblically examine this issue. These factors do not require knowledge or training in psychotherapy. Further, he demonstrates that any serious Bible-studying layman can correctly determine biblical principle and practice.

This brief presentation on masturbation demonstrates one specific example in which a basic principle of interpretation is ignored by Christian psychotherapists. Although masturbation is not explicitly called sin similar to homosexuality (1 Cor. 6:9; 1 Tim. 1:10), the spirit of the law does clearly cover it as a sinful practice. Widespread failure to understand biblical solutions to such problems continues to plague psychotherapists.

Powers and Dangers of Psychiatry

The father of a junior high school student called to ask if I would counsel his daughter. She had attempted suicide by taking an overdose of pills. Emergency treatment had been simple and effective with little threat to her life since neither the kind nor the quantity of pills was lethal. After the first counseling session, he told me that the school required a statement that she would not make this attempt again. I sent the school a letter in which I stated that the daughter was involved in counseling and thought it was best for all concerned that she return to school. I assured them that I thought it was highly unlikely that she would attempt suicide again. At that point, the parents were informed that she could not re-enter school until she had been evaluated by a psychiatrist whom they had wanted to avoid in the first place! Thus, the school adminstration by their policy forced her to see a psychiatrist who did not hold the same values as the family. By implication the "omniscience" of the psychiatrist could be trusted, where other authority could not. The parents had *no alternative* if they wished to keep their daughter in school, so they complied.

The power of modern psychiatrists and psychologists should not be underestimated.[45] Their authority extends into the legal system, the family, personal freedom, schools, and the Supreme Court.

About sixty percent of admissions to psychiatric units in this country are involuntary.[46] The prevalence of such admissions varies from state to state, but in California a psychiatrist can order an extra fourteen days of confinement after the initial period. On that basis 75,000 patients are kept for that two weeks in institutions every year in that state. Although extensions can be challenged in court before the end of that time, only a minority request hearings. Of these, fewer than half are released. During that time psychotropic drugs can be given involuntarily. Thus psychiatrists have powers which places limits in our "free society." Practically, Dr. Morse reasons against this practice: involuntary patients are less likely to be amenable to change, legal problems tie-up the courts, lawyers, patients and doctors, and the average time now available for hospital-based psychiatrists to treat inpatients in only fifteen minutes per week.

Most schools of psychotherapy undermine self-responsibility. From Freud's unconscious drives to Skinner's mechanistic behavior, they all seek a cause that will place the responsibility somewhere else. Each person is completely limited by his genetic endowment and his social milieu. Such denial of personal responsibility is a denial of the Christian faith.

> . . . so long as you remain bitter and resentful, so long as you cannot accept yourself without resentment, you do not confess what you are to God; you only complain about it. Complaints never lead to healing. Confession does. . . . This is hard for many of us. We prefer to find reasons for what we are, reasons that diminish our own responsibility. Yet whether it makes sense or not we are responsible for what we are, as well as what we do. And the tragedy is that until we accept our responsibility we cannot be helped.[47]

The Bible nowhere excuses irresponsible behavior. Everyone is accountable for their thoughts and behavior (Rom. 1:18-2:16). Such personal responsibility distinctly contrasts psychotherapies and the Bible. Searching the indexes of psychiatric texts for references to self-responsibility and the will is pointless— there are no such references. If the will is mentioned, it is frequently treated negatively and in the individual is considered incapable of responsiblility. If self-responsibility were explicit the particular theory would fall. The Bible clearly and forcefully proclaims that personal choice to do God's will is the highest achievement for man (Matt. 7:21; Rom. 12:2; Phil. 2:12-13) and all of us are responsible to God for our choices.

"Cope" is common in the language of psychotherapy and has proliferated among Christians in the field. Its contrast with biblical texts demonstrates it is not clearly understood by those of biblical reality. Webster defines "cope" as the "ability to *maintain* a contest or combat usually on even terms or with success; to deal with and *attempt* to overcome problems and difficulties." Its application to life's problems involves one's ability to be equal to whatever challenge is encountered in life. Perhaps one could say that Christ "coped" at the cross and at the resurrection; or that Christ came that we might be able to "cope," rather than have the abundant life (John 10:10) or "Consider it joy, my brethren when you encounter various trials, knowing that . . . "You are able to cope (James 1:2-4) or "Do not be overcome by evil, but . . ." cope with evil by good (Rom. 12:21)? Reworked that way, these texts sound ridiculous, but they are the stated goal of those Christian therapists who try to help their patients cope. Any believer who uses the word, "cope," in such contexts has not adequately understood Christ's great sacrifices and the indwelling power of the Holy Spirit.

Lawyers frequently advise their clients to plead insanity or mental illness. Americans are familiar with accounts of criminals who are tried and sent to a mental institution instead of a prison. One such example involved the man who attempted to assassinate President Reagan. One authority has stated, ". . . data shows psychiatrists to be poor predictors of violence, and the vast majority of violent criminals are not mentally ill."[48] Fortunately, forensic psychiatry seems to be beginning to lose its influence in the courts, and the trend exists among psychotherapists to be less inclined toward the explanation that criminals are not fully responsible to stand trial for their crimes. Jonas Robitscher who has doctorates in medicine and law, has written extensively on the influence of psychotherapists in the courts in his book, *The Powers of Psychiatry.*

Without doubt, psychiatry was instrumental in the Supreme Court decision of 1973 which legalized abortion. Such a causal relationship is simple. Less than five percent of abortions fall under the reasons of rape, incest, and the threat of physical harm to the mother. That leaves more than ninety-five percent which must be justified in another manner.

> In attempting to legislate the legal availability of abortions, Congress and to a lesser extent, the state legislatures have recognized their lack of expertise in drafting criteria for the performance of therapeutic ("medically necessary") abortions. After being prodded by the courts, the legislatures have included that they must leave the answering of medical questions to the medical profession. . . . According to the Supreme Court . . . 'appropriate medical judgment' may include physical, emotional, psychological, familial, and personal factors. . . .[49]

In other words abortions may be performed for any reason considered "appropriate medical judgment." Psychiatric reasons may predominate, but then, psychiatry is a medical science!

History records the role which psychiatrists and other physicians played in the Nazi holocaust:

> Even before the Nazis took open charge in Germany, a propaganda barrage was directed against the traditional compassionate nineteenth century attitudes toward the chronically ill. . . . Sterilization and euthanasia of persons with chronic mental illnesses were discussed at a meeting of Bavarian *psychiatrists* in 1931. By 1936 extermination of the physically or socially unfit was . . . openly accepted. . . . The first direct order for euthanasia was issued by Hitler on September 1, 1939. . . . The decision regarding which patients should be killed was made entirely on the basis of . . . brief information by expert consultants, most of whom were professors of psychiatry in the key universities. These consultants never saw the patients themselves.[50]

Readers who refuse to believe that abortion, with its denigration of human life, has opened the same destructive forces which degenerated into the Nazi holocaust do not understand the extent of utilitarian ethics or the tenacity with which physicians and others will protect themselves at others' expense.

All physicians bear the responsibility, but most physicians acquiesce to psychiatric theory and practice. In a previous chapter I demonstrated that the personal philosophical or metaphysical values of the physician are the very essence of the practice of medicine. This reality is more disturbing by the degree to which nonpsychiatic physicians look to their psychiatric colleagues to define such values. Many psychiatrists are willing to do so:

> Because psychiatry has in the past had the main responsibility for educa-
> tion in, broadly speaking, the psychological and social aspects of medicine,
> it is widely assumed, especially by psychiatrists, that to psychiatry properly
> belongs the task of teaching the new approach in the future. History and
> practice give strong support to such a claim.[51]

In other words physicians are willingly allowing psychiatrists to define right
and wrong behavior and to be taught by them. Psychiatry is a godless science.
An easy proof of this statement is to review the literature and seek specific
statements that traditional, orthodox Chrisitanity has a place in the mental
health of patients. More commonly, the opposite is true: Christianity is
denigrated. Since psychiatrists have the legal power to determine the reality
in which a person believes, the only step which remains for the incarceration
of Christians is the thorough application of the current "science" of psychiatry.
Psychiatry, with its several hundred theories, is generally an enemy of the Christian faith.

Do Christian Psychotherapists Have A Place?

I decided to counsel Mrs. Jones because I was convinced that God has effective principles for a spiritual change. I was decidely nervous because several
family members and our church members would be observing me closely. I
directed her in scheduling daily activities which included personal care and
housekeeping with recognition of her physical limitations. She was to have daily
time in meditation and prayer, attend Sunday school and worship services on
Sundays. Basics of salvation and forgiveness were covered. I prayed at the end
of each session. I explained that choice, not feelings, was the basis for carrying
out these responsibilities. I talked of the present hope of Christians.

A significant part of the process was instructing family members. Previously,
they had tried to console and "baby" her during the crying spells. Now, they
were to change their response during these by directing her toward responsible thought and activity. They had taken away most of her daily responsibilities,
criticized many decisions which she made, and only allowed her a few personal toiletries. I directed them to let her resume household responsibilities.
They were to assist in instances where physical risk was present. They were
instructed to seek forgiveness from their mother for removing responsibilities
and integrity as an adult. And they did!

I had seven counseling sessions with Mrs. Jones. During this period of time
she began to carry out these activities and to feel better. Eventually, her in-
house help moved out. It has been six years since that time. She has not had
to see another counselor or take any "nerve" medications. The family has been
freed to live their own lives. During this time she has not been depressed again,
even while going through two major trials: additional surgery and the loss of
someone very close to her.

The son indicated those principles which he considered the most significant:
forgiveness allowed all family members to make a new start; their demeaning

support for their mother left her without value to herself and to others. Hindsight has shown two other strengths: (1) Mrs. Jones had led a responsible life as a committed Christian prior to her husband's death. (2) The son was faithful during these years to question the use and approach of non-Christian psychotherapists. For example, during the first episode of depression the Christian physician who was treating Mrs. Jones referred her to a non-Christian psychiatrist, but the son insisted that she see a Christian. For the second episode he drove her to a town several hours away in order to see a Christian counselor. God was faithful to them and to me in His management of our lives when our effort was to honor Him and His Word.

From our discussion one wonders whether psychotherapy has any place for Christians because their practices are derived for naturalistic presuppositions. Non-Christian psychotherapists have no more wisdom than any other human being to direct changes in others' lives. The Christian psychiatrist has a place within well-defined guidelines. My only reason for this allowance is for those Christians who are occupied in these professions. On the one hand instant acceptance of these concepts is unlikely and decisions about future vocation will require time and study. One the other hand any true believer who progressively understands the whole of Scripture, and on that basis is progressive in sanctification, will recognize the necessity of these narrow guidelines.

1. Evangelism must be the highest priority when dealing with an unbeliever. The offer of salvation is what every unbeliever needs before he will desire right behavior and be able to live it.[52]

2. If a patient chooses not to accept Christ, then he must be informed that he has rejected the ultimate answer to his problems and that anything else is by comparison, worthless (Phil 3:7-8). Counseling may continue if the patient is still willing, since the possibility of helping the patient temporarily may allow the opportunity for evangelism to be pursued at a later session.

3. Counseling should never compromise an explicit or clearly implicit biblical principle.

4. Every problem encountered must be examined to determine its biblical definition and solution.

5. If the patient is a Christian, and biblical counseling is available at the patient's church, counselors must refer the patient there.[53]

6. A Christian who plans to enter a counseling career should have thorough, formal theological education rather than secular training. Counseling should then be done only under the authority of a church—preferably as a pastor or elder.

7. A counselor should have read and essentially agree with *Competent to Counsel* because its analysis of the place and content of counseling is biblical; and is a complete development of these concepts.[54]

8. An evangelical committment is minimal to a pursuit of this field.

9. The counselor should be committed to the principles of the balanced Christian life or a similarly comprehensive approach to the Christian life, both its attitude and its activities.

10. The real work of the Holy Spirit in biblical counseling must be acknowledged.[55]

These criteria are narrow, but biblical. Disagreement can come only on a biblical basis: empiricism or naturalistic theory has insufficient views of metaphysical reality to be in realistic disagreement. Since biblical counseling is not yet widely available, some exigencies might occur; for example, counseling of the member of one church by a member of another. The biblical goal for all counseling to be done under the aegis of the church should remain clear.

The argument might be posed that the various fields of psychotherapy represent an evangelistic opportunity. More opportunities would be available by increasing the number of biblical counselors; an additional benefit of an increased number of biblical counselors would be their availability to those Christians who need biblical answers to their problems. The church of Jesus Christ must begin to demonstrate the reality that Christ and His Word provide solid answers to life's problems *far* beyond the possibilities a secular approach offers.

Who should a Christian with psychological problems seek for help? First, he should see his pastor or that person who counsels *under* the authority of his church.

Beyond the governing leadership of the church, the most knowledgeable and experienced Christian should be sought. In some rare instances medication or hospitalization may be necessary. Both the counselor and the counselee should be certain that all spiritual resources have been tried and specifically identifiable physical causes have been investigated. Even if one or both these sources become necessary, the pastor or someone else (as described above) must remain involved to prevent any compromise of clear biblical principles. Realistically, medication or hospitalization *may* be necessary, but I fear that even my mention of these will enhance their use to the neglect of spiritual resources. Perhaps it is a manifestation of our sinful natures that we will escape personal responsibility and confrontation under Christ's Lordship by any avenue left open. Both laymen and pastors must work diligently toward the full application of spiritual resources while remembering that a fallen world both prevents perfect understanding and its application.

NOTES

1. The basic distinction between psychologists and psychiatrists is that the latter have training as physicians and are able to prescribe medications. The theories of both overlap widely with adherents to common schools within both fields. In a discussion of their approach to psychotherapy, it is really not necessary to distinguish between them. The terms, psychotherapist and psychotherapy, embrace both and will be used here to avoid repetitious use of both names. The specific name will be used where the context primarily refers to one or the other.

I must affirm my awareness that many Christians in these disciplines are true evangelicals, and therefore, are brothers and sisters in Christ. In addition many are effective in changing lives and leading people to Christ. I am convinced, however, that most give too much credence to their disciplines. Their effectiveness could be greater if they used a thorough and consistently biblical approach. Modern Christianity is weakened because the spiritual ability of the Christian to live abundantly, joyfully, and peacefully in difficult trials, is minimized. I would ask them to make a serious effort to read entirely, and evalute objectively, the content of this chapter and other critiques. The matter is extremely serious!

2. "Task force Report on Religion and Psychiatry of the American Psychiatric Association: Phase III," *American Journal of Psychiatry* 13 (1978): 775-778.

3. I will use the term "psychotropic" to designate such drugs that are used to treat "mental illness."

4. Arthur Guyton, *Basic Human Neurophysiology* (Philadelphia: W. B. Saunders Co., 1981), pp. 177, 182, 192, 198-199, 202-203.

5. L. E. Hollister, "Tricyclic Antidepressants," *New England Journal of Medicine* 299 (1978): 1106-1109.

6. Ibid., p. 1107.

7. Ibid.

8. M. R. Littleton," Depression: The Chemical Side," *Moody Monthly* (October, 1981), pp. 127-129.

9. F. J. Ayd, "Social Issues: Misuse and Abuse," *Psychosomatics*: Supplement 10 (1980) 21:21-25.

10. National Institute of Mental Health: "Mental Health Services in Primary Care Settings," Report of an Institute of Medicine Conference, Washington D. C., (April 2-3, 1979), Series DN 2, DHHS Publication ADM 80-995. (Government Printing Office, 1980).

11. D. A. Regier, I. D. Goldberg and C. A. Tabue, "The DeFacto U. S. Health Services System," *Archives of General Psychiatry* 35 (1978): 685.

12. J. Hankin and J. S. Oktay, "Mental Disorder and Primary Medical Care: An analytic Review of the Literature," *National Institute of Mental Health* (Rockville, Maryland): Series D, No. 7, DHEW publication No. (ADM) 78-661, (Government Printing Office, 1979).

13. J. D. Stoeckle, et. al., "The Quantity and Significance of Psychological Distress in Medical Patients," *Journal of Chronic Disease* 17 (1964): 959.

14. J. P. Geyman, "Mental Health Care in Family Practice," *Journal of Family Practice* 12 (April 1981), pp. 615-616.

15. Orville S. Walters, "Psychiatry," in *Baker's Dictionary of Christian Ethics*, ed. Carl F. Henry (Grand Rapids: Baker Book House, 1973), pp. 550-552.

16. T. C. Manschreck, "Schizophrenic Disorders," *New England Journal of Medicine* 305 (Dec. 31, 1981): 1628-1632.

17. "Endorphin-Mental Illness Link Far From Proved," *Journal of the American Medical Association* 247 (Feb. 5, 1982): 570-577.

18. Nouthetic counseling is a type of biblical counseling, as developed by Dr. Jay Adams. See *Competent to Counsel* (Phillipsburg, N.J.: Presbyterian and Reformed Pub. Co., 1970).

19. Ibid.

20. Jay Adams, *Christian Counselor's Manual* (Grand Rapids: Baker Book House, 1973).

21. Jay Adams, *More Than Redemption* (Phillpsburg, NJ: Presbyterian and Reformed Pub. Co., 1970).

22. I am only using these authors to illustrate the essentially metaphysical nature of psychotherapy. I do not endorse their writing because they generally do not develop adequate biblical approaches, in spite of such recognition.

23. Paul Tournier, *The Meaning of Persons* (New York: Harper and Row, 1957), pp. 107-108.

24. Orville S. Walters, "Psychiatry," in *Baker's Dictionary of Christian Ethics*, pp. 550-552.

25. Haddon W. Robinson, ed., "Psychiatry and Christianity," *Journal of the Christian Medical Society*, vol. 6 (4) 1975:1-28.

26. Dr. Malcolm Beck, "Christ and Psychiatry," *Journal of the Christian Medical Society*, vol. 6 (4) 1975:7-12.

27. J. R. Runions, M.D., "Toward a Christian Psychiatry," *Journal of the Christian Medical Society*, vol. 6 (4) 1975:13-19.

28. Dr. Mansell Patterson, M.D., "The Christian Psychotherapist: Yes/No," *Journal of the Christian Medical Society*, vol. 6 (4) 1975:26-28.

29. A. M. Nicholi, *The Harvard GLuide to Modern Psychiatry* (Cambridge: Belknapp Press, 1978).

30. John White, *Flirting with the World* (Wheaton: Shaw Publishers, 1982), pp. 116-117.

31. Morris B. Parloff, "Can Psychotherapy Guide the Policy Maker?" *American Psychologist* 34 (April, 1979): 296-306. Dr. Parloff is Chief of the Psychotherapy and Behavioral Intervention Section, National Institute of Mental health, Clinical Research Branch. His position would naturally cause him to accentuate the positive and minimize the negative. Thus, his largely negative comments are more significant.

32. Ibid., p. 299.

33. M. B. Parloff, "Psychotherapy and Research: An Anaclitic Depression," *Psychiatry* 43 (Nov. 1980): 279-293.

34. Ibid., p. 280.

35. Ibid., p. 284.

36. Ibid., p. 286.

37. Ibid., pp. 286-293.

38. Ibid., p. 288.

39. Ibid., p. 292.

40. M. B. Parloff, "Can Psychotherapy Guide the Policy Maker?", p. 303.

41. James Dobson, *Preparing for Adolescence* (Santa Anna, CA: Vision House, 1978), pp. 86-87.

42. M. O. Vincent, *God, Sex, and You* (Philadelphia: Holmán, 1971), pp. 174-176.

43. Jerry White, *Honesty, Morality, and Conscience* (Colorado Springs: Navpress, 1979), pp. 199-210.

44. The reader may conclude that I have a preoccupation with the pronouncement of sin. I hope that that is correct to the extent that the Bible, as God's voice, also denounces sin for which God's solution is found through forgiveness in Jesus Christ. I would remind the reader that my discussion of the balanced Christian life involved more positive practices, and showed no preoccupation with sin (chapter 6. Cf. my discussion on p. 71, note 58).

45. J. Robitscher, *The Powers of Psychiatry* (Boston: Houghton Mifflin Co., 1980).

46. S. J. Morse, "Hospital Lockups Serve Neither Mental Patients Nor Their Doctors," *Medical World News* (Nov. 9, 1981), p. 107.

47. John White, *Daring to Draw Near* (Downers Grove: InterVarsity Press, 1972), p. 59.

48. S. J. Morse, "Hospital Lockups Serve Neither Mental Patients Nor Their Doctors," p. 107.

49. T. D. Harper, "State-funded Abortions: Judicial Acquiescence in the Sanctity of a Physician's Medical Judgment," *Journal of the Medical Association of Georgia* 69 (April, 1980): 313-315.

50. Leo Alexander, "Medical Science Under Nazi Dictatorship," *New England Journal of Medicine* 241 (July 14, 1949), pp. 39-47.

51. G. L. Engel, "The Psycho-Biophysical Modeland Medical Education," *New England Journal of Medicine* 306 (April 1, 1982):802-805.

52. The basics of salvation are frequently, erroneously discussed by psychotherapists. The seriousness of this fact should be apparent. If the basics of salvation cannot be clearly and succinctly stated, the psychotherapist cannot effectively communicate about the most important issue for anyone—his eternal destiny.

53. Jay E. Adams, *Competent to Counsel*, pp. 59-77.
54. Ibid.
55. Ibid., pp. 20-25.

REFERENCES

Alexander, Leo. "Medical Science Under Nazi Dictatorship." *New England Journal of Medicine* 241 (July 14, 1949):39-47..

Ayd, F. J. "Social Issues: Misuse and Abuse." *Psychosomatics*, Supplement no. 10. (1980) 21:21-25.

Dobson, James. *Preparing for Adolescence*. Santa Anna, Calif.: Vision House, 1978.

Engel, G. L. "The Psycho Biophysical Model and Medical Education." *New England Journal of Medicine* 306 (April 1, 1982):802-805.

Geyman, J. P. "Mental Health Care In Family Practice." *Journal of Family Practice* 12 (April 1981):615-616.

Guyton, Arthur. *Basic Human Neurophysiology*. Philadelphia: W. B. Saunders Company, 1981.

Hankin, J. and Oktay, J. S. "Mental Disorder and Primary Medical Care; An Analytic Review of the Literature." In National Institute of Mental Health (Rockville, Md.): Series D, No. 7. DHEW publication No. (ADM) 78-661, Government Printing Office, 1979.

Harper, T. D. "State-Funded Abortions: Judicial Acquiescence in the Sanctity of a Physician's Medical Judgment." *Journal of the Medical Association of Georgia* 69 (April 1980):313-315.

Hollister, L. E. "Tricyclic Anti-depressants." *New England Journal of Medicine* 299 (1978):1106-1109, 1168-1172.

Littleton, M. R. "Depression: The Chemical Side." *Moody Monthly*, October 1981, pp. 127-129.

Manschreck, T. C. "Schizophrenic Disorders." *New England Journal of Medicine* 305 (December 31, 1981):1628-1632.

"Medical News, Endorphin-Mental Illness Link Far From Proved." *Journal of the American Medical Association* 247 (Feb. 5, 1982):570-577.

Morse, S. J. "Hospital Lockups Serve Neither Mental Patients Nor Their Doctors." *Medical World News*, November 9, 1981.

National Institute of Mental Health: Mental Health Series in Primary Care Settings. Report of an Institute of Medicine Conference, Washington, D.C., April 2-3, 1979. Series DN #2. DHHS Publication # (ADM) 80-995.Government Printing Office, 1980.

Nicholi, A. M. *The Harvard Guide to Modern Psychiatry*. Cambridge: Belknap Press, 1978.

Parloff, M. B. "Can Psychotherapy Guide the Policy Maker?" *American Psychologist* 34 (April 1979):296-306.

Parloff, M. B. "Psychotherapy and Research: An Anaclitic Depression." *Psychiatry* 43 (Nov. 1980):279-293.

Regier, D. A. Goldberg, I. D. Tabue, C.A. The De Facto U.S. Mental Health Services System. Archives of General Psychiatry 35 (1978):685.

Stoeckle J. D. et al. "The Quantity and Signficance of Psychological Distress In Medical Patients." *Journal of Chronic Disease* 17 (1964):959.

Task Force Report on Religion and Psychiatry of the American Psychiatric Association: Phase III. *American Journal of Psychiatry*, 13 (1978):775-778.

Tournier, Paul. *The Meaning of Persons*. New York: Harper and Row, 1957.

Vincent, M. O. *God, Sex, and You*. Philadelphia: Holman, 1971.

White, John. *Flirting with the World*. Wheaton: Harold Shaw, 1982.

White, Jerry. *Honesty, Morality, and Conscience*. Colorado Springs: Navpress, 1979.

White, John. *Daring to Draw Near*. Downers Grove: InterVarsity Press, 1972.

SUGGESTED READING—SECULAR CRITIQUE

Glasser, W. *Reality Therapy*. New York, Harper and Row, 1965.

Robitscher, J. *The Powers of Psychiatry*. Boston: Houghton Mifflin Company, 1980.

Szasz, T. *The Myth of Psychotherapy*. Garden City: Anchor Press, 1978.

Torrey, E. F. *The Death of Psychiatry*. Radnor, PA: Chilton Book Co., 1974.

SUGGESTED READING—CHRISTIAN CRITIQUE

Adams, J. E. *Competent to Counsel*: Philadelphia, Presbyterian and Reformed Publishing Company, 1970.

Bobgan, M. D. *The Psychological Way/The Spiritual Way*. Minneapolis: Bethany Fellowship, 1979.

Brownback, P. *The Danger of Self-Love*. Chicago, Moody Press, 1982.

Erricsson, S. E. *Clergy Malpractice: Constitutional and Political Issues*. Center for Law and Religious Freedom (Christian Legal Society), P.O. Box 2069, Oak Park, Illinois 60303.

Lloyd-Jones, Martyn D. *The Doctor Himself and the Human Condition.* London: Christian Medical Fellowship, 1982.
Vitz, P.C. *Psychology as Religion: The Cult of Self Worship.* Grand Rapids: Eerdmans, 1977.

11 | Priorities in Dying, Death, and Grief

John Murray, writing on the sanctity of life, states, "Nothing shows the moral bankruptcy of a people or of a generation more than the disregard for the sanctity of life."[1] This backruptcy is apparent in the churches' lack of applied biblical principles on dying, death and grief. The Bible is centrally a book about life and death and provides insights through meditation or investigation. Christ overcame spiritual death for all regenerate people, yet Protestant thought has not been "very helpful in the present quest" for medical ethics.[2] The application of biblical principles and priorities will yield much fruit (Isa. 55:11).

Dying, death and grief are experienced by everyone.[3] Our culture tries to obscure death, yet a clearer focus on its finality provides an opportunity to proclaim the Christian hope of eternal life. Even so, the difficulties of determining, defining and predicting death are complex.

> Argumentation tends to take the form of questioning the moment we tackle the borderline problems—problems which cannot be resolved by casuistic definition but demand that we venture to make decisions. . . . One must simply run the risk of making the decision—and be prepared in so doing to err, and thereby to incur guilt. As a Christian, I would say that whoever hopes to come through it all without illusions or repressions will have to live in the name of forgiveness.[4]

Mrs. Susie Johnson, 60 years of age, developed an increasing shortness of breath over a period of several days. She had no chest pain, but severe nausea. Her electrocardiogram suggested a myocardial infarction, or heart attack, so she was admitted to the hospital. Subsequently, her workup revealed a diagnosis of a cardiomyopathy, an enlargement of the heart due to any process which progressively destroys heart muscle until pumping of blood is no longer possible.

When such a diagnosis is certain, most patients die within five years. Upon improvement in her symptoms, she was discharged from the hospital without being told of her shortened life span. Her family physician was convinced that she and her husband needed to know her prognosis and scheduled a thirty minute interview. During that time he quietly informed them of her prognosis. It took them and their family several weeks to accept her prognosis. On two occasions their physician witnessed to them, offering forgiveness in Jesus Christ as the means to hope and comfort. Although they were church members, their vague profession did not give much credence to salvation, nor did they ever make a clear profession of faith. Unexpectedly, within eighteen months of the onset of her cardiomyopathy, she developed cancer of the pancreas and died within a month.

The case illustrates several pivotal points and represents an unsuccessful attempt at evangelism.[5] That Adam and Eve were created to live forever is strongly implied in the threat of death upon their disobedience of the one prohibition (Gen. 2:7) which God had placed upon them.[6] As the whole Scripture is reviewed it becomes apparent that more than one concept of death exists. A paradox seems to exist when the offer of salvation in Jesus Christ is "eternal life"(John 3:16; Rom. 6:23); yet both believers and unbelievers will experience physical death. Further the Bible states that death has lost its "sting" for believers and "death is swallowed up in victory" (1 Cor. 15:54-55). This apparent paradox is explained by biblical anthropology, that is, that man consists of two elements: body and spirit. Both are subject to a type of death (see Figure 1).

A progression within the Old Testament, and the clear emphasis of the New Testament is the permanence of spiritual reality over physical reality. Thus, the predominant reference to life in the New Testament involves spiritual and eternal life for those who are freed from the power of spiritual death through belief in Jesus Christ (John 3:36, 6:40; Rom. 5:17-21, 8:23; 1 Cor. 15:26, 51-57). Spiritual death is called the "second death" (Rev. 2:11; 20:6, 14: 21:8) and has an inseparable association with sin as did the sin of Adam and Eve (Rom. 5:12, 17, 6:23; 2 Cor.5:21-22; James 1:15).[7] Jesus' illustrations include "outer darkness" (Matt. 22:13), "weeping and gashing of teeth" (Matt. 2:13), "eternal punishment" (Matt. 25:46), "agony . . . flame . . . torment . . . fixed chasm" (Luke 16: 19-21). Thus, physical death becomes inconsequential in comparison to spiritual death. The Christian's priority in situations of physical death must be that of the rich man's request to warn others of the "second death which is final and without hope."

In view of these consequences, an attitude of timidity and misdirected priorities needs changing in many evangelical efforts that do not reveal the obscuration of death in Western society. Funerals are elaborate arrangements of

Figure 1

	Death	*Life*
1. *Physical*	*Body — Soul*	*Body* + Soul
2. Spiritual	Soul—God	Soul + God
3. Eternal	Body + Soul—God forever	Body + Soul + God forever

flowers and contrived eulogies. Usually, death is removed from the family and close friends and occurs in an institution. Words such as ''expired'' and ''passed away'' blur the finality of death. These above biblical descriptions cannot be understood without the association between sin and death. If physical death was the only spectre, it might be a reasonable option to alleviate suffering, e.g. intactable pain, deep loneliness, or bodily mutilation. Man's fear of death results not from physical death but from his created awareness of banishment from an omnipotent God who gives no recourse from the ''second death.''[7]

As physical death approaches, God's sovereignty is a great comfort to all believers and a thorough study of God's sovereignty demonstrates that life and death are in His hands. This great truth pushes to the periphery most issues which are discussed in dying and death. It is the most important understanding necessary for the believer in these situations.

Dangers of the Death and Dying Movement

Spiritual reality demands that evangelicals counter in every possible way a subtle, but very prominent trend away from our cultural denial of death: the death and dying movement and its associated teaching of near-death experiences. These trends are subtle because in fairness they intend to help people and to bring into the open the cultural avoidance of death and dying. Many Christians support this movement, but such teaching is erroneous and antithetic to the basic Christian message of hope. Regretfully, these movements entered the vacuum which was created when Christian preaching, teaching, and caring neglected and shunned dying and death. Elisabeth Kubler-Ross has identified five stages of experience through which a patient goes after he has been informed that death is imminent. These stages are: denial and isolation, anger, bargaining, depression, and acceptance.[8] These stages have become standard teaching for medical personnel and have found their way into chaplaincy and seminary programs. These stages, by her own admission are not always identifiable or sequential. She persistently maintains, however, that acceptance is the desirable final stage, even that ''death is the final stage of growth.''[9] The biblical position is opposed to acceptance, as it teaches that unbelievers are doomed to a horrible eternity. The Christian is the true realist; and Kubler-Ross' goals are not biblical.

An outgrowth of Kubler-Ross' results is the thanatology movement which focuses upon people who have had near-death experiences—including supposed out-of-the-body observation of resuscitative efforts by emergency personnel. Other descriptions include a verbal inability to describe the experience, the hearing of the message of their own death, feelings of peace and quiet, a buzzing noise, a dark tunnel, meeting others, a white being, a life review, a border or limit, and the process of coming back.[10]

Superficially these descriptions seem consistent with Christian beliefs: a being of light, a confirmation of life after death, and positive life changes which result from the experience. Thus, many Christians have been led astray. Both biblical and medical teaching, however, are opposite to these supposed consistencies: (1) Almost always the experience is pleasant; heaven will be ineffably pleasant—*but* those who are not regenerate will experience an eternity in an anguish unknown on earth,'' . . . it is appointed for men to die once, and after this comes judgment'' (Heb. 9:27).[11] (2) People who report these experiences were not dead. Physical life and physical death are states of existence and nonexistence. Although the moment of passage from life to death may not always be clear, no one confuses their inseparability as states. Those people who have had near-death experiences did not truly die. It is dangerously deceptive to apply the physiologic changes which constitute the process, to the final state. (3) Many people who are prominent in thanatology are also involved in the occult. Kubler-Ross herself has described talking with spirits and leaving her body.[12] Other practices are combinations of Eastern mysticism, parapsychology, and spiritism.[13] (4) A kind of universalism is commonly accepted. "In the decades to come, we may see one universe, one humankind, one religion which unites us all in a peaceful world."[14] (5) Death should not be feared and at times should be welcomed! Why not, if death is described as pleasant and peaceful states which are difficult qualities to find in earthly existence with its economic, political, and ecological woes. Such acceptability would inevitably enhance the practice of euthanasia.[15] On the basis of clear biblical teaching, the thanatology movement is incompatible with Christianity and directly opposed to it.

A Biblical View of Death

All the above has been introductory to a development of biblical priorities in dying, death, and grief. Death is inextricably related to sin, salvation and eternal life. A distinctive throughout this book has been the antithesis between Christian and non-Christian. If the patient is not a believer, a clear presentation of the gospel becomes a necessity. Obviously this presentation should be made with sensitivity, gentleness, and concern for the patient's physical status. The Christian physician should assume this responsibility personally or delegate it; unless he is certain that the patient's pastor or someone else will do so. Further, any Christian involved in the care of a terminally ill patient should attempt to evangelize the patient. A patient who is a Christian will rejoice to talk of heavenly things and the patient who does not know Christ will have a final opportunity to avoid eternal death.

Other principles apply when the impact of death causes problems of guilt, fear, worry, secrecy, and despair for the individual, his family and others who are close to him. Some problems will be solved through evangelism; but all problems have biblical solutions which provide the possibility to turn tragedy into blessing. One question is whether the terminally ill patient should be told the truth. Lying or withholding information in the face of imminent death creates problems and compounds others because in every conversation around the patient, this emotionally laden topic must be guarded with care. Moreover, forgiveness and reconciliation cannot be sought without exposure of the avoided topic. The solution to these problems is the Ninth Commandment which forbids lying and allows open discussion of serious issues at a time when there will be no second opportunity.

Frequently, guilt is associated with the death of someone close, especially a spouse, but guilt can be minimized and even become an opportunity of enhancing relationships *if* forgiveness and reconciliation occur. Although the pastor or elder is primarily responsible to encourage discussion which leads to biblical solutions in troublesome areas, in his absence the physician or any other knowledgeable believer should take the initiative. Time suddenly becomes precious between intimates and additional guilt will occur if the time is lost.[16] Thus, the emotional pressure of dying can lead to biblical communication and healed relationships. Joy, not despair, is the goal of believers' trials, "that you may be perfect and complete, not lacking in anything" (James 1:2-4).

Following death, the physician will have or must provide opportunity to discuss the thoughts and emotions which the family is experiencing. Most people who are close to the grieving person naturally avoid potentially sensitive issues, yet resolution of conflicts will need to occur. The presence of guilt, anger, and resentment should be probed in a sensitive manner. Denial or morbid preoccupation with thoughts or possessions of the deceased may occur. Always, a significant reorganization of the surviving person's life needs to occur. Most teaching about death and dying stops with the death of the ill person even though the survivors have problems and will need help to rebuild their lives. Close observation is needed to prevent unhealthy, sinful patterns from becoming established.[17]

Obstacles are prevalent in the practical application of these principles. Christians, primarily physicians, will need to consider alternatives to these obstacles. The case of Jeffrey James illustrates the problem. In his mid-thirties, J. J. was admitted to the hospital for chemotherapy of his chronic leukemia. The admission was considered routine. Complications occurred when he developed a lung infection because of a low number of white blood cells. As his breathing became more difficult, J. J. was admitted to the Intensive Care Unit. For approximately two weeks he was stable and remained communicative. He delighted in hearing the Bible read since he was unable to do so himself, yet he was limited to the five minutes each hour that the hospital allowed for visitors. His family members were given priority to visit him, but most of them were unbelievers who could not discuss Christian beliefs. Numerous Christians desired to minister to him but were unable to do so because of this restricted visitation. After a total of six weeks in the hospital, he developed an overwhelming infection, other complications, and died. His pastor and Christian friends spoke of their frustration in ministering to him because of hospital regulations. Could their frustration have been avoided, and J. J. comforted to a greater extent?

Dr. Everett Koop said, "I don't think a medical student is ever told what his mission in life is."[18] Great efforts are made to give all possible medical care to all people for as long as possible. Physicians may go to these extremes because they are "afraid of death in greater proportion than experimentally controlled groups of patients."[19] A portion of this fear may result from the obvious fact that all physicians will eventually fail with all their patients! The medical mission must include acceptance of this inevitable reality. From the other side, patients and their families need to be aware of these prevalent attitudes within the medical profession which can result in unnecessary procedures and expense in the care of the terminally ill. In addition, physicians' belief in the medical system will isolate patients from their families, pastors, and friends. As with Jeffrey James, this isolation frequently involves the patients' last days because of the seriousness of the illnesses which places them there. Such isolation is frequently not medically necessary but occurs as a matter of hospital routine.

If the reality of the pneumosomatic effect is believed, then exposure to spiritual influence, prayer, Bible reading and study, anointing with oil, etc., has physical, as well as spiritual benefit. The physical effect is secondary to the biblical injunction that spiritual care not be neglected for any reason. Again, responsibility for this care falls first on pastors and elders who are responsible for spiritual oversight of their congregation—especially those members who are hospitalized because of serious illness. This oversight should include attempts to convince hospital staffs to make regulations which allow these ministrations. The situation in the future may worsen as medical care becomes more inclusive and comprehensive. Christian physicians can contribute significantly, attempting to influence hospital policies from within and they can personally or by delegation, provide a spiritual ministry to patients.[20] Both physicians and church officers can be alert to vacancies in hospital chaplain positions. When the opportunity occurs, every effort should be made to bring in an evangelical chaplain. This person would be an invaluable resource, but should not replace the duties of pastors and elders.

Inappropriate prolongation of death can be another hindrance to biblical principles because many physicians are inhibited by their fear of failure. Another hindrance is the use of mind-influencing drugs, such as tranquilizers, antidepressants, and analgesics. The patient's pain should be adequately treated, but the presence of pain does not automatically require heavy doses of these drugs.[21] With the families' help a balance must be sought between the lucidity of the patient's thinking and control of pain. In many instances a more complete application of biblical principles may reduce or even obviate the need for analgesics.

Lying and withholding of information (already shown to be forbidden by the Bible) are other hindrances to full care of terminally-ill patients. Remaining days can be used to seek reconciliation with family members, as well as the enrichment of facing this trial with the comforts and strengths of the Christian faith. Final matters must be decided concerning financial estate, especially if a family is left behind (John 19:25-27; 1 Tim. 5:8).

> Families that could spend weeks (months or years) making the most of their last earthly hours, drawn more closely together, resolving tensions and differences, and planning for the future, instead grow apart, become cold and fearful of one another because of the great secret that is covered by a thousand lies.[22]

To remove these hindrances the Christian who recognizes this sin must inform the family that he is willing to inform the patient. The believer's primary obligation is to God who has commanded truth.[23]

Another hindrance to the realization of biblical priorities is the obsuration of death by our American culture. Expensive caskets, makeup, and floral arrangements obscure the stark reality of a dead body. Eulogies emphasize the best and minimize the worst. It is accurate to say that these are attempts by society to remove the "sting of death." In changing these practices, "an ounce of prevention is worth a pound of cure." Christian preaching and teaching should denounce such sham and proclaim the biblical realities of death and its hope, "But we do not want you to be uninformed, brethren, about those who are asleep . . . (1 Thess. 4:13-18).

Teaching medical students and residents that they should be detached from their patients is another hindrance to the full care provided by biblical principles. This teaching stems from the instability of a non-Christian philosophical position in the presence of death. Spiritual resources to the believing physician allow him to "rejoice with those who rejoice and weep with those who weep" (Rom 12:15); to accept that an appropriate time exists for "every event under heaven" (Eccl. 3:1-8); and not to carry the burden alone. The physician is biblically directed to be intimately involved with his patients, commit himself to excellent medical care, and rest in the outcome which is primarily determined by Another.

Physicians' aggressiveness and overconfidence is a problem which may result in extensive and costly procedures which have little chance of affecting the course or outcome of the illness. Without reflective discernment, choices will be presented to the patient and/or his family in a manner which will not reflect the involved ambiguities. Families should ask questions: What are the chances that your proposal will prolong life or ease suffering? Do the majority of physicians agree with you? What would be the arguments against this proposal by those who do not favor it? What is it likely to cost?[24] Would you advise having it done to yourself, your spouse, or your mother? Do you mind if I get a second opinion?[25] All concerned should weigh their decisions and carefully pray for wisdom. Usually these decisions are not urgent and are best decided over several days, even weeks. More than one consultation with the physician is reasonable to allow time to ask those questions which were not thought of initially, and to meditate and pray. The counsel of elders and pastors should be sought as well.

A hindering misconception is the concept that certain diseases are terminal and others are not. Almost everyone makes this association with cancer, yet some cancers are only slowly progressive and otherwise of little consequence. On the other hand, many heart diseases, when initially diagnosed or as they progress are predictably terminal.[26] Death from diseases of the liver, brain, lungs, and other organs or systems is predictable, also. Although all physicians will err significantly, these predictions will assist the patient and families in their planning. Thus, physicians should be consulted about the possibilities of death in any serious illness. Otherwise, time or disability may prevent them from doing all that needs to be done in these circumstances.

God's sovereign care of the believer can become obscured in the maze of medical technology. God is the final and only arbiter of life and death. The presence of fear in a believer indicates an inadequate grasp of this truth. Careful biblical study should be undertaken to enable him to grasp the numerous biblical texts which pertain to God's care and omnipotence. All Christians should prepare themselves with biblical understanding before they face the inevitable circumstances of death.

Perspectives in Physical Suffering

Phyllis, Joan, and Marie are sisters who have muscular dystrophy. All have lost the ability to walk and are confined in wheelchairs or bed. Currently they are in their fifties and need help with most daily routines. Their mother is in her eighties, has had one leg amputated and thus is also confined to a wheelchair. They all live together without live-in help. Numerous people and agencies contribute to their needs and care for them in various ways. Their lives are severely restricted, exemplifying physical suffering. Although this family has fought institutionalization to maximize their independence, on a physical level little purpose appears to exist in their circumstances. The spectre of imminent death adds a unique dimension to suffering. The Christian has not been granted immunity to such situations, but he does have the spiritual resources to develop a right attitude, and in many instances to understand some of the purposes in suffering.[27]

The first awareness in suffering involves an awareness of causality. Genetic defects occur, inflict harm upon others, and Satan causes physical suffering (Job. 2:2-7; 2 Cor. 12:7). Personal sinfulness may result in suffering through neglect, defiance, or ignorance. Ultimately, however, the believer must see suffering as a part of God's plan. The truth of Romans 8:28 is not a cliche, but it is assured by an omnipotent and perfect God of love. The sufferer's faith is the key issue ". . . for he who comes to God must believe that He is . . ." (Heb. 11:6). Of course, time, study and meditation are also required for someone to reach this attitude, but suffering will never be effectively overcome without acceptance.

The second awareness in suffering involves its purpose. Thus suffering should be divided into that which is self-engendered and that which is not. This division determines the necessary response, either repentance (1 John 1:9; James 5:15) or acceptance. Suffering which results from a consequence of a particular sin must be acknowledged and put off before God's purpose can be worked out.[28]

Numerous Bible verses demonstrate the New Testament emphasis that God is more concerned about eternal values that are determined by the Christian's handling of such situations in life, than His concern for physical comfort. Ultimately, the purpose of suffering is the believer's reflection of the glory of God. His glory results when the person shows His power to overcome and His deliverance of His people through trying circumstances (Job. 42:1-6; Ezek. 20:9, 14, 22, 33, 39; 2 Cor. 24-33). Even nonbelievers will notice the person who has joy, peace, and fulfillment in the presence of physical suffering and thus demonstrates the hope of a nonsuffering existence beyond this life and the reality of the Spirit in this earthly life.

Specific purposes may be revealed to the sufferer. A spouse may find God through the serious searching which occurs at the time of disability or death of a mate. Illness may confine a person to a place that provides opportunity to minister to another or be ministered to himself. Suffering may result in a benefical change of employment or geographical location. Suffering may provide an opportunity for two people to meet and marry. Examples are endless. On the other hand a clear purpose may not be forthcoming or a recognized purpose may not be the deeper purpose which God intends.[29] In both instances purpose is certain because God is sovereign in his care of His children. Thus, the best approach would not involve an intensive search for specific purposes because Christians are often required to trust God by faith alone without revealed purpose (John 20:29).

Some guidelines may be helpful:[30]

1. Don't be surprised when it comes.
2. Self-pity is a wrong response. One's responsibilities should be continued within the limits of the physical illness.
3. Time should be used for serious reflection. Is there a sin which is clearly related? Am I balanced in my Christian life?
4. A thorough Bible study on suffering and God's sovereign care is necessary.
5. Pray diligently and without ceasing. Involve loved ones in this

attitude. A request for healing and anointing with oil is appropriate, but the more important emphasis should be upon the fulfillment of God's purposes.

6. Specific causes may be sought but always rest in God's grace.
7. Suffering should not be taken lightly; do not present a false front to others.

Pain is the most serious fear and concern related to suffering. Certainly, most disease processes involve a degree of pain at one time or another, but its absence or minimal presence is more the rule than the exception. Another aspect of pain is its necessity. Dr. Paul Brand has spent his entire life studying the physiology of pain. For his leprosy patients the absence of pain sensation as an effect of the disease results in repeated injury to fingers and toes.[31] Eventually, these injuries cause the loss of these digits. Pain is protective, and it is truly a rare event when it becomes an enemy rather than a friend.

Another characteristic of pain is its degree of subjectivity. Pain is worse at night than during the daytime because of the nocturnal reduction of sensory stimulation of sounds, smells, touch, taste, and sights. Pain has essentially unhindered access to one's consciousness. Music, television, visitors, reading, massage and many other modalities can be used to increase sensory input and possibly reduce pain.[32]

Since pain threshholds vary greatly, attitudes play roles. This factor points out the need for a thorough biblical and physiological understanding of pain that can control the fear and anxiety that exacerbates pain perception. A real decrease in pain perception will result from the inner peace and joy of the experienced Christian life and the care and support of the Christian community.

A final comment about management of pain medications. Narcotics can reduce and stop pain perception or make the patient unconcerned. Problematically, conscious awareness and other brain functions, particularly respiration, are also reduced. Pain and depression of the nervous system must be balanced against each other. In most situations, pain medications should be given as needed, not regularly. The latter is more likely to result in untoward drug effects. However, the patient and the family should not assume that the physician has the same goals that they do. These should be discussed openly with the physician so that the priorities in terminal illness are honored.

The most important factor in one's approach to suffering is attitude toward and knowledge of God. Is He all-loving, but unable to fulfill that love because of a lack of power? Is He all-powerful, but sadistic? Is he aware at all? Does He really know what I am going through? These questions are not only basic to the issue of suffering, but to life in general. Suffering makes them more urgent and intense. The Christian rests upon God's omniscience, omnipotence, omnipresence, perfect wisdom and an infinite love that can only work for the highest good of the believer. The believer himself might have chosen other circumstances and all his questions may not be answered, but God has promised never to overwhelm (1 Cor. 10:13) or forsake (Heb. 13:5); and promises to work every detail of our experience in life for good (Rom. 8:28).

Caring Alternatives

Mrs. James was admitted to the hospital because of her increasing short-ness of breath. She had been previously diagnosed as having cancer of the colon with metastasis (blood-borne tumors from the primary location of the cancer to other sites in the body) to the liver, lungs, and brain. She was only vaguely aware of where she was, but responded to conversation or touch by a slight squeeze of her hand. Her general condition had deteriorated rapidly over the past several weeks. Her primary reason for shortness of breath was pneumonia and respiratory depression from the tumors in her brain. Usually patients whose main problem is severe lung disease are intubated and placed on a respirator. However, because of her spreading cancer, the decision was made in consulta-tion with her husband not to use a respirator. She was given antibiotics and intravenous fluids and fed through a nasogastric tube. With these procedures and general nursing care, she lived five days after admission. Her husband was with her most of the time and did some of the nursing care. In this case, all that could have been done was not done because of her obviously terminal condition.

Paul Ramsey entitled a chapter of one book, "On (Only) Caring for the Dying."[33] He argues that a moral position may be taken to limit treatment in cases of terminal illness for which medical science is unable to offer effective treatment, but it may prolong life. On that basis he pleads for alternatives to the use of extraordinary means. Dr. Ramsey directs us to consider what medical education does not teach effectively—the care of the terminally ill. We cannot moralize and criticize without offering alternatives and becoming a part of the solution of this serious problem.

Hospices grew out of the death and dying emphasis of the 1970s. They consist of special care for the terminally ill in a shelter such as hospital, nursing home, or private home. Family and friends may visit freely and assist with the patient. Certainly, this concept is an improvement over the isolation that is present in most hospitals and nursing homes, but should not Christians first consider their own homes as a place for their dying? This question is asked with the realization of the limitations that may result without certain provisions of medical and/or nursing care. Many terminal illnesses involve problems for which specialized care and institutions are needed, but the care of most pa-tients involves daily routines that could be learned by lay people with little instruction. Through prayer and open discussion, terminal patients could be cared for at home. A patient who could not be managed at home is one whose presence would be so demanding physically by his illness or behaviorally by his actions, that the responsibilities of the husband, wife, and children to each other would be significantly compromised or prevented.

Advantages to the patient and the family argue strongly for home care. The patient spends his/her last days surrounded by family and close friends. The reality of death becomes intimate and experiential, not theoretical. The necessary communication during final times together is enhanced by proximity, atmosphere, and necessary interaction. A witness is provided to the community that the Christian family is capable of facing dying and death and shows love for its members in this extraordinary manner. Economically, costs would be markedly reduced. With the prevalence of insurance companies and third-party payers, costs may not seem significant; but the increasing cost of medical care means that less costly alternatives must be sought. Physicians, nurses, and other health personnel within one's congregation could assist in training the family in patient care. Many churches have medical professionals who would be willing to contribute in this way.

These advantages exceed the few hours, days, or even weeks of survival, which otherwise might be gained by the technical, but isolated care within an institution.

> Desertion is more choking than death, and more feared. The chief problem of dying is how not to die alone. To care, if only to care, for the dying is, therefore, a medical-moral imperative. . . . (A case is cited of a man whose) want of his friends and familiar circumstances . . . should have been an imperative and taken precedence over any and all technical matters.[34]

Particularly to enhance biblical priorities and to demonstrate self-giving love, home care of the terminally ill calls for serious consideration. Even further, patients who are not relatives may be cared for in Christian homes.

Another innovative alternative could be a hospice run by evangelicals whose purposes included both personalized care and the presentation of the gospel. Technically, medical care would be equal to that provided anywhere. Although this alternative is attractive and an important means of ministry, it is not a priority for most evangelical bodies primarily because of the high cost of time, energy and money. Even so, God may lead some Christians to this type of medical ministry and priorities in the future may enhance this opportunity.

One resource book which discusses these alternatives is *Death and the Caring Community* by Larry Richards and Paul Johnson. Its strength is its movement into an area which has largely been neglected by modern evangelicals. Its weakness is a heavy reliance upon secular models without a discernment of biblical priorities: for example, the home as an alternative is absent. Specific strengths include the priority of evangelism, the seriousness of death, assurance of God's sovereign care, a right view of faith healing, the use of Scripture and truthfulness among patients, families, and medical people. Negatively, God's condemnation of those outside Christ is never mentioned and a false hope to many is implied; directions for the management of resentment and guilt are inadequate; secular organizations are relied upon rather than the church; and the book does not mention the serious biblical problems which are associated with near-death experiences. The book is a shallow beginning with deep potholes to be avoided. A more thorough biblical development is needed, but this book does attempt a Christian response to dying and death. For that reason it deserves reading.

In summary, dying, death, and grief involve the essence of biblical truths. Evangelism of nonbelievers is the highest priority. For believers, God's sovereign care needs explicit and serious attention to produce the blessings of peace and joy. Obstacles which may interfere with these priorities include: extraordinary medical measures, separation of the patient from spiritual fellowship, pain medications, lying, and cultural obscuration of death. A thorough biblical view of pain and suffering is necessary. Finally, Christians need to consider alternatives to the secular system to enhance these spiritual priorities and to provide a unique witness to the unbelieving community.

NOTES

1. John Murray, *Principles of Conduct* (1957; reprint ed., Grand Rapids: Eerdmans Pub. Co., 1978), p. 122.

2. Paul Ramsey, *The Patient as Person* (1970; reprint ed., New Haven: Yale University Press, 1979), p. 119.

3. Those people alive at Christ's Second Coming will not die a physical death (1 Thess. 4:13-18), yet unbelievers will still face spiritual death (*infra*).

4. Helmut Thielicke, "Ethics in Modern Medicine," in *Who Shall Live?*, ed. Kenneth Vaux (New York: Harper and Row, 1964), pp. 164, 166.

5. For balance, I have presented this case to demonstrate that all situations do not turn out as we would hope.

6. John Murray, *Principles of Conduct*, p. 107. Louis Berkhof, *Systematic Theology* (1938; reprint ed., Grand Rapids: Eerdmans Pub. Co., 1969), pp. 669-671.

7. Carl F. Henry, *Christian Personal Ethics*, (1957; reprint ed., Grand Rapids: Baker Book House, 1977), p. 177.

8. Elisabeth Kubler-Ross, *On Death and Dying* (New York: Macmillan, 1969), pp.38-137.

9. Elisabeth Kubler-Ross, *Death: the Final Stage of Growth* (Englewood Cliffs: Prentice-Hall Inc., 1975).

10. Raymond Moody, *Life After Life* (Atlanta: Mockingbird Books, 1975), pp. 21-76.

11. These passages are only a very few of those which might have been selected. Systematic theologies should be consulted for a thoroughly developed argument.

12. J. H. Lavin, "Has Elisabeth Kubler-Ross Really Flipped?" *Medical Economics* (August 4, 1980), pp. 62-80.

13. Mark Albrecht and Brooks Alexander, "Thanatology: Death and Dying," *Spiritual Counterfeits Journal* (April, 1977).

14. Elisabeth Kubler-Ross, *On Death and Dying*, p. 3.

15. Jay E. Adams, *More Than Redemption* (Phillipsburg, NJ: Presbyterian and Reformed Pub. Co., 1979), pp. 297-300.

16. The chief reason for these processes is not to avoid guilt or other complications, but because it is biblically correct to resolve conflicts, e.g. Eph. 4:26, "do not let the sun go down upon your anger."

17. For a fuller discussion of practical methods of biblical principles of dying, death, and grief see Jay E. Adams, *Shepherding God's Flock*, vol. 1 (Philadelphia: Presbyterian and Reformed, 1974), pp. 128-156.

18. C. Everett Koop, *Right to Live, Right to Die.* (Wheaton: Tyndale House, 1976), p. 97.

19. Charles D. Aring, "Intimations of Mortality: An Appreciation of Death and Dying," *Annals of Internal Medicine* 69 (July 1968):139.

20. Many members of the patient's own congregation may be available. At some time he/she would want to sit down with his pastor and make a list of these people. Often, members may be found employed in the hospital who can drop by to minister to patients.

21. R. M. Marks and E. J. Sachar, "Undertreatment of Medical Inpatients with Narcotic Analgesics," *Annals of Internal Medicine* 78 (Feb. 1973): 173-181.

22. Jay E. Adams, *Shepherding God's Flock*, p. 130.

23. Ibid., pp. 130-134.

24. One patient spent $250,000 going from one hospital to another without definite benefit. His life savings were exhausted and the widow was left with an enormous debt. Studies of physicians have shown their lack of awareness of costs, especially in the hospital. With terminally-ill patients costs are huge although results may be minimal (see next chapter).

25. Physicians who are reluctant or opposed to second opinions are not aware of the gross ambiguities and uncertainties of medical care.

26. Heart diseases are much more frequent causes of death than cancer (see table, chapter 6).

27. Howard E. Dial, "Sufferology: Counseling Toward Adjustment in Suffering," *Journal of Pastoral Practice* 3 (2) 1979: 19-24.

28. General purposes of suffering are abundant in the Bible: spiritual growth (Heb. 12:4-12), wisdom (James 1:5-8), humility (James 1:9-11), proof of faith (1 Peter 1:6-8), contentment (Phil. 4:11), experience to share with others (2 Cor. 1:3-2:4), obedience (Heb. 5:8), guidance (Acts 8:4), reward (Matt. 5:10-12), and Christ-likeness (Rom. 8:29).

29. James I. Packer, *Knowing God* (Downers Grove: InterVarsity Press, 1973), pp. 89-97.

30. Howard E. Dial, "Sufferology: Counseling Toward Adjustment in Suffering," pp. 19-24.

31. Paul Brand, *Escape From Pain* (London: Christian Medical Fellowship, 1970).

32. Dr. A. E. Wilder Smith has suggested, not unreasonably, that this diminuation of pain is one reason that Paul and Silas were singing and praying at midnight in the Philippian jail. They would have been in severe pain after being flogged (Acts 16:22, 25).

33. Paul Ramsey, *The Patient as Person* (1970; reprint ed., New Haven: Yale University Press, 1979), pp. 113-164.

34. Ibid., pp. 134-135.

REFERENCES

Adams, Jay E. *Shepherding God's Flock.* vol. 1. Philadelphia: Presbyterian and Reformed, 1974, pp. 128-156.

Albrecht, Mark and Alexander, Brooks. "Thanatology: Death and Dying." Berkley: *Spiritual Counterfeits Project Journal*, April 1977.

Aring, Charles D. "Intimations of Mortality: An Appreciation of Death and Dying." *Annals of Internal Medicine* 69 (July 1968):139.

Brand, Paul. *Escape from Pain.* London: Christian Medical Fellowship, 1970.

Dial, Howard E. "Sufferology: Counseling toward Adjustment in Suffering." *Journal of Pastoral Practice* 3 (2):19-24.

Koop, Everett C. *Right to Live, Right to Die.* Wheaton: Tyndale House, 1976.

Kubler-Ross, Elisabeth. *Death: The Final Stage of Growth.* Englewood Cliffs: Prentice-Hall, Inc., 1975.

Kubler-Ross, Elisabeth. *On Death and Dying.* New York: Macmillan, 1969.

Lavin, J. H. "Has Elisabeth Kubler-Ross Really Flipped?" *Medical Economics,* (August 4, 1980), pp. 62-80.

Marks, R. M. and Sachar, E. J. "Undertreatment of Medical Inpatients with Narcotic Analgesics." *Annals of Internal Medicine* 78 (Feb. 1973):173-181.

Moody, Raymond. *Life after Life.* Atlanta: Mockingbird Books, 1975.

McQuilkin, J. Robertson. Suffering as a Means of Grace. Class Notes: Theology 509 and 401. Columbia Bible College, Columbia, S.C.

Packer, James I. *Knowing God.* Downers Grove: InterVarsity Press, 1973, pp. 89-97.

Rawlings, Maurice. *Beyond Death's Door.* 1978. Reprint. New York: Bantam Books, Inc., 1981, pp. XI-XIV, 1-8, 85-103.

Richards, Larry and Johnson, Paul. *Death and the Caring Community: Ministering to the Terminally Ill.* Portland: Multnomah Press, 1980.

12 | Euthanasia and a Definition of Death

It is now appropriate to direct our attention toward practical clinical problems, the sanctity of life, and a growing emphasis upon euthanasia.

"We are not dealing with a condemnation of death, we are dealing with two appropriate methods of treatment for a very sad case," stated the parents' lawyer concerning their mentally-retarded newborn with Down's Syndrome. Baby Doe was born April 9, 1982 with esophageal atresia, a congenital blockage of the esophagus. The condition was correctable by surgery, but Baby Doe died April 15, 1982. She died of starvation because parents and physicians agreed to withhold corrective surgery. Their decision was upheld by a local judge and the Indiana State Supreme Court. A *Chicago Tribune* columnist remarked, ". . . in at least one state it is now permissable to do to a deformed, retarded infant what would be illegal if done to a dog or a cat."[1]

Sanctity of human life is the central issue to both abortion and euthanasia. In abortion the critical question is whether this sanctity is given to the unborn baby, but euthanasia concerns life which has independent existence. Such sanctity must not be removed before that life has ceased.

Orthodox Christianity has consistently based its sanctity of life position upon the Sixth Commandment: "You shall not murder" (Ex. 20:13).[2] The NASV accurately reflects that "the term used in the commandment is the specific one to denote what we call murder . . . the prohibition of violent, *willful*, malicious assault upon the life of another" (emphasis added).[3] The commandment is applied to specific situations in other parts of the Mosaic law, e.g. Numbers 35:6-34 and Deuteronomy 19:1-11. Even earlier the seriousness of the offense is seen in the curse upon Cain for the murder of Abel (Gen. 4:6-15) and in God's instructions to Noah (Gen. 9:6). The divine image constitutes man's uniqueness (Gen. 1:27) in contrast to animals.

Some confusion may arise when the sanctity of life is perceived as an absolute.[4] Under the Mosaic law, Israel had the right to take the life of another after due process, "on the evidence of two or three witnesses" (Deut. 19:15). Examples of crimes which exceeded the right to life were intentional murder (Deut. 19:11-13), a rebellious son (Deut. 21:18-21), adultery and immoral sexual behavior (Deut. 22:20-30), false prophecy (Deut. 18:20), and war (Deut. 20:1-20).

With the passing of the theocracy, these requirements for capital punishments changed. By implication, Jesus abrogated the Mosaic death penalty for adultery when He instituted divorce (Matt. 5:31, 32; 19:9).[5] Under the New Testament's organizational structure, the church can only inflict spiritual punishment. (Matt. 18:15; 1 Cor. 5:1-13). Other punishments are transferred to governments: "The prerogative of the civil magistrate carries with it, express warrant for the infliction of death . . . the sword (Rom. 13:14; 1 Peter 2:14).

Sanctity of life rests solidly on the fact that human life was created in the very image of God and by God. By extension, biblical principle related to terminal illness is established. *Any activity which is initiated to kill a terminally ill patient is never justifiable.* This principle is a key to the following definitions, prescribes, and proscribes.

Euthanasia denotes "good death" and connotes death without suffering. Two general categories are active euthanasia and passive euthanasia. Active euthanasia is the intentional use of medical technology to induce or hasten death.[6] The action may be voluntary, with the patient's consent, or involuntary, without the patient's consent. Passive euthanasia involves the withholding or withdrawal of medical means and allowing the terminally ill to die as a consequence of the "natural" course of his disease process. A subdivision of active euthanasia is "managerial" euthanasia whereby individuals or groups are selected to be put to death for "medical" reasons. Limited medical and economic resources may make this action moral, but it may easily be broadened for immoral purposes.[7] Most people choose to believe that the latter would never occur in the United States, but a parallel is already present in this country.

By our biblical ethic of the sanctity of life, active euthanasia is prohibited since intentional killing is limited to the state in war and criminal punishment. In addition the ambiguity of a physician who both preserves life and ends it is a contradiction of a purely medical ethic: "The doctor's role is healing, not to be the suspected purveyor of death."[8]

At this point an additional distinction between active euthanasia and passive euthanasia where "brain death" has occurred is necessary. A Christian position seems to be that the cessation of life support falls under the division of active euthanasia.[9] The cessation of such treatment should not be placed under the category of active euthanasia where brain death has occurred. The distinction is between withdrawal of support from a patient who is still alive, as opposed to a body which is dead. The presence of life or death is established by specific, detailed criteria. That withdrawal of support as an active step cannot be denied, but in this instance death has already occurred. Respirators may keep hearts beating and other organs functioning for years. The situation is both economically and psychologically taxing on the family. This distinction involves the establishment that (brain) death has occurred, so the cessation of mechanical processes allows organs to die or be transplanted. It does not fall into the category of active euthanasia.

Two specific applications of this principle should be made because of inappropriate distinctions that are commonly made. First, patients on respirators are used as examples of situations where a decision must be made to continue or discontinue life support because of brain death. In so doing, the more common examples, such as IV's, feeding tubes, and antibiotics are overlooked. Based upon the above discussion, these measures could be withheld or stopped. They are not as obvious or as likely to result in immediate death as respirators, but they are no less life-sustaining in patients who are dependent upon them. Optional remedies should be defined "in terms of what would be 'extraordinary' for this individual."[10]

Second, the irreversibility that characterizes brain death also characterizes terminal illness where brain death has not occurred. The patient, his family, his physician and all others concerned have the moral option to discontinue any medical measures that prolong the occurrence of death. Emergency situations and incomplete information on patients in the course of a work-up may result in the initiation of measures that later are recognized to prolong the patient's and family's suffering. . . . "a decision to stop 'extraordinay' life-sustaining treatments requires no greater and in fact the same moral warrant as a decision not to begin to use them."[11] To begin or to stop treatments causes death to occur sooner, so the effect is inevitably the same. Using or not using treatments should be based solely upon the ethical principles of the situation and the medical condition of the patient. The Golden Rule (Matt. 7:12), as qualified by the biblical world view in the same manner that situational ethics are qualified, provides some guidance for these agonizing decisions. The necessary point here is that the concept of active euthanasia does not apply to this cessation of so-called ordinary or extraordinary treatments. Sometimes, the withholding of ordinary treatments may be life sustaining as in the case of Baby Doe, for without corrective surgery, any food given her would have gone into her lungs and suffocated her . Emphatically, however, all relevant biblical principles must be applied since temporal life is being shortened and accounts must be settled while one has the mental capacity for moral responsibility.

Commonly, passive euthanasia is equivalent to euthanasia when the word is used without adjectives. Thus, the following involves what most simply designate as euthanasia. Even passive euthanasia, however, is not sufficient to clearly describe the situation where a means of life support is withheld. To withhold water from someone whose only problem is deyhdration commits him to death as surely as a lethal dose of morphine. Thus, to withhold certain necessities for life can hasten a patient's death in a manner that is unethical as withdrawal of mechanical support may or may not be ethical. Terminal illness is too complex to use simple designations without each decision to treat, withhold or withdraw treatment individually evaluated in each situation.[12] Technically, from an ethical, legal, or biblical base, the withholding of life support (passive) which is clearly necessary to maintain life is not equivalent to murder (active). But the simple designation "passive euthanasia" does not convey appropriately the possibility that a choice may be clearly unethical.

Sometimes passive euthanasia is used synonymously with voluntary euthanasia, but the former may be voluntary or involuntary. Involuntary euthanasia would refer to those comatose or mentally-incompetent patients who were clearly not aware of reality, for whom the decision to withhold medical treatment was made by someone else, e.g., the family, the doctor, or other.[13] Voluntary euthanasia means the patient makes the final decision himself or herself at the time of, or previous to, the decision. Planning for the likelihood that a person's medical condition will necessitate such decisions is increasingly taught and accepted, to the extent that at least eight states have passed "right to die" legislation and at least forty-two others have had it introduced. The underlying intention in this movement is a sincere, moral attempt to prevent the prolongation of death in patients who are hopelessly terminal and subject to extreme cost and prolonged family agony. Clearly, this prevention is necessary and Christians should be innovative, but these issues are not so simply solved.

The voluntary euthanasia advocates desire the achievement of legislation which will give legal status to "living wills." These wills state that extraordinary means are not to be used in the event of a loss of rationality by the patient during a terminal illness. The definition of ordinary and extraordinary varies among medical professionals and medical crises do not allow the needed time for reflection on these proposed desires of the patient nor do they allow for changes in treatment as the patient's condition changes. For example, a patient may arrive at an emergency room with a cardiac arrest. All would agree that every attempt must be used acutely to save this patient's life. Subsequently, the patient may remain in a coma with severe, permanent brain damage after the cause of the cardiac arrest has been treated effectively. The patient may not have desired a respirator, but its use was initially unavoidable. How can a man decide the degree of distress that he is likely to tolerate at some future date?[14]

> . . . a woman in respiratory failure . . . after several days of intensive care withdrew her endotracheal tube with the balloon inflated in order to remark that she had "had enough of tubes," and "why did we not just write her off?" Intensive care was stopped forthwith. It so happened that she survived. Later, she recollected none of the therapy, but thanked everyone cordially for it . . .[15]

The patient is incapable of predicting his future attitude and the physician is incapable of predicting future medical conditions of individual patients. This argument holds against a growing movement in Great Britain and in the United States to allow and provide instructions for terminally ill patients to commit suicide. Also, a judgment must be made about the rationality of the patient. If he has a living will, it is only effective when he is no longer able to make decisions about himself. His physician(s) must decide when that condition has developed. The decision has not been removed from the physician after all! And he may find himself at odds with the family!

The nature of medicine prevents precise prognoses. Many physicians are familiar with examples of patients who were thought to be incurably terminal, but who survived. Some opportunity must be provided to allow for such unexpected recovery.

Living wills do not offer a solution to one's future medical dilemmas. The physician must still consider the situation and the family where such dilemmas exist. The great danger with living wills is the "thin edge of the wedge" because decisions about quality of life are made legally . It can be demonstrated clearly from history that a moral standard, in this instance the sanctity of life, further degenerates if even once it is altered legally. Eventually, quality of life becomes the standard of the group that is in control. Baby Doe is a poignant example, but in reality this event is nothing new. In one report over a period of 2½ years, in only one hospital 43 babies were allowed to die following discussion between the physicians and the family that this was the right course.[16] The complexity of these issues should be apparent. Definitions must be carefully used without overlooking the particulars of each situation. Both patients and physicians can be inaccurate in their judgments. This inaccuracy and uncertainty requires guidelines which will allow for the variability of times, medical conditions, patients' and family attitudes, and other pertinent information.

"Death with dignity," leads one to think that the dying should be treated with great care. The phrase entails significant problems which should not be overlooked. On a Christian basis, death is never dignified. Death is inseparably related to sin. Death is a symbol and result of rebellion against God; death is the "last enemy" (1 Cor. 15:26). "Death with dignity" is used as though the management of the dying is simple. The phrase does not allow the necessary flexibility. An earlier use of this phrase appeared in a book published in Germany in 1920 as a motto for a movement to legalize the killing of those who had "the right to the complete relief of an unbearable life."[17] Despite its "catchiness," the term *death with dignity* is a subtle but distinct departure from the biblical position of the sanctity of life.[18]

The words "quality of life" have similar problems. Its hidden agenda is brought out by the questions, "What are the criteria of quality and who determines those criteria?" That quality is already being decided in newborn nurseries. The beginning of the Nazi Holocaust involved the elderly and mentally ill who were considered not to have a "quality" which gave them a right to life. In a very short time, Jews and others had lost their "quality," as well. A "life not worthy to be lived" is less subtle, but this euphemism is similarily applied to people with various problems.

"Right to die" is another current euphemism. No one needs a right to die because death is inevitable. What is needed is maximum discernment of the time when all hope for recovery is lost with the cautious attitude that allows for the particulars of each case. When this phrase is applied to the terminally ill, it is easily broadened to justify anyone who desires to commit suicide. Facetiously asked, why shouldn't any depressed or anxious person be given the "right to die" and escape their distress?

Deceptive and demeaning words and phrases are used by Christians. Dr. Norman Geisler, an ethicist who is a respected evangelical, describes some lives as "prehuman" or "subhuman." He states, as one of his points, that taking a prehuman, subhuman, or posthuman life is less serious than taking a fully human life.[19] That thinking is biblically inadequate and morally inferior to current laws which would say that a person who shot and killed a Mongoloid child must be tried for murder. Such thinking and terminology will diminish the effectiveness of Christian persuasion. Unfortunately we as Christians have, not had our "senses (faculties of our minds) trained to discern good and evil" (Heb. 5:14).

Since abortion is now legal and widely prevalent, it provides a parallel in the use of euphemisms which blur distinctions and generalize moral issues. The unborn baby has been termed "fetal tissue," "product of conception," and "potential human life." Abortion is called a "termination of pregnancy." The brainwashing effect which occurs can be summarized: "Since the old ethic has not been fully displaced, it has been necessary to separate the idea of abortion from the idea of killing, which continues to be socially abhorrent."[20] These euphemisms about the terminally ill are the beginning of the devaluation of life; if so, then, is not the devaluation of any time of life, i.e., all of mankind, only a step further?

The abortion issue is perhaps the watershed to prevent the liberalization and/or legalization of euthanasia, because both involve the sanctity of life. Possibly, the greatest prevention to stop liberalization of euthanasia would be the enactment of federal legislation to reverse the Supreme Court decision which legalized abortion. Laws reinforce positively or negatively the values of a society. Thus, legal establishment of life at conception would strengthen society's attitude toward the sanctity of human life at all stages. Euthanasia cannot be separated from the abortion issue, and those who oppose euthanasia, to be consistent, must oppose abortion, as well.

Other euphemisms are: "vegetable," "parasite," "living cadaver," "gork," "living shell," and "life devoid of value." As Christians, we should not minimize the complexities of the management of the terminally ill, but we should be able to identify those terms which detract from the biblical sanctity of life.

Life and Brain Death

In December 1979, "Mack," an on duty policeman, was shot three times. Complications of these injuries included aspiration (inhalation of the contents of his stomach into his lungs) and cardiac arrest. These events resulted in severe brain damage and for seven months, Mack did not respond to stimuli. No hope was given by his physicians that he would regain consciousness. At that time with the agreement of his doctors and family, the respirator was turned off, and his anticonvulsant medications and antibiotics were stopped. Surprisingly, Mack was able to breath on his own. In October 1981, a physician making rounds in the nursing home routinely ordered, "Breathe deeply." To the doctor's amazement, Mack did! He could also open and shut his eyes. More intensive rehabilitation was begun. Today, he is back to 95 percent of his preinjury intellectual ability, but he is unable to use his arms and legs. His physician concluded that Mack's recovery is "the biggest surprise I've had as a neurologist . . . virtually everything in the medical literature suggests patients in a vegetative state three to six months after anoxic (without oxygen) ischemic injury to the brain have an essentially hopeless prognosis."[21]

Clearly, this case is unusual and illustrates the relative unpredictability of coma and death. Emotionally, the decisions which concern the presence or absence of life are the most difficult. Technical competence has required that well-accepted criteria, and confidence that life has ceased and death has occurred, be updated. Two points must preface a more detailed review of this issue. First, "these questions have to do with the nature of human existence . . . (and as such) is too serious a matter to be entrusted exclusively to physicians."[22] Second, "In these areas there are no easy solutions. Whichever way we turn, we come up against borders which give us no peace."[23] As we have previously asserted, the medical profession is essentially devoid of any recognition of a transcendent nature of man. Thus, Christians must increasingly bring the biblical view of man into these issues. Although difficulties and imprecision will remain, an emphasis upon the sanctity of life hopefully will retard any further development of the quality of life ethic.

Life and death will refer to the presence or absence of *physical* life respectively unless otherwise noted. Dying is a process of transition from the state of life to the state of death. No confusion exists about the characteristics of each state. The supreme problem is deciding when the process of dying has progressed over the boundary which separates one state from the other.[24] Until the respirator became widely available, the presence of one state or the other was rarely in question. However, the evidence shows that the numbers of patients who fall into the gray area is increasing.

The determination that life has ceased is primarily a medical decision, not a moral decision—the absence of physiological criteria in an individual patient is determined medically. Those criteria themselves, however, are determined primarily upon a moral basis. An ethicist cannot evaluate respiration, heartbeat, etc., but he can contribute to, and determine the morality of those criteria.

The role of the physician will be clearer if it is kept in mind that he functions primarily as a supplier of the needed information. As the final arbiter in individual situations, however, he may interpret such information as to conform to his own moral purposes.

Man's spiritual nature is not measurable and cannot be perceived through the five physical senses. So the presence or absence of life can only be measured in its physical or physiological manifestations. That physicians are the most knowledgeable people about the body is without question. However, Christians must require physicians to make only those physiological evaluations which are appropriately limited in moral judgment.

The simplicity of death pronouncement in the past is more relevant than one might expect.[25] Those criteria were essentially the absence of spontaneous respiration and heartbeat. Today, a third criteria of brain death has been added. Respiration, however, is primarily dependent upon brain function, as the muscles of respiration are stimulated by a lower center of the brain.[26] Respiration reflects a functioning brain, and coupled with a condition in which consciousness co-exists with nonfunction of the respiratory center is rare. Conscious response to all of the five senses and electroencephalographic waves can be absent and the respiratory center still function. These circumstances present medical dilemmas, such as Mack's condition. In the past the activity of the brain was being measured indirectly by respiratory function. There are more sophisticated means used to measure brain function today.

Death occurs primarily as a result of the failure of the functioning interrelationships of the heart, lungs, and brain. The heart rate may be increased or decreased by the brain, but its ability to contract repetitively is inherent within the organ itself. Thus, one mode of death occurs when oxygen is not taken to the brain and it ceases to function. Respiration ceases without the brain function. Another mode occurs as a diseased or injured brain ceases to function causing respiration to cease—without oxygen the heart ceases. A third mode of death is when the diseased or crushed lungs cannot transfer sufficient oxygen into the blood to maintain function of the heart and brain.

This interrelatedness of the heart and respiration is essential to an understanding of brain death. The terminology is new, but it is merely an update of defining death which is based upon newer technology which requires more detailed criteria. The brain is the receiver, transmitter, and clearing station of the nerves of the body. Its functioning can only be determined by some response of the physical body: a voice, a hand raised, eyelids blinked, withdrawal from pain, respiration, EEG waves, etc. Although thought may continue within one's spirit, its lack of physical manifestation where brain death has occurred prevents any determination that thought continues in that dimension. Thus, the absence of any physical response is equivalent to death, assuming irreversibility of the brain's condition.

In July 1981, a report was approved and sent to the president, as the latest update on brain death.[27] The signatories were medical consultants to the

President's Commission for the Study of Ethical Problems in Medicine and Biomedical and Behavioral Research. Their task was the diagnosis of death. Their report was entitled, "Uniform Determination of Death Act:"

> An individual who has sustained either (1) irreversible cessation of circulatory and respiratory functions, or (2) irreversible cessation of all functions of the entire brain, including the brain stem, is dead. A determination of death must be made in accordance with accepted medical standards.[28]

The act is proposed as a model jurisdiction. It is endorsed by the American Bar Association, the American Medical Association, the National Conference of Commissioners on State Laws, and the President's Commission. In the journal in which the act appeared, advisory guidelines followed in the text. Every reasonable precaution is included to insure that these criteria are met.

Such criteria for brain death, however will not remove a worrisome mystery:

> It is conceivable that a person who is dying may stand in a passageway where human communication has long since been left behind, but which nonetheless contains a self-consciousness different from any other which we know.[29]

This mystery alone should preclude anything other than a prayerful, serious and humble determination that death has occurred by whatever criteria.

The decision to discontinue a respirator, medications, or other forms of treatment, based upon statements #1 and #2 of the "Death Act" and its guidelines, is consistent with previous criteria of death: (1) involves no change. (2) is synonymous with cessation of spontaneous respiratory function, and subsequently cessation of the heartbeat. The definition has changed to include brain function since the heart and lungs may now be kept functioning artifically after brain function has ceased.

The "Death Act" is consistent with biblical criteria since the ability to physically express moral responsibility of an individual has ceased. Thus, biblical principles allow for respirators, medications, and other treatments to be stopped where brain death has occurred. The reluctance by Christians to accept this position probably results from their determined effort to guard life. The criteria of brain death establishes the state of death. If that establishment is ethical, then the disposal of the body or its use for organ transplantation is ethical.[30]

Although it should be apparent, the body which meets the criteria of brain death is distinct from the person who is hopelessly, terminally ill. The latter may be the same as the former, but the large majority of the latter are not the same as the former; *the criteria for brain death is absent.* These two situations must be distingushed because their similarity may cause confusion when a decision must be made whether to initiate treatments or withdraw modes already begun. "Rightly declaring a patient to be dead is not the same as no longer to oppose his death."[31]

With the exception of situations where donor organs are needed, the current policies and practice of medicine in the determination of death are compatible with a biblical position. This circumstance is encouraging in view of many ethics and practices that are not. If anything, the aggressiveness to do all that can be done in medical practice and the view that death is a failure of medical care is more of a problem than protection of existing life.

Since the courts are sometimes involved with death determination and the withdrawal of means of organ support, the problem is not only medical. In addition the growing movement toward social acceptance and legalization of voluntary euthanasia is a harbinger of events which may result in a weakening of these criteria of determining death.

Possible exceptions to the above conclusion are situations which involve a need for organ transplantation. A characteristic of a scientist is the strong desire to do all that is technically possible. In this case two additional pressures are present. Available donor organs are always less than the demand; so the patient, his family, and his doctor are anxious to obtain them. In many cases, death may be imminent without those organs. Second, decisions must be made quickly to prevent deterioration of the donor organs and to allow time to make the complex arrangements for operating rooms and teams to make the transplants. Many physicians and ethicists have proposed that the determination of brain death be done by physicians entirely different from those who are involved with the recipient. Although the above pressures coupled with the nonavailability of separate teams make practical implementation difficult, that standard must be sought with predetermined arrangements for practical implementation. Paul Ramsey does not equivocate:

> If no person's death should *for this purpose* (organ transplantation) be hastened, then the definition of death should not *for this purpose* be updated or the procedures for stating that a man has died be revised as a means of affording easier access to organs. . . . This ought to be a judgment and an agreement in medical science and practice that is also independent of whether organ transplantation is bedeviled, impeded, or assisted thereby (his emphasis).[32]

Anyone who recognizes the above pressures to proceed with organ transplantation and the serious necessity that a patient's death be determined solely upon the criteria of physical evidence, will realize the potential for danger. The general compliance with, or violation of, this standard is not known, but individual violations are likely to occur.

In conclusion, the formal criteria for brain death is compatible with a biblical position. The distinction between life and death can be more clearly maintained if each is recognized as a state of existence or nonexistence. This distinction is entirely physical. Situations in which brain death criteria must be applied are uncommon, but are likely to become more prevalent. The greatest current danger which violates the sanctity of life in the determination that death has occurred involves organ transplantation. Based upon the physiological inter-dependency of the lungs, the heart, and the brain, it can be demonstrated that the criteria for death has not been changed, but appropriately updated for the application of newer technology that has made possible the preservation of function of the heart and lungs when the function of the brain has ceased.

Guidelines for Casuistry

"Mother" realized her worst fears when she developed a cancerous brain tumor. A family decision was made that she not be told that she had cancer, but her eyes betrayed that she knew. We were told that surgery was necessary. The night before surgery, she was anointed with oil. Following surgery she was given two months to live. Her doctor recommended that she not be made miserable with radiation and chemotherapy during her final days. At his suggestion we took her home to be with the family. Questions came from time to time whether "everything" should be done. The experience was difficult: convulsions occurred, her eating stopped, and her breathing became labored during the three days preceding her death. God was faithful and gave Mother a "peace and serenity in place of the fear that had always been part of her personality" during these last days—now she has an eternal and perfect peace.[33]

Are practical guidelines possible? They are, although these guidelines may lack the precision and comprehensiveness which some might desire.

Surprisingly, present care of the terminally ill has much that is acceptable, even favorable. Professionals and lay people are examining and wrestling with better approaches: dying and death guidelines, hospices, and nursing homes. As stated, the most frequent problem seems to be an unwillingness to let patients who face certain, imminent death, die peacefully.

Dr. Everett Koop has argued that the decisions concerning what procedures are to be used, and for how long, must be "tailored to the problems at hand, the background and experience of the physician, the depth of understanding of the family, and the relationship which exists between the patient and physician and family and physician."[34] In addition he states that laws must not be enacted to govern these situations because of these specific, individual variations. Perhaps Christians can develop these conclusions further, and base them upon principles under consideration here.

The church has the resources and responsibility to be involved in the care of its members. The pastor or elders should develop experience in the biblical and practical approach to the terminally ill. One or more physicians could be consultants. Even better, one of the elders may be a physician, assuming that he is otherwise biblically qualified. Another solution would be care by a Christian physician who is wise in these and other situations. Where a patient is known to be a Christian, and the physician is not, the family, pastor, or elders may have to be assertive to prevent unnecessary procedures and expense. Christians should consider caring for the dying in their homes. Anointing with oil, serious prayer, and other means are assumed to be applicable.

It has been stated that Christians have the moral freedom to choose not to accept certain modes of treatment in cases in which there is virtually no medical hope, in which the complications of treatment may hasten death or in which intended treatment is not clearly effective. These circumstances are more common than most people realize. Detailed questioning of medical personnel will often reveal that extensive, expensive procedures have uncertain benefit and may hasten death. As is being stressed, many individual variables must be considered, but the moral freedom not to comply with recommended medical treatment should be a clear option. This point is very important.

Under the past and present system the physician is the final arbiter in the sense that his/her directions are those which result in what is actually done, or not done, to patients. This situation is the most ethically practial assuming Christians fully apply other biblical ethics. However, two problems need to be addressed. First, is there not a better way for these decisions to be made? Might not a selected panel be a better approach because of accumulated experience and objectivity? Might an immoral physician do less than is indicated ethically, even hasten the patient's death? These questions are serious objections to the physician role, but they are insufficient to supplant him. Further, the physician is not "free" to do whatever he wants. Nurses and many others participate in and observe the care of patients, and frequently are vocal in their disagreements. Also, the family members are close observers. Other physicians are commonly involved as consultants. Although it is not absolute, an awareness of observation causes a person to be more careful to do the right thing.

The threat of malpractice poses a second problem with the physician's role. Many physicians will do more than they really think is necessary on the probability that a malpractice suit may be brought later. One realization, however, minimizes this possibility. The courts are extremely lenient in cases which involve the obviously terminal patient. Since the Christian physician trusts God's sovereignty, he should be minimally affected by the threat of malpractice.

The central role of the physician should not be assumed to be the best approach in the future. No guarantee exists that physicians will appropriately care for the terminally ill. Western morals have been declining. Previously considered evidence shows pressure toward the enactment of euthanasia and the availability of means to commit suicide. Economic pressures are increasing. Physicians cannot be depended upon to act according to the Christian ethic. Abortion, infanticide, and other issues have demonstrated that fact. With the erosion of the sanctity of life, diligent attention must be given to changes which threaten to result in inappropriate care for the dying.

Although economics seems out of place when human lives are involved, expenditures for medical care are a staggering reality and continue to increase. For example, in 1980 a patient presented to an emergency room with a ruptured abdominal aneurysm. In spite of heroic measures including surgery, he died within sixteen hours. His bill was $10,302.[35] In a study from 1977-1979 of admissions to medical intensive care units and coronary care units and subsequent follow-up, mortality of patients who were older than 75 years was 44 percent; 65-74 years was 33 percent; 55-64 years was 22 percent within 1 year.[36] Hospital charges for these were $6,096, $8,489, and $13,653 respectively, and would be considerably greater today.

Balance is necessary at this point. On the one hand, sanctity of life cannot be lessened on the basis of economics. On the other hand, many situations do not necessitate these expenditures. The example of "Mother" is an illustration in which nursing homes, even intensive care, could have been used, but in her case death was certain. All that can be done does not have to be done, and should not necessarily be done. With a biblically directed value system, Christians should be aggressive to discover new alternatives with little or no compromise to the appropriate care of patients.

In the final analysis only one guideline is necessary. Final decisions are left to the physician with input from the patient, family, pastor, and elders. Preferably, a Christian physician with experience and study concerning these issues should care for the patient. Where a Christian physician is not caring for the patient, this role for the physician is less certain with no guarantee that biblical principles will be applied. The current status of moral values will not allow for complacency. The most important role for Christians is to make every effort to establish and implement biblical values and priorities with dying patients and to protect the sanctity of life from an increasing movement toward active euthanasia and voluntary suicide.

NOTES

1. *Chicago Tribune*, quoted in "Action Line," the newsletter of the Chrisitan Action Council, May 14, 1982.

2. John Murray, *Principles of Conduct* (1957; reprint ed., Grand Rapids: Eerdmans Pub. Co., 1978), pp. 107-122.

3. Ibid., p. 113.

4. We recognize the disagreement which exists among conservative believers concerning capital punishment. The argument here is directed to those who do consider that some situations allow for the intentional killing of another.

5. John Murray, *Principles of Conduct*, p. 119.

6. Duncan Vere, *Voluntary Euthanasia — Is There An Alternative?* (London: Christian Medical Fellowship Publication, 1971), p. 50. The concepts in this paragraph are mostly from Vere, chapter 3. His entire book is devoted to the fallacies and dangers of voluntary euthanasia and living wills and to the development of alternatives.

7. Robert W. White, Moral Issues in Medicine. Unpublished Paper.

8. Duncan Vere, *Voluntary Euthanasia*, p. 50.

9. C. Everett Koop, *Right to Live, Right to Die* (Wheaton: Tyndale House, 1976), pp. 105, 107.

10. Paul Ramsey, *The Patient as Person* (1970; reprint ed., New Haven: Yale University Press, 1979), p. 120.

11. Ibid., p. 121.

12. See Guidelines for Casuistry, infra.

13. It is an interesting moral inconsistency that a Mongoloid child, such as Baby Doe, can have treatment withheld and be allowed to die legally in the sterile atmosphere of a hospital but similar action invoking a Mongoloid child in his home would result in a murder trial. The medical environment seems to exist under a separate set of rules.

14. Duncan Vere, *Voluntary Euthanasia*, p. 18.

15. Ibid., p. 19.

16. R. S. Duff and A. G. Campbell, "Moral and Ethical Dilemmas in the Special Care Nursery," *New England Journal of Medicine* 289 (1973): 890-894.

17. Francis A Schaeffer and C. Everett Koop, *Whatever Happened to the Human Race* (Old Tappan, NJ: Fleming H. Revell Co., 1979), p. 90.

18. Paul Ramsey, "The Indignity of Death and Dignity;" In: *Death Inside Out*, eds. Peter Steinfels and Robert M. Weatch (New York: Harper and Row Publishers, 1974), pp. 81-96.

19. Norman Geisler, *Ethics: Issues and Alternatives* (Grand Rapids: Zondervan, 1971), p. 234.

20. Everett C. Koop, *Right to Live, Right to Die* (Wheaton: Tyndale House, 1976), p. 48.

21. *Medical World News* (May 24, 1982), pp. 8, 13.

22. Helmut Thielicke, "The Doctor As Judge of Who Shall Live and Who Shall Die," in: *Who Shall Live*, Kenneth Vaux, ed., (New York: Harper Row, 1964), p. 147.

23. Ibid., p. 164.

24. The word "body" may sound callous, but a person, especially from the Christian viewpoint, is not present in a body without physical life. Thus, to say that a person may exist in a state of life or death is inaccurate. A dead boy is not a person. Also, technically, to say a person is alive or dead as it is usually meant, is inaccurate. A person is alive in a body, or he departs the body to the spiritual realm, but he never ceases to live.

25. I am grateful to the clarity with which Dr. Paul Ramsey has presented these issues in his book. The reader is urged to review his chapters on dying and death for a clarity which rarely enters into these discussions.

26. *Lower* means the part of the brain that lies below conscious thought.

27. Report on the Medical Consultants on the Diagnosis of Death to the President's Commission for the study of Ethical Problems in Medicine and Biomedical and Behavioral Research. "Guidelines for the Determination of Death," *Journal of the American Medical Association* 246 (Nov. 13, 1981): 2184-2186.

28. Ibid.

29. Helmut Thielicke, "Ethics in Modern Medicine," in *Who Shall Live?*, ed. Kenneth Vaux (New York: Harper and Row, 1964), p. 163.

30. Someone may think that these criteria might be used to justify abortion. Although consciousness is not present, spontaneous heartbeat, respiration, and brain activity are present. Besides, the state of the fetus is one of an expected increase in all its functions, not unexpected recovery.

31. Paul Ramsey, *The Patient as Person* (1970; reprint ed., New Haven: Yale University Press, 1979), p. 99.

32. Ibid., p. 104.

33. The Presbyterian Journal (July 28, 1982), pp. 9-11.

34. Everett C. Koop, *Right to Live, Right to Die*, p. 101.

35. W. M. Hendricks, "If This Is How Doctor's Families Are Treated," *Medical Economics* (January 4, 1982): pp. 46-48.

36. E. W. Campion, A. G. Mulley, et al, "Medical Intensive Care for the Elderly: A Study of Current Use, Costs, and Outcomes," *Journal of the American Medical Association* 246 (Nov. 6, 1981): 2052-2056.

REFERENCES

Campion, E. W., Mulley, A. G. et al. "Medical Intensive Care for the Elderly: A Study of Current Use, Costs, and Outcomes." *Journal of the American Medical Association* 246 (Nov. 6, 1981):2052-2056.

Duff, R. S. and Campbell, A. G. M. "Moral and Ethical Dilemmas in the Special Care Nursery." *New England Journal of Medicine* 289 (1973):890-894.

Geisler, Norman. *Ethics: Issues and Alternatives.* Grand Rapids: Zondervan, 1971.

Hendricks, W. M. "If This Is How Doctor's Families Are Treated . . ." *Medical Economics* (January 4, 1982), pp. 46-48.

Koop, Everett C. *Right to Live, Right to Die.* Wheaton: Tyndale House, 1976.

Ramsey, Paul. The Indignity of 'Death and Dignity.' In: *Death Inside Out*, eds. Peter Steinfels and Robert M. Weatch. New York: Harper and Row Publishers, 1974.

Report of the Medical Consultants on the Diagnosis of Death to the President's Commission for the Study of Ethical Problems in Medicine and Biomedical and Behavioral Research. Guidelines for the Determination of Death. *Journal of the American Medical Association* 246 (Nov. 13, 1981): 2184-2186.

Thielicke, Helmut. "The Doctor As Judge of Who Shall Live and Who Shall Die." in *Who Shall Live*, Kenneth Vaux, ed., New York: Harper Row, 1964.

Vere, Duncan. *Voluntary Euthanasia — Is There an Alternative?* London: Christian Medical Fellowship Publications, 1971.

White, Robert W. Moral Issues in Medicine. Unpublished paper.

13 | Where To Now?
Practical Considerations

Any physician who would pursue correct biblical/medical ethics faces an awesome task. Such activities are an addition to the heavy intellectual and physical demands of professional competency and personal maturity. With any task a foundation must be laid and an organized approach developed. Directions for immediate and continuing involvement will allow current active participation for those who pursue a consistent and thorough biblical ethic.

When my study of Christian evidences began, their quantity and quality were more objective than I could have imagined! Study became a springboard to increasing investigation of scientific evidences, as well as the biblical definition and description of the Christian and his calling.

Contrary to this experience, naturalistic philosophies of medical schools train physicians to think and behave in patterns which are variously inconsistent and opposed to biblical principles. Subconsciously, this training has a strong and lasting influence on one's mind. Without a study of the evidences for the Christian faith, a full commitment is unlikely because the counter-balancing principles are not consciously present in the believer's mind. Any believer who understands the relationship between his faith and the natural sciences can be certain that his position is more consistent with the scientific evidence than that of the unbeliever. A study of this evidence will strengthen one's faith.

Along with the scientific evidence as a necessary precedent to the foundation of both personal and professional ethics, is thorough and systematic Bible study. Medical students and residents are encouraged to attend Bible college or seminary. For many graduate physicians such formal training may not be possible, but many other opportunities exist today to acquire biblical understanding. The most important is the selection of a local church which teaches the "whole counsel of God" in a thorough and consistent manner. Obviously, many other desirable qualities will be inherent to such a church, fellowship, worship, encouragement, etc., but such teaching is a prerequisite. This type of church is so necessary that it should be the highest priority in choosing where to live. The difference that such a church can make in the lives of family members is exciting, but unfortunately too many Christians will not experience the difference because such churches are uncommon. Other resources for biblical teaching are seminars, conferences, cassette tapes, home study courses, extension programs, and books. No Christians in history or in modern times have had such resources: thus, "to him whom much is given, much is required" (Lk. 12:48).

An emphasis upon Bible study would be incomplete without emphasis upon obedience. Biblical knowledge is not equivalent to wisdom or to holiness. Many theologians and laymen are thoroughly knowledgeable about the Bible and claim to love God, but they do not obey God in living righteous lives. Jesus said, "If you love me, you will keep my commandments" (John 14:15). The experience of obedience gives an understanding and insight into the Bible which is impossible otherwise. Thus, personal ethics (morality) is another prerequisite to an increasing understanding of ethics. Progress in the former with continued Bible study will increase the latter and effective Christians must have both.

I once asked Dr. Robert White why so few Christian physicians are involved in medical-ethical issues so clearly contrary to biblical teaching. His letter to me included this response:

> Let's face it, this is simply a very tough intellectual exercise . . . When we start to talk about life issues . . . we find ourselves not only isolated sometimes, socially and spiritually, but professionally. . . . It is simply easier to choose to be ignorant or indifferent. . . . By the very nature of these issues, we are on the attack. . . . Churches, even evangelical churches, have not generally been supportive. . . . Many physicians don't have any direct knowledge of what is going on because of their particular practices, but this is an unacceptable excuse.[1]

Thus, these issues are not to be avoided, but neither are they to be undertaken lightly. A biblical-medical ethic is a strenuous, costly task.[2]

But what approach should those take who are willing to study diligently? The beginning should involve a study of Christian ethics in general, then scientific and medical ethics written by Christians. Unfortunately, not much biblical work has been done in this latter area. Several books are listed in the bibliography and references. Since the Bible rarely speaks specifically about scientific or medical issues, principles and practices will vary. Discernment is needed to allow freedom where freedom exists and to post limits where the Bible explicitly restricts.

A key attitude in the development of a biblical-medical ethic is an unwillingness to accept traditional or common medical ethics without biblical scrutiny. Medical ethics has not grown out of the Christian world, but the secular world. The whole of Scripture is clear that the thinking of the unregenerate is opposed to God's thinking. Medical ethics must not be "conformed to this world," but "transformed by the renewing (biblically) of your (Christian physicians') mind" (Rom. 12:2) by which Christ's glory can be manifested (2 Cor. 3:18). If Christians cannot discern God's morality, no hope exists that the non-Christian world will discover it!

> . . . we have been carried along by the shifting, sinking sands of our social morals . . . taught by pseudomedical weirdoes and their studies, surveys, polls, noncommittal, nonjudgmental, in order that just as a body of water will seek its own level so human behavior will sort itself out and new norms will help me understand, get with it, and glory in a new age of liberation of the human spirit.[3]

Only the "renewed" mind is able to offer anything better.

Is it too late? Are the forces against such a change too entrenched to overcome? The answers to these questions depend upon God's sovereign will. This much is certain. Christians are His agents of proclamation and reform. If He does choose to stay or reverse the immoral trend in the United States, it will only be through "renewed minds." In every area of life, a great need exists for knowledgeable *and* committed Christians. Most of the Christian church and all of non-Christian thought is bankrupt for these characteristics. Logically, biblical philosophy has a stronger argument and can easily refute its oppositon. However, this refutation requires a biblically-trained mind which results from study and reflection. For such a mind it is an opportue time.

For any who are willing to pursue a biblical-medical ethic—do something today to begin implementation: make some change(s) in your life. Doctors should pray with their patients; patients should pray with their doctors; both should pray for each other. Read booklets with biblical answers to life's problems, schedule more time for study, and examine the balanced Christian life for ommitted areas in your life. Do not omit the latter, because God requires it of every believer. Act now, for this day of opportunity may not last. Christians are literally fighting for their freedom in the United States. Our only hope is for "judgment, recognition, then biblical change to begin with the household of God" (1 Peter 4:17).

In the December 1981 issue of the *Journal of the Medical Association of Georgia,* an editorial appeared which portrayed the Christian faith as being one way among many; and quoted Scripture to develop this position! In the past, the Journal balanced their editorial policy, so I responded with a letter which they published. It follows.

COUNTERPOINT TO THE CHRISTMAS EDITORIAL

Dear Sir:

Paul Kuntz (*JMAG*, December, 1981) speaks of "a way to God through reason above all particular faiths of mankind . . . a universal way." Jesus Christ's own words conflict with Kuntz's analysis: "I am the way, the truth, and the life. No one comes to the Father except through me" (John 14:6, NIV). In addition, Kuntz speaks of "one society with one code of laws."

Jesus Christ speaks of two societies in Matthew 25: "you who are blessed" (v.34) and "you who are cursed" (v. 41). Each group has a different destiny: "eternal punishment" and "eternal life" (v. 46).

The issue needs more comprehensive explanation than either Mr. Kuntz or I have presented. Jesus Christ, however, by His own words spoke of His being the only way. On that basis, He is not compatible with other ways. There are only three options. First, He spoke the truth sometimes and lied sometimes. Second, He may have been demented. If these possibilities are correct, all Christians follow and worship either a liar or a lunatic. The third possibility is that He always spoke the truth. In this case, Christians worship and follow Him as Lord, Savior, and God.

Mr. Kuntz is misrepresenting Christ Himself to state that He is one of several ways. A choice must be made between Jesus Christ and any other way. His (Jesus) own words confront every person with (the necessity of making) that decision.

This letter is presented as one example of a method by which an opportunity exists to speak to others through existing means. Many editors will publish letters which are written responsibly. These allow counterpoints to previously published positions, and even statements of opinion that are not responses. Many publications, e.g., *New England Journal of Medicine, American Medical News, Journal of the American Medical Association, and Medical World News,* are distributed to physicians of all specialities. Explicit Christian positions may be edited out or not accepted for publication, but it is important to reinforce in reader's minds a conservative ethical position. Begin sending letters this week!

Many who are in academia should consider longer editorials, articles, and books. Today, articles on medical ethics are commonly included in many major medical journals and some are devoted entirely to this subject. Thus, medical ethics are a valid form of publication for academic recognition. Major changes in the area of one's involvement may be necessary, but no greater need exists in the practice of medicine.

Political opportunites also exist. Currently, the primary thrust must be against abortion. Anti-abortion legislation and action groups, such as the Christian Action Council, should be supported. Such involvement is also an opportunity to learn about the political machinery of American democracy since Christians must use this process to protect Christian freedom and attempt true reform. At the same time Christians should demonstrate creativity and willingness to contribute to practical needs. Crisis pregnancy centers which help women with unexpected pregnancies are examples for this kind of contribution. Christian alcohol and drug treatment centers are other possibilities.

A great need exists within Christianity to disarm the role of psychiatry and psychology. In any involvement of a biblical-medical ethic, psychotherapeutic issues will be involved. Again, a secularly-developed system is an antithesis of a biblically-developed system. Psychiatrists and psychologists should read Christians' critiques of their fields to discover the points of conflict with biblical theology. If pastors have these professionals in their congregation they should take the opportunity to teach these men and women. Other physicians could also be discipled.

Physicians can begin to practice biblical, wholistic medicine. Examples of that practice have been presented, but more innovation is possible. For example, Dr. Hilton Terrell has a wholistic approach in his office which includes non-acceptance of third party payment. Dr. Paul Brand revolutionized the surgery and management of leprosy patients because he did not accept the traditional approach. Dr. Richard Stewart has developed the use of midwives in an outlying hospital to allow more natural childbirth and decreased physician involvement in Douglasville, Georgia. The Christian physician can give better medical care than the non-Christian, but only if he begins to question traditional concepts. Christians should be pioneers, not followers.

Dialogue and criticism are needed in a pursuit of the biblical practice of medicine because so little work has been done. Many topics need to have a biblical/medical ethic developed: artificial insemination, cloning, in vitro fertilization, "right" to medical care, economics and the practice of medicine, organ transplantation, birth control and sterilization, use of medications, and genetic engineering, etc. All of these are pressing issues with little or no biblical substance.

The cost of a truly biblical/medical ethic is great. Fewer patients can be seen, decreasing one's viable practice and income. Both Christian and non-Christian friends or colleagues may not understand or even be critical. Many articles may be rejected, even by Christian publications. The time and money spent on vacations and pleasurable pursuits will have to be examined. Medical practices will need to be examined and changed. The cost must be counted (Luke 14:25-35). Such committment is self-denying and cross-carrying (Luke 9:23); but "for what is a man profited if he gains the whole world, and loses or forfeits himself?" (Luke 9:25). Dr. White has these thought-provoking comments:

> As physicians we have three choices, but not four. We can become activists. We can be indifferent. We can be ignorant. But we cannot be neutral . . . at least some of us must with utmost vigor and cool-headedness come down hard on the side of reviewing and renewing our interests and activism. . . . Otherwise . . . we further abandon the battle to those whose humanistic utilitarian motives continue to torpedo the moral underpinning of any viable and vibrant society with resultant inevitable and eventual collapse.[4]

NOTES

1. Personal Letter, February 8, 1982.

2. Such statements are likely to seem arrogant, but one tires of professing Christians who are biblically ignorant through a lack of disciplined effort; yet they consider themselves able to disagree with those who have made the effort. Certainly this book is imperfect, but it has been preceded by hundreds of hours of study and review by both physicians and theologians. Critics should at least make similar preparation and consultation.

3. Robert White, Moral Issues in Medicine, Unpublished paper.

4. Robert White, Moral Issues in Medicine, Unpublished paper.

Appendix

Biblical Priorities for the Physician and Medical Student

My involvement in medical education begin in 1965, my freshmen year of medical school and continues to the present, excluding three years of miltary service. This time includes four years of medical school, one of internship, two years of family practice residency, and ten years as a faculty member. I have observed the lives of peers and other students from their initial exposure to medicine, through continued training, and eventually into private practice or academia. A common pattern with most Christian medical students has been an increasing involvement in medicine and a decreasing involvement with other areas of Christian responsibility.

Medical school begins after four years of college and consists of four additional years. Specialty training (residency) is another three to seven years. By then, most physicians are approximately thirty years of age and, since the age of six years, have been in formal education. Still ahead is a practice to be established or academic recognition to be achieved. The whole process is arduous and demanding. Little time is available for a serious reflection upon the totality of one's life.[1]

To graduate from medical school with a sound faith in itself is an achievement because of naturalistic philosophies that assail one's faith. Even so, many do survive with a faith intact, and many become Christians during those trying years. Once in medical school, however, the above-mentioned pattern begins. The first two years of medical school are similar to college with its regularity of class structure, so Christian students often remain active in their churches and Christian organizations on campus. As clinical training with patients (in most institutions) begins during the third and fourth years, however, the students appear less frequently in Christian contexts. Most are irregularly active or entirely absent. Days are filled with rounds, workups, laboratory studies, conferences, and other aspects of patient care. Nights involve on call duty. Neither their churches nor campus fellowships, however, show much concern because these students are legitimately involved in a high calling of service to mankind, the practice of medicine. Unfortunately in many instances, they continue in this pattern for the remainder of their lives, allowing their professional activities to exclude other spiritual obligations.

Indeed, medicine is a high calling, but it must be placed within a biblical system of priorities; that is, it must be placed within the whole will of God. The believer must seek God's will in *every* area of his life for his own spiritual growth and that of others. In addition chapter 6 provided evidence that optimal physical health is promoted by a right relationship and right response to the Great Physician. On this basis the inclusion of spiritual activities, e.g., prayer, evangelism and counseling, is an essential ingredient of a sound medical practice. Not only should God's will be lived out because He is God, but His way (will) is always the best for all concerned (physical health being no exception). "For what will a man be profited, if he gains the whole world and forfeits his soul? (Matt. 16:26). What will a physician be profited if he is a great physician in every other way except the establishment of God's will in his practice to the neglect of his own soul and that of his patients?

There is much confusion about the will of God. Often the phrase is equated with choosing a career. Certainly, the will of God includes a career, but a career is only a part of the whole, In fact, if a Christian does not seek to practice the whole of God's will in a balanced way, his vision concerning vocations will be limited by experience. God's will for the believer is synonymous with those activities which govern one's relationship to God and others, as prescribed in the Bible. Four general *characteristics* are certainty of salvation (an understanding of justification by faith), right attitude (voluntary submission), obedience (in attitude and activities), and perserverance (a persistance through times of trial and peace). Eight *activities* are worship, prayer, Bible study, fellowship, physical health, elimination of sin, ministry, and daily necessities. (Since these characteristics were discussed generally in chapter 6, only those activities particular to the physician and the medical student are emphasized here.)

Christians need to study time management in order to make allocations that are determined by biblical priorities. These priorities are common to all believers but specific allotments require individualization. The goal is adequate time to do these activities in a quality way, but it cannot be reached without an organized, preplanned schedule. Businesses do not function smoothly without schedules, and neither will individual lives. A sobering thought is the realization that we will reach those goals which we truly value. Thus, our daily activities with whatever degree of organization *do reveal what we value*.

The greatest concern for the Christian should be his relationship with God the Father through the Son, Jesus Christ, and the indwelling Holy Spirit. God is not a person with whom we can talk verbally and hear physically, but He has willed the means by which His children are to fellowship with Him. *These means are the activities of the Christian life,* performed according to the above characteristics. Significant involvement in these activities is necessary to the Christian life to experience the abundant life of joy, peace, and blessing. Some imperfections always will remain, but increasing knowledge and experience will progressively refine and balance these activities.

Worship, prayer, and Bible study are the most direct means by which a believer relates to God. *Worship* should be both corporate (Heb. 10:25) and personal (Matt. 6:9-10; Ps. 1:2). *Prayer* includes worship (Matt. 6:9-10), but it is a means of cleansing (1 John 1:9), thanksgiving and supplication (Phil. 4:6) also. The importance of the devotional time is recognized by most Christians, but the need for its *daily* observance often is overlooked (Ps. 1:2, 5:3; Luke 9:23; Matt. 6:34). In addition the best time is early morning (Ps. 5:3; Matt. 6:11; Ps. 57:8; Luke 4:42). *Bible study*, as meditation, should be a part of the devotional time, but it should be pursued *systematically* at other times on an ongoing basis. Spiritual growth is dependent upon biblical knowledge and understanding which only comes through diligent effort. The New Testament is clear in its description of such effort when it uses such words as work, discipline, disciple, slave, armor, wrestle, diligent, persevere, and strive. It is my conviction that the lack of study and application of Scripture are major reasons for the defeated and impotent lives of individual Christians and the universal (true) church. The moral consciousness of the believer is little, if any, better without the light of Scripture than that of the unbeliever. I issue a challenge to the Christian physician to study the Bible with the same diligence and effort that he studies medicine. I am convinced that his care of patients will only be enhanced as God redeems the time he gives to His priorities.

The Bible is not an easy book to study, but many excellent tapes, books, seminars, courses, and other means are available to assist the Christian. Concurrently, skills for personal study of the Bible should be developed as one studies the interpretation and teaching of others. Professional and personal ethics are severely needful of such study since God "has granted to us everything pertaining to life and godliness" (2 Peter 1:3).

Physicians and medical students will need to examine their areas of ministry, which primarily include their spouse, children, local church, and career. The marital relationship is designed to reflect the relationship within the Trinity (1 Cor. 11:3) with the husband loving his wife as "Christ also loved the church" (Eph. 5:25). Principally the responsibility for love in the home falls not on the wife, but on the husband.[2] On the other side, if the wife is the physician, she is still to be subject to her husband, "as to the Lord" (Eph. 5:22). The professional role of either spouse should not interfere with the biblical roles for marriage; for example, neither the husband's nor the wife's body belongs to himself or herself, but each belongs to the other (1 Cor. 7:3-5). From the beginning (Gen 2:18) the unity of husband and wife ("one flesh" Gen. 2:24; Matt. 19:5) has been the basic building block of the church and society (except when individuals have the gift of celibacy (1 Cor. 7:7). Leadership in the church is based on qualities of leadership in the home (1 Tim. 3:4-5). Thus, the biblical priority within the home is the marital relationship, not the parent-child relationship. Often this truth is overlooked because of cultural influence. Children, however, are not to be neglected but are to be brought "up in the discipline and instruction of the Lord" (Eph. 6:4), as a way of life (Deut.6:4-9). Certainly, this plan requires a significant effort by the parents.

Practically, the husband (or the wife) who is a physician must be certain that time is scheduled (not left to chance) for his/her spouse and their children. This scheduling will require *complete* call-coverage by other physicians and specific hours for patient care. Irregular and interrupted schedules can be devastating to family relationships. The priority of a physician's practice over his family is frequently where he fails biblically. Patient care should not prevent responsibilities to wife and children. Actually, neither has to exclude the other. An accurate barometer to determine whether the quality and quantity of time at home are adequate for both the spouse and the children may be the nonphysician spouse: ask him or her! The physician-spouse is not able accurately to make that determination. No exception exists in Scripture which allows neglect of the home, even for the care of patients. No doubt, it will be difficult for such scheduling because of the demands of medical practice, but there are physicians who do accomplish this balance. This priority is so necessary that changes in practice arrangements, e.g., off-duty coverage, geographical location, and even partners, should be made to allow for family time. If the neglect of the spouse (first) and the children (second) is present, the physician will have chosen a secondary area of ministry, and worse that choice involves continuing sin because of its improper balance.

Another area of ministry to which the physician must allocate time is the local church. Every Christian is a part of the body of Christ (Rom. 12:6; 1 Cor. 12:1-7) and his ministry is essential to his own growth toward maturity and that of the local church (Eph. 4:11-16). Thus, the maturity of both individuals and the whole will be less than what God has planned (and gifted) without active participation of *all* members. Gifts are given for the numerical and spiritual growth of the church body, not for the community or place of employment (Eph. 4:12). Believers have a special obligation to other believers, an obligation which they do not have to unbelievers (Gal. 6:10). A specific point of conflict may be Sunday. Obviously, patient care must continue seven days a week, but the physician who realizes that Sunday has been ordained by God as a day of worship and rest (Ex. 20:9-11) will make rounds and schedule his calls to allow for active participation in his church on this special day.

An activity to which all Christians are biblically directed, but one which physicians should personally emphasize, is that of physical health (1 Cor. 3:16-17, 1 Cor. 6:19). This activity is a special opportunity for the physician to demonstrate, by example, the maintenance and preventive care necessary for physical welfare. If physicians do not consider it worthwhile to expend effort for health, other people and particularly his patients, will be less inclined to give attention. A lack of such effort will imply, as well, that after-the-fact medical care is in reality more important to the physician than health maintenance and prevention. Role modeling is probably the strongest means of teaching (Mark 3:14; Luke 6:40; Acts 4:13). Paul was not afraid, nor was he boastful, in pointing to himself as an example (Phil. 3:17; 2 Thess. 3:7) and directing others to be an example (1 Tim 4:12).

Fellowship, mortification (the progressive but never complete process of putting off sin), and daily necessities will be left to the reader's investigation and study. Readers are encouraged to read other books and articles about personal Christian ethics, a number of which are referenced in this book. Only by the renewing of our minds will our lives and practices be transformed according to God's will, rather than conformed to the world's life and practice.

The activities which have been discussed here will not occur without planning by the physician or medical student. The time to develop these patterns is as early as possible. Medical school or residency training does not exempt one from these biblically prescribed activities. The physician's spiritual life, family life, church life, and medical practice will be less than what God would have it to be, if these areas are neglected. Jesus said that His followers must count the cost. For the physician this cost may include less income, fewer patients, less availability to patients and, possibly, a lesser standing among peers. The medical student may sacrifice better grades, and from that, less chance of acceptance into the more prestigious residency programs. To the medical student or physician, however, who chooses God's ways and means, "If God is for us, who is against us. He who did not spare His own Son, but delivered Him up for us all, how will He not also with Him freely give us all things" (Rom. 8:31-32). Initially, these things may appear to be sacrifices, but in reality they are only our "reasonable service" (Rom. 12:1, KJV) which is "producing for us an eternal weight of glory far beyond all comparison (1 Cor. 4:17). Even now, in this life, peace and joy are promised (Rom. 5:1; James 1:2-4).

The central issue is priority. No profession or vocation is so important that it may supercede those activities to which every Christian is directed by the Scriptures.[3] The important role of medical care that has been ascribed by society and exists within the medical profession tends to blur God's priorities. Until Christian physicians rearrange their priorities, a clear and progressive understanding of the modern relationship of medicine and the Christian faith is not likely to occur. Worse, preoccupation with medicine can become excessive, even to the point where one violates the First Commandment (Ex. 20:3; Matt. 22:37-38). Some physicians might object to these directives on the grounds that their burdened lives will be further burdened. But they must be reminded that God never places more responsibilities upon us than those which can be competently managed (1 Cor. 10:13; James 1:2-4). When demands are excessive, we have placed them upon ourselves (Prov. 14:12).

Evangelism

The physician cannot take advantage of the vulnerability of the sick patient
to advance his own, or even his nation's social and political philosophy.
This is a first principle derived from the fact of illness, the act of profession, the principle of non-harm, and the ethical axiom of vulnerability.[4]
 . . . it needs to be said again and again, that the doctor's task is first and
last, and all along, to a good doctor—not an evangelist.[5]
To argue that people should be left to their original religions reveals both
disbelief in the historic Christian claim to be the only true religion and
a fundamental misunderstanding of evangelism.[6]

It is apparent that the first two quotes contrast with the third, yet the former
are consistent with the common position of many Christian medical ethicists.
There is a great reluctance, even unwillingness, among Christian physicians
to evangelize their patients. In the third quote there is an emphasis upon the
centrality of evangelism in all Christian endeavors. These statements as they
stand, contradict each other. However, they can be synthetized into a balanced
position.

Abuses in evangelism in medical settings can and do occur. As Pellegrino
points out in the first quote, because of physical illness the patient is vulnerable
physically and mentally. Also, the doctor's role is to be the best possible physician as Vale underscores. Still the command is "go and make disciples of all
nations" (Matt. 28:18) so the Christian physician cannot exclude evangelism
from his practice. He must, however, realize the patient's vulnerability and
develop a gentle, caring approach which respects the patient and considers his
comfort. Time and place are important factors, and the physician should not
persist if the patient, verbally or nonverbally, indicates disinterest or opposition. Medical needs, as one kind of physical need, give the physician an opportunity to demonstrate his professional art and science as an avenue for
evangelism (James 2:15-18). And, since as I have shown in earlier chapters,
spiritual health is a prerequisite to physical health, evangelism is essential to
good medicine. Thus, the Christian physician has the duty to witness in
medicine, to be the best possible physician, and to approach the patient in a
sensitive, considerate manner. None of these elements can be omitted.

Are patients willing to hear the gospel? At a recent conference on evangelism,
sponsored by the Christian Medical Society, two speakers stated that patients
are almost always open; usually, they are more willing to hear than physicians
are to speak. My own experience confirms this. To avoid misunderstanding,
the physician should develop some method to let his patients know of this Christian faith when they enter his practice, and that he may discuss it at some time
in the course of his care for them. This acknowledgement could be a brochure
which describes the practice, a brief explanation during an early visit, or a
letter to all new patients. Such acknowledgement may be considered by some
to be ethically unnecessary, since all physicians bring their philosophical biases
into their practices. Ultimately, each physician should weigh what that ethical
position should be for his practice.

Does evangelism involve deception, since the patient comes to the physician for medical help? Much content of this book answers that question. Medical problems have been shown to be related directly and indirectly to spiritual problems. For example, treatment of the cause of the problem may be unavoidably spiritual, as in a sexually transmitted disease. Further, all physicians treat what they discern to be the etiology, which may be entirely unrelated to the patient's presenting problem. The patient who sees a physician for stomach pain and is found to have appendicitis, will not be sent away with only pain medication, but he will have surgery recommended. The patient has no idea of etiology, so the physician's task is to determine it. Often, the etiology will be found to be of a spiritual nature. Patients want the best treatment available and Christian physicians should comply! Further, the most effective medical treatment will never bring the peace that can only be given by the Great Physician.

An encouragement for physicians to evangelize their patients is the respect which physicians retain in society among all the professions—often exceeding the respect given to the clergy. Although all professions have declined in respect over the last twenty years, physicians appear at, or near, the top of all surveys. "When physicians speak, people listen." Because of this respect, non-Christian patients are likely to consider seriously what physicians believe. Thus, Christians in the medical profession have a unique opportunity.

Two factors do limit physicians' opportunities to evangelize their patients. First, patients have a high expectation for a medical solution which is quick and complete, as this attitude is enhanced by the media. Failure to realize this expectation may cause patients to lose respect and trust in their physicians. Second, the Holy Spirit prepares persons to receive spiritual truth. Even though most patients will listen politely, many will not respond. Others will respond purely on the hope that somehow their physical condition will be helped.[7] The physician needs to clearly understand the Spirit's role. As finite beings, we cannot discern the openness of another's heart. We are only His instruments to present the gospel, but God has promised that His Word will not return empty (Isa. 55:11). Many patients will not accept the truth, but some will so opportunities must be seized.

Tom and Mary illustrate the need for patience and recognition of the Spirit's work. I had provided medical care to their family (two children) for three years when Tom hit Mary with his fist one night during one of their frequent arguments. She came for counseling, but he was unwilling to come, even though he had professed a conversion experience several months earlier. I was frustrated. How could I encourage his wife, an unbeliever, to submit to her husband and actively demonstrate her love for him when he had progressed to physical abuse? After a few sessions I shared the message of salvation and she trusted Christ. About the same time he began to come for counseling, but he was still rebellious concerning any change. Gradually, they became influenced by a Pentecostal community, learned biblical roles in marriage, and began to practice them. Over the six years since, their home has been increasingly harmonious with demonstrated love. This outcome, however, did not develop clearly or predictably, yet the Spirit was at work and even harmonized the efforts of believers of different persuasions.

Time and energy given to evangelism should include an evaluation of spiritual gifts, although a detailed review is not possible here.[8] Biblical texts for the examination of gifts are Romans 12:6-8; 1 Corinthians 12-14; Ephesians 4:8-13; and 1 Peter 4:10-11. In the contexts of these passages it is clear that gifts are given by the Holy Spirit to individuals for the purpose of the qualitative and quantitative edification (building up) of the church, as the body of Christ. Although all believers are to evangelize, evangelism is only one specific gift. The presence of this gift in a physician places a responsibility upon him to orient his practice to allow for frequent opportunities to witness to patients. One method could be a slow paced schedule of office visits to allow for the time necessary to talk to individuals. A physician who does not have this gift is still obligated to witness, but his time may involve other emphases. For example, I believe that one way in which my gifts are manifested is counseling. Because of that, I plan one-half day per week for time to counsel. Specific gifts will affect the emphasis and structure within a particular practice and facilitate an individualized outline of a practice that is suitable for every Christian physician.

A plan, however, should be devised to provide an opportunity for every patient to hear the gospel. Office personnel may be assigned this function. Christians who have been through a similar circumstance that the patient is experiencing, may be used to establish identity, and may be even more effective. Literature may be made available in the waiting room. Mailings allow for contact with every patient. To personalize his witness, the physician could write a brief summary of his own conversion and the importance of Christ in his life and publish it for distribution to his patients. In this way, he could make himself vulnerable, as the patient is vulnerable. As someone has said, "Witnessing is one beggar telling another where to find bread." Physicians need to be open, as patients are open. A spiritual history could be included as a part of the medical history. One opthalmologist has devised eye charts which contain the lines of a simple gospel tract! With some time for creative thought, a physician could make evangelism a natural part of his medical practice.

To summarize, the Bible is clear that every Christian should seek opportunities to witness in every area of life. Although patients have a certain vulnerability to which the physician must be sensitive, the medical context cannot be excluded from the Great Commission. On the other hand the physician's faith cannot be used as an excuse for failure to become the best possible physician.

Most, but by no means all, patients will willingly discuss spiritual matters. Because of the unity of the physical and spiritual dimensions of man, medical treatment must involve the spiritual dimension. Evangelism is not simple and straightforward, but involves the sowing of seeds which may sprout in the course of time. Spiritual gifts will individualize practice. Creativity should be given to evangelistic approaches. Although many Christian medical ethicists have tried to minimize or eliminate evangelism from the medical arena, the needs of patients, and more importantly, the directions of Scripture, dictate a central role for evangelism.

The Physician And His Practice

For some Christians a false dichotomy exists between the spiritual and the secular realms. Jesus Christ, however, unified the two when He prayed, "I do not ask Thee to take them out of the world, but to keep them from the evil one" (John 17:15). Paul directed, "Whatever you do, do your work heartily as for the Lord rather than for men. . . . It is the Lord Christ whom you serve" (Col. 3:23-24). Various errors in thought and behavior can result if it is not realized that Christ is Lord over all daily activities. When the truth is realized, each area is not seen to be competitive with others, but harmonious when a balance according to the general directives of Scripture and the personal distinctives of each believer is achieved.

Denis Burkitt, famous in the medical world for his work with a type of cancer (lymphoma) which carries his name, provides some thoughts for consideration:

> I find my attention . . . is directed to increasingly costly, and to a lesser degree increasingly successful, provisions made and measures adopted, to cater to the physical needs of the biological component of man (p. 4).
> Even on a purely scientific level we have probably grossly over-estimated the achievements of medical science, yet when one considers man in his true proportions, it is humbling to realize (and more so to acknowledge) how relatively little we have benefited many of our patients . . . to consider Christ's challenging question 'What is a man profited even though he gains the whole world and loses himself? . . .' To what extent do I profit my patients or others if I treat them exceedingly well; but do nothing whatever to improve the welfare of their true selves? (p. 12).
> With all its creditable achievements the overscientific approach to medicine can easily turn pathetic patients into consecutive cases, and care-ridden mothers into clinical material (p. 5).
> So often our patients have a problem that is not removable and sometimes only slightly alleviable. In those circumstances the all-important factor is the ability to accept and even triumph by the aid of inward resources (p. 15).[9]

In his concluding remarks Dr. Burkitt presents the example of the man in Jesus' parable who lived a totally biologically-oriented life (Luke 16:19-31). His food, his clothes, his home bore eloquent testimony to his priorities. He asked for, but was not granted, a return to physical existence to warn others. His message "would have been a plea to concentrate on the spiritual, to take earnest regard to their standing before God and their eternal well being."[10] In all the technology and sophistication of modern medicine, are Christian physicians too concerned with the limited existence of the physical body compared to the immortal soul?

The Christian physician's goal should be to determine what constitutes success.[11] A sobering thought in this regard is the reality that ultimately we will fail with every patient: he/she will die. This point is obvious, but how many medical students and physicians ever seriously ponder this fact? How is ultimate failure reconciled with successful medicine? To what extent should the physician blame himself each time his patients die? With every patient the greatest wisdom and technology that medical science can offer, at some point will fail. Perhaps, the concerns which would direct one's meditation to find a balance between successful care and ultimate failure, are the specific medical practices for which Jesus Christ will say, "Well done, thou good and faithful servant" (Matt. 25:23 KJV). It may be helpful to ponder often the difference between caring and curing and the frequency with which the physician is involved in the practice of one or the other. All physicians become uncomfortable when they cannot cure or significantly affect the course of a patient's illness. Concerning the spiritual dimension, the following guidelines suggest means by which to make a practice more fully Christian.

The physician should be careful to think of patients as people and to call them by their names.[12] An expression such as "the cirrhotic in room 212" denotes a disease entity and will be considered a thing rather than a living person with an immortal soul. Words such as "crock," "troll," "dirtball," "gomer," and "spos" (disposable) are common expressions which are used to label patients and are heard repeatedly from the earliest experience of medical students on the wards. Patients are labeled "interesting" if they have some disease process or finding which is unusual or represents a good example for teaching purposes. Otherwise, they may be seen as inconveniences. We must remember God's intimate care for people (Matt. 10:30) whose eternal destinies are determined by their physical existence (Heb. 9:27).

The physician should seek opportunities to pray with his patients, especially during times of severe illness or major surgery. Many patients who are not believers cherish prayer and it may open an opportunity, then or later, for the physician to share Christ. Patients may be informed that prayer is available using any of the means for evangelism which were mentioned in the previous section. The Great Physician is readily available through prayer. His supplication is a resource for comfort with the possibility of His supernatural intervention (see Healing, chapter 8).

God's sovereignty should become a great comfort to the believing physician. A simple, but not simplistic, summary of the concept is "And we know that God causes all things to work together for good to those who love God, to those who are called according to His purpose" (Rom. 8:28). Any reader not fully acquainted with God's sovereignty should study the concept. The Westminister Confession of Faith, for example, discusses God's plans and purposes in a full and complete way. Today, malpractice is prevalent as a real source of worry for physicians who, out of fear, do many things with, and for, patients that otherwise would not be done. The Christian physician does not have to be subject to this pressure. He is free to exercise his best judgment and rest upon God's sovereignty whenever he has managed the patient to the best of his ability, realizing his finite knowledge and skills. Then any complications or unexpected events are within His will. God's sovereignty is not an excuse for incompetent medical care, obviously, but it does guarantee freedom for the physician to rest the patient's outcome with the Great Physician. The unbeliever faces the stark reality that his own fallibility is the only hope he has to offer his patient. No wonder the suicide rate for physicians is one of the highest of any profession!

Physicians face temptations which are unique to their profession.[13] (a) Financial prosperity is essentially guaranteed, but the Scriptures are clear that riches present one of the major temptations to be overcome (Matt. 6:19-24; Matt. 13:22; Matt. 19:23, 24; 1 Tim. 6:6-10). (2) Sexual problems head almost every New Testament listing of sins (Matt. 5:28; Mark 7:20-23; Gal. 5:19-21; Col. 3:5-11). The physician is privileged to examine the naked body and must be careful to minimize all temptation. (3) Pride results from the prestige and status that society bestows upon the physician e.g., (Prov. 16:8; James 4:6; 1 Peter 5:5; 1 John 2:16). (4) The care of patients during the night is exhausting and increases the liability that sin may result (Ps. 127:2). (5) Drugs which relieve pain and tension are accessable, making the physician vulnerable to self-medication. The rate of addiction to drugs and alcohol among physicians is estimated at twenty percent! (6) Patient demands which abuse a physician's time and professional peer pressure are other problems. Other particulars might be named, but these are sufficient to indicate the severity and constancy of temptations for the Christian physician who carries the defeated, but still present, old nature (Rom. 6:1-23, 7:14-25). If the above temptations result in sin (James 1:13-15), guilt naturally results. Sadly, too many Christians do not understand how God has provided for guilt. "Where the guilt complex remains, it paralyzes moral effort.[14] Much more could be said here, but hopefully three basic principles will result in a clearer understanding. The first principle is justification by faith. If one does not understand the fullness and finality of forgiveness and purity in a relationship with God through Jesus Christ, he/she is impotent to progress in the Christian life and to experience joy and peace. A detailed study of Romans 1-8 should result in an adequate understanding. Second, the burden of guilt is unnecessary for the Christian (Rom. 8:1). Christ provided forgiveness of sins through His blood sacrifice (Heb. 9:22). "If we confess our sins, he is faithful and just to forgive us our sins, and to cleanse us from all unrighteousness" (1 John 1:9). His great sacrifices and our commitment to repentance removes the spiritual reality of guilt. Feelings of remorse, sadness, and shame may persist, but time, right thinking and right action will markedly diminish them. Third, repetitive sins are the most crippling because of cumulative guilt feelings. For the reader who continues to be frustrated and burdened by guilt, Dr. Adams has thoroughly developed the biblical concepts of guilt and forgiveness.[15] In another book, he has detailed the practical application of those concepts.[16] A balanced effective understanding cannot be accomplished without *serious* study and meditation, but the Christian life is intended by its Creator to be a life of joy, peace, and growth in righteousness. Any Christian who is not experiencing these should further examine his entire understanding of his relationship to God, the freedom of activity which flows from that relationship, and the power to overcome sin.

Physicians are sometimes unaware of their biases, as they are taught to be "objective" with patients. That goal is desirable, but it is impossible to put into practice. In particular, Christians should, as they mature, become increasingly aware of the deceitfulness of their own hearts (Jer. 17:9). In managing patients, the physician's and the patient's attitudes and biases should be kept in mind by both:

> On the one hand, consider the physician with an aggressively interventionist philosophy. . . . In situations that could be expected to improve spontaneously, intervention would nevertheless be undertaken to promote a more rapid or comfortable return to health. . . . On the other hand, consider the more passive physician with a non-interventionist approach. . . . This physician would view the body as a sort of sacred entity that should be manipulated only under exceptional circumstances.[17]

For example, surgery for atherosclerosis of the cerebral (brain) arteries remains highly controversial. The first physician would urge the patient to have surgery; the second physician would direct his patients not to have surgery. The patient could not avoid being influenced by the physician's medical judgment and would probably never be aware of the equivocal nature of the surgery in either case.

Another example demonstrates *patient bias*. Healthy volunteers were placed in the circumstance of having cancer of the larynx.[18] Their choices were: (1) laryngectomy (removal of the larynx) with a three-year survival of 60 percent or (2) radiation therapy with a 30-40 percent three-year survival. One out of five chose radiation with its lesser longevity in order to preserve their voices. Such choices are not predictable, so there must be an effective communication between patient and physician.

The respect, and often awe with which patients may view their physicians is powerful and often inhibits them from freely expressing themselves.[19] The physician needs to develop a conscious awareness of this attitude as well as his own biases as he explores values with his patients. Medical decisions involve much subjectivity by both patient and physician as these two examples (above) illustrate. The patient's best interest will be reached more likely by reciprocal communication.

Christian physicians should consider other modifications with patients. The resources of the Christian (counseling, prayer, anointing, pneumosomatic strengthening, and the local community of believers) are much greater than those of the non-Christian. The Christian physician should strive to develop those resources. Some may be available through contacts with the patient's pastor and/or church. Many Christian patients are already aware of these resources. This situation is strategic! Since many liberal and conservative churches fail to teach the strengths available to the believer, the physician can counsel the patient or direct him to a pastor who can counsel. Floundering Christians, then, will have an opportunity to experience the abundant life through these spiritual resources and then, to contribute to the advancement of the kingdom.

Christian patients may *cause* particular problems for physicians. For example, their views on healing may differ from those of the physician, resulting in a conflict. Lengthy explanations may be necessary to explain why healing did not occur, even though the ritual of their particular fellowship was carried out. Expectations from a Christian physician may exceed his resources, ability, or even be impossible to meet. Simple, quick remedy may be expected when a lengthy, persevering process is the only alternative. As in counseling, a series of questions will help to clarify patient's expectations. "What is your problem?" "What have you done about it?" "What do you want us to do?"[20] Even with these problems, Christian patients are mostly a joy!

The physician should seek a method to determine the presence or absence of Christian belief in his patients. A practical opportunity occurs during the history taking portion of a complete examination. What else contributes more to the health or disease of the patient? At this time the physician can be aware of an open or closed atttitude toward Christianity, if belief is not already present. Particular denominational doctrine may enhance or impede the patient-physician relationship. All this information can be kept in the patients' record for future reference. A distinctive approach can be maintained according to this information. Such distinction is rare, even among Christian physicians and ethicists, but it has been suggested at least once.[21]

Primary care physicians (mostly family physicians, pediatricians, obstetrician-gynecologists, and general internists) who desire a truly Christian practice may face serious financial limitations. The practices described here involve more time with some patients and considerable time away from medical practice to fulfill the "balanced" life. One physician, whom I know personally, has limited his practice for these reasons even though the respect that he has by other physicians, has resulted in their referral of themselves and their families to him. Even further restrictions may occur if biblical evaluation of the "third party" payer concept (private insurance, industrial, and governmental programs) reveals that this removal of primary responsibility from the patient is inconsistent with biblical accountability. Another physician of whom I am aware is convinced that such payment is unbiblical and has established his practice on that basis. He *has* had considerably less income than most physicians in situations similar to his own. This result reflects the cost of commitment (Luke

14:24-35) to *distinctive* Christian principles. His example should stimulate others in the profession to such committment.

In summary, the Christian physician should help his patients aim toward spiritual goals, realizing their tendency toward preoccupation with the physical body. He should reflect seriously upon the balance between caring, curing, and the ultimate death of every patient. Euphemisms relating to patients should be avoided. Prayer should be a natural response with patients. The physicians'fallibility rests in God's sovereignty. Temptations must be avoided, but where conscious sin occurs, a clear understanding of guilt, forgiveness, and change can be sought. Although objectivity in medical decisions is a reasonable goal, the impossibility of achieving it should be recognized. Practical use of the resources of the Christian community can be extremely helpful. The particular beliefs in Christian patients may enhance or impede care. These beliefs may be obtained during the patient history. Other distinctives may be developed by the thinking Christian physician.

Some Words to the Medical Student

Having survived the premedical grind, the vast majority (of medical students) genuinely desire to be helpers. As they spend more of their waking hours in classroom, laboratory, and later in high pressure clinical settings among patients who are in and out of the hospital and whom they can only marginally help, they set aside . . . " their own humanity to learn the science and technology of medicine." In a sense they cultivate a persona that is more professionalized and narrowed. In so doing, there is a danger of becoming "we" not "they"—the people served. . . . In the process insidious changes in personality may occur.[22]

This description and the one which began this chapter should be red flags to medical students.

The time for the Christian to develop right patterns of life is *now*. Pressures will *increase* over the next several years with further training and the likelihood of a family. A tendency of the sinful nature is to think that the future somehow will be more manageable than the present. Such deception is common, since the physician has many "wait-untils" (graduation, residency, practice, etc.). It is not an overstatement to say that the medical student who cannot manage the priorities which have been briefly presented, should reconsider any continuation with a medical career.

One means to attain an increased biblical understanding is a period of time in a Bible college or seminary. Probably, the easiest time to pursue any formal training is the earlier period of adult life when a family is not yet established, the habits of study are familiar, and one is adjusted to a lower level of income. An opportune time is upon completion of an internship and prior to specialization. The physician can obtain a state license to allow necessary income to be earned with only a few hours per week of "moonlighting." Also, this juncture allows further evaluation of future plans, including the possibility of missionary service since the greatest need for medical care remains in the Third World countries. The medical problems of the Western world are primarily of a direct spiritual nature, but other countries lack basic medicine and hygiene. No doubt, the physician who truly desires to be most effective in medical care will consider Third World needs.

The Christian medical student needs to consider seriously that in many instances a truly Christian medical practice will not yield the financial income that other physicians receive. He must be careful to avoid the attitude that he has a right to a large income. Biblically, the lure of money is a frequent cause of compromise of principle. By developing clear principles for his practice and an expectancy of less income, the temptation for compromise will be much decreased.

A special plea is made to the medical student or young physician who is interested in the fullest development and definition of a biblical approach to medical care. He should seriously consider a full seminary education with the inclusion of Greek and Hebrew. Not only are much greater developments in biblical/medical ethics needed, but the study of the biblical words that describe diseases, treatments, and other medically-related matters is needed. The understanding of these words could be enriched by a comparison of the historical usage with modern concepts of human physiology. Perhaps, such a physician would be able to assist translators. An example is the word *leprosy* (Hebrew-*zarath* and Greek *lepra*). The modern disease, known as leprosy, constitutes only a small portion of those skin diseases which are included in the words of the original languages.[23]

The medical student must begin to think and act on biblical priorities. God's will in all areas of the Christian life concerns much more than any career, even the practice of medicine. The diligent pursuit of a balanced Christian life will result in a more competent and caring physician than time and energy focused almost exclusively upon the study and practice of medicine.

NOTES

1. Similar problems exist in other careers. It is a narrow perception by physicians that only we face such rigors in our professional development. My observations, however, are limited to my profession. I suspect that the same general problems of biblical priorities exist in other vocations.

2. Jay E. Adams, *Christian Living in the Home* (Philadelphia: Presbyterian and Reformed Pub., 1972), p. 100.

3. D. Martyn Lloyd-Jones, *The Doctor Himself and the Human Condition* (London: Christian Medical Fellowship Publications, 1982), pp. 51, 63.

4. Edmund D. Pellegrino and David C. Thomasma, *A Philosophical Basis of Medical Practice* (New York: Oxford University Press, 1981), p. 275.

5. J. A. Vale, *Medicine and the Christian Mind* (London: Christian Medical Fellowship Publications, 1975), pp. 62-63.

6. Donald Tinder, "Evangelism, Ethical Aspects," in *Baker's Dicltionary of Christian Ethics*, ed. Carl F. Henry (Grand Rapids: Baker Book House, 1973), p. 225.

7. D. Martyn Lloyd-Jones, *The Doctor Himself and the Human Condition*, p. 103ff.

8. Bobby Clinton, *Spiritual Gifts* (World Team Publications, 1975).

9. Denis P. Burkitt, *Our Priorities* (London: Christian Medical Fellowship Publications, 1976), pp. 4-5, 12, 15.

10. Ibid., p. 18.

11. D. Martyn Lloyd-Jones, *The Doctor Himself and the Human Condition*, pp. 12, 76ff.

12. Ibid., p. 18.

13. Ibid., p. 9.

14. Carl F. Henry, *Christian Personal Ethics* (1957; reprint ed., Grand Rapids: Baker Book House, 1977), p. 381.

15. Jay E. Adams, *More Than Redemption* (Phillipsburg, NJ: Presbyterian and Reformed Pub. Co., 1979), pp. 184-232.

16. Jay E. Adams, *The Christian Counselor's Manual* (Grand Rapids: Baker Book House, 1977), pp. 63-70.

17. A. S. Brett, "Hidden Ethical Issues in Clinical Decision Analysis," *New England Journal of Medicine* 305 (Nov. 5, 1981):1150-1152.

18. B. J. McNeil, R. Weichselbaum, and S. G. Pauker "Speech and Survival: Tradeoffs between quality and quantity of Life in Laryngeal Cancer," *New England Journal of Medicine* 305 (Oct. 22, 1981):982-987.

19. D. Martyn Lloyd-Jones, *The Doctor Himself and the Human Condition*, pp. 18, 64.

20. Jay E. Adams, *The Christian Counselor's Manual*, p. 274.

21. C. Everett Koop, "The Ill Child, the Family and the Physician," *Christian Medical Society Journal* 3 (4) 1972:4-9.

22. Cato 6 (a pseudonym), "Dirtball," *Journal of the American Medical Association* 247 (June 11, 1982):3059-60.

23. R. A. Braillie and E. E. Baillie, "Biblical Leprosy as Compared to Present Day Leprosy," *Southern Medical Journal* 75 (July 1982):855-857.

REFERENCES

Adams, Jay E. *Christian Living In The Home*. Philadelphia, Presbyterian and Reformed, 1972.

Baillie, R. A. and Baillie, E. E. "Biblical Leprosy as Compared to Present Day Leprosy." *Southern Medical Journal* 75 (July 1982):855-857.

Brett, A. S. "Hidden Ethical Issues in Clinical Decision Analysis." *New England Journal of Medicine* 305 (Nov. 5, 1981):1150-1152.

Burkitt, Denis P. *Our Priorities*. London: Christian Medical Fellowship Publications, 1976.

Cato 6 (a pseudonym). "Dirtball." *Journal of American Medical Association* 247 (June 11, 1982):3059-3060.

Clinton, Bobby. *Spiritual Gifts*. Worldteam Publications, 1975.

Koop, C. Everett. "The Ill Child, the Family and the Physician." *Christian Medical Society Journal* 3 (4):4-9.

NcNeil, B. J., Weichselbaum, R., Pauker, S. G. "Speech and Survival: Tradeoffs between Quality and Quantity of Life in Laryngeal Cancer." *New England Journal of Medicine* 305 (Oct. 22, 1981):982-987.

Pellegrino, Edmund D. and Thomasma, David C. *A Philosophical Basis of Medical Practice*. New York: Oxford University Press, 1981.

Vale, J. A. *Medicine and The Christian Mind*. London: Christian Medical Fellowship Publications, 1975.

INDEX

Abel, 197
Abortio, 140
Abortion, 4, 8, 55, 82, 202
  210n
  AMA and, 2
  Bible and, 1
  Catholicism and, 6
  CMS Statement on, 8
  criminal, 141
  elective, 141
  ethics and, 28, 31, 56, 58-60, 68,
  110, 202, 208
  Hippocratic Oath, 2
  historical - legal aspects, 2, 139-151,
  171
  law and, I, 57, 119-120, 140, 143-
  151, 216
  physicians and, 59
  psychiatrists and, 55
  sanctity of life and, 197
  spontaneous, 141
  statistics, 3, 36, 47n, 58, 139-142,
  150-151, 151n, 172
  Supreme Court and, 2
  teenagers and, 119
  therapeutic, 141, 172
  throughout pregnancy, 141, 151n
Abortionist, 59, 141, 143
Abrreibung, 141
Absolutes, 25n
Accidents, 110
  alcohol use and, 92
  death statistics, 90-92
Acts
  1:7-8; 168
  3:1-10; 114
  3:11; 103
  4:9; 103-104
  4:10; 104
  4:13; 225
  5:15-16; 104
  6:1-6; 128

  8:4; 194n
  9:37; 104
  10:38; 103
  14:8; 105
  16:11-18; 102
  16:22, 25; 194
  16:28; 105
  19:12; 105
  20:5-16; 102
  21:1-19; 102
  23:24; 103
  27:1 and 28:16; 102
  28:1; 103
  28:5; 105
  28:8; 103
  28:9; 103
  28:27; 103
Adam, 81, 84, 112, 130, 146-147,
  152n, 163, 182
Adams, Jay E., 71n, 96n, 121n, 136n,
  162, 176n, 178n, 193n, 194n, 232,
  236n
Adenoidectomy, 44
Adiaphora, 107
Adultery, 67, 198
Adunatos, 105
Advertisements, 41, 54
Aesclepius, 4
Aging process, 54, 79, 88
Agnew, Spiro, I
Ai, 118, 123n
Alameda County, Calif., 93-94
Albrecht, Mark, 193n
Alcohol
  use of, 88
  Bible and, 106
  disease and, 91-93, 135
Alcoholism,
  among physicians, 231
  as disease, 40
  as sin, 92
  Bible and, 82

prayer of, 115
science and, 28-30, 168, 213
suffering and, 188
Fallopian tube, 142
Falsehood, 19
Family, the
   biblical structure for, 120, 223-224, 228
   children and, 120
   church and, 214
   communication and, 120
   death and, 184-187, 191-192, 199-201, 207
   definition of, 119
   disintegration of, 20
   home care and, 191-193
   hospital policy and, 186
   medical care and, 112-121, 130-134, 187-188, 207-208
   psychotherapy and, 170, 173
   stress and, 88, 131
   suffering and, 188
Fantasies, 169
Farmer, Betty, 129
Fantasies, 169
Farmer, Betty, 129
Father, headship of, 120-121
Fats, 93
Fear, 35, 167, 207
   of death, 183-185
   of pain, 190
Fellowship, 84, 95, 122n
   isolation from 193
   medical care and, 130
   of church, 214, 222, 225
   on campus, 222
Fertilization, 147-148, 151n, 152n, 217
Fetus,
   abnormal, 1, 59, 148
   birth and, 147
   death of, 3, 141, 150
   development of, 144-145, 147, 210n
   ectopic, 142
   ensoulment and, 145-146
   viability and, 144, 146, 151n
Fever, 103-104
Finances, 55
First Commandment, 129, 225
First National Conference on Emotional Stress and Heart Disease, 88

Flesh, weakness of, 78, 104
Fletcher, Joseph, 6
"Focus on the Family" series, 169
Food and Drug Administration, 44, 56
Foods,
   See Diet
Forceps, 142
Forgiveness, 59, 82, 163
   biblical concept of, 181-182, 185, 230-231, 234
   mental health and, 173-174
Forker, Alan D., 97n
Fornication, 67
Fourth Commandment, 65
Freedom,
   Christians and, 214-216
   conscience and, 64
   See also Liberty
Freud, 161, 170
Friedman, Howard S., 47n
Friedman, M., 97n
Fries, James F., 97n
Friends, 186, 191
Fruits, 93
Fundamentalism, 25n
Funerals, 183

Galatians,
   4:13; 104
   5:17; 19
   5:19; 169
   5:19-21; 231
   5:22-23; 87
   5:23; 94
   6:1; 131
   6:10; 224
Galilee, 102
Gametes, 146
Ganz, Richard L., 70n
Garden of Eden, 81, 95
Gastritis, 116
Gastroenterologist, 75
Geisler, Norman, 71n, 202, 210n
Genes, deleterious, 149
Genesis,
   1:27; 76, 197
   2; 152n
   2:7; 143, 146-147, 182
   2:18; 223
   2:24; 120, 223

Pneuma, 77-78, 83
Pneumonia, 90-92, 191
Pneumosomatic health,
  achieving, 85-90
  principles and practice, 75-96
  See also Health, Medicine
Politics, 216
Preus, Robert D., 121n
Poisoning, 92
Pollock, John, 70n
Pollution, 80
Pope, the, 6
Porneia, 169
Positivism, 24n
Postulates, 13, 30
The Powers of Psychiatry, 172
Practice, medical
  See Medical practice
Prayer, 64, 66, 133, 168, 173, 186
  between doctors and patients, 215, 234
  for healing, 105, 114-115, 129-132
  suffering and, 189-191, 207
Pregnancy, 3, 59, 110
  abnormal, 1, 150
  abortion and, 140-141, 144-145
  crisis centers for, 216
  ectopic, 142
  ensoulment and, 145
  incest and, 150
  minors and, 119, 139
  rape and, 150
  See also Abortion
Premises, 30
Prenatal care, 44
Prenatal life,
  See Life, prenatal
Preparing for Adolescence, 169
Prescriptions,
  See Drugs
President's Commission for the Study of
  Ethical Problems in Medicine, 205
Presuppositions, 29-30, 69
Preventive medicine,
  See Medicine
Pride, 231
Priests, 56, 105
Primum non nocere, 42
Principles,
  biblical, 64, 67, 69, 77, 83, 106-108,
    113, 127, 155-156

  ethical, 59-60, 66
  practice and, 68
  worldly vs. biblical, I, 6
Prison, 171
Pro-life position, 148, 151
Problems,
  behavioral, 119
  marital, 120
  medical, 75
  physical, 52, 108-109, 115
  psychiatric, 52
  solution of, 75
  spiritual, 52, 108-109, 115
Prophecy, false, 198
Propoxyphene, 41
Proverbs,
  3:7-8; 85
  3:16; 85
  3:21-26; 85
  4:10; 85
  9:11; 85
  10:27; 85
  14:12; 225
  16:8; 231
  17:22; 87
  20:1; 92
  22:7; 120
  23:20; 92
  23:20-21; 106
  23:29-35; 92, 106
  31:4-6; 92
Psalms,
  1; 129
  1:2; 223
  5:3; 84, 223
  8:5; 56
  38; 85
  48:10; 116
  51:5; 152n
  51:10; 128
  57:8; 223
  90:10; 86-87
  103:8-14; 84
  127:2; 94, 231
  139:13-16; 152n
  139:14; 113
  139:16; 150
  139:23-24; 107, 131
Pseudoreligion, 56
Psyche, the, 11, 51, 53, 78, 88

DATE DUE